Advanced Fitness Assessment & Exercise Prescription

Third Edition

Vivian H. Heyward, PhD
University of New Mexico

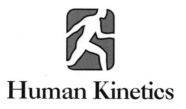

Human Kinetics

Library of Congress Cataloging-in-Publication Data

Heyward, Vivian H.
    Advanced fitness assessment & exercise prescription / Vivian H.
    Heyward. -- 3rd ed.
        p.   cm.
    Includes bibliographical references and index.
    ISBN 0-88011-483-5
    1. Physical fitness--Testing.   2. Exercise tests.   3. Health.
    I. Title.
    GV436.H48   1997   97-17557
    613.7--dc21   CIP

ISBN: 0-88011-483-5

Acquisitions Editor: Scott Wikgren; **Developmental Editor:** Elaine Mustain; **Assistant Editors:** Sandra Merz Bott, Erin Cler, Melinda Graham; **Editorial Assistant:** Amy Carnes; **Copyeditor:** Brian Mustain; **Proofreader:** Sarah Wiseman; **Indexer:** Craig Brown; **Graphic Designer:** Stuart Cartwright; **Graphic Artists:** Yvonne Winsor and Angela K. Snyder; **Photo Editor:** Boyd LaFoon; **Cover Designer:** Chuck Nivens; **Illustrator:** Keith Blomberg; **Mac Illustrations:** Craig Ronto; **Printer:** Edwards

Printed in the United States of America   10   9   8   7   6   5   4

Human Kinetics
Web site: http://www.humankinetics.com/

United States: Human Kinetics, P.O. Box 5076, Champaign, IL 61825-5076
1-800-747-4457
e-mail: humank@hkusa.com

Canada: Human Kinetics, 475 Devonshire Road, Unit 100, Windsor, ON N8Y 2L5
1-800-465-7301 (in Canada only)
e-mail: humank@hkcanada.com

Europe: Human Kinetics, P.O. Box IW14, Leeds LS16 6TR, United Kingdom
+44 (0)113-278 1708
e-mail: humank@hkeurope.com

Australia: Human Kinetics, 57A Price Avenue, Lower Mitcham, South Australia 5062
(08) 82771555
e-mail: humank@hkaustralia.com

New Zealand: Human Kinetics, P.O. Box 105-231, Auckland Central
09-523-3462
e-mail: humank@hknewz.com

In memory of Mom—for her gentle encouragement
and unwavering confidence in me.

Contents

Acknowledgments   ix

Preface   xi

Chapter 1   Physical Activity, Health, and Hypokinetic Diseases   1

Physical Activity, Health, and Disease: An Overview   1

Cardiovascular Disease   4

Hypertension   5

Hypercholesterolemia   7

Cigarette Smoking   7

Diabetes Mellitus   8

Obesity and Overweight   8

Musculoskeletal Diseases and Disorders   8

References   9

Chapter 2   Preliminary Health Screening and Risk Classification   13

Health Evaluation   14

Lifestyle Evaluation   28

Informed Consent   28

Sources for Equipment   29

References   29

Chapter 3   Principles of Assessment, Prescription, and Exercise Program Adherence   31

Components of Physical Fitness   32

Purposes of Physical Fitness Testing   33

Testing Order and the Testing Environment   33

Test Validity, Reliability, and Objectivity   33

Evaluating Prediction Equations   34

Administering and Interpreting Physical Fitness Tests   37

Basic Principles for Exercise Program Design   38

The Art and Science of Exercise Prescription   39

Exercise Program Adherence   41

Certification and Licensure   42

References   44

Chapter 4   Assessing Cardiorespiratory Fitness   47

Exercise Evaluation   48
Maximal Exercise Test Protocols   52
Submaximal Exercise Test Protocols   65
Field Tests   73
Exercise Testing of Children and Older Adults   76
Sources for Equipment   78
References   78

Chapter 5   Designing Cardiorespiratory Exercise Programs   83

The Exercise Prescription   83
Essentials of a Cardiorespiratory Exercise Workout   92
Aerobic Training Methods and Modes   92
Personalized Exercise Programs   95
References   103

Chapter 6   Assessing Strength and Muscular Endurance   105

Definition of Terms   105
Strength and Muscular Endurance Assessment   107
Calisthenic-Type Strength and Muscular Endurance Tests   115
Muscular Fitness Testing: Sources of Measurement Error   116
Additional Considerations for Muscular Fitness Testing   117
Sources for Equipment   119
References   120

Chapter 7   Designing Resistance Training Programs   121

Application of Training Principles to Weight Resistance Exercise   122
Types of Resistance Training   122
Comparison of Resistance Training Methods   127
Developing the Resistance Training Program   129
Designing Resistance Training Programs for Children   133
Designing Resistance Training Programs for Older Adults   134
Effects of Resistance Training Programs   134
Muscular Soreness   137
Common Misconceptions and Questions About Resistance Training   139
References   141

Chapter 8   Assessing Body Composition   145

Classification and Uses of Body Composition Measures   145
Body Composition Models   146
Laboratory Methods for Assessing Body Composition   148
Field Methods for Assessing Body Composition   152

Sources for Equipment   171
References   172

Chapter 9   Designing Weight Management and Body Composition Programs   177

Types of Obesity   178
Causes of Overweight and Obesity   178
Weight Management Principles and Practices   181
Well-Balanced Diet   182
Designing Weight Management Programs: Preliminary Steps   186
Designing Weight-Loss Programs   189
Quick Weight-Loss Diets and Precautions   195
Designing Weight-Gain Programs   196
Designing Programs to Improve Body Composition   197
References   199

Chapter 10   Assessing Flexibility and Designing Stretching Programs   203

Definition and Nature of Flexibility   203
Factors Affecting Flexibility   204
Assessment of Flexibility   205
Designing Flexibility Programs   215
Designing Low Back Care Exercise Programs   220
Sources for Equipment   221
References   221

Chapter 11   Assessing and Managing Stress   223

Physiological Response to Stress   223
Stress and Disease   224
Assessment of Stress and Neuromuscular Tension   224
Exercise and Stress   225
Relaxation Techniques   226
References   227

List of Abbreviations   229

Appendix A   Health and Fitness Appraisal   231

A.1 Glossary of Medical Terminology   231
A.2 Physical Activity Readiness Questionnaire (PAR-Q)   234
A.3 RISKO: A Heart Health Appraisal   235
A.4 Medical History Questionnaire   239
A.5 Medical Clearance   241

A.6 Sample ECG Tracings   242
A.7 Lifestyle Evaluation   251
A.8 Informed Consent   253
A.9 Analysis of Sample Case Study in Chapter 5   254

Appendix B   Cardiorespiratory Assessments   257

B.1 Summary of GXT and Cardiorespiratory Field Test Protocols   257
B.2 Rockport Fitness Charts   259
B.3 Step Test Protocols   261

Appendix C   Muscular Fitness Exercises and Norms   263

C.1 Average Strength, Endurance, and Power Values for Isokinetic
     (Omni-Tron) Tests   263
C.2 Basic Static (Isometric) Exercises   265
C.3 Dynamic Resistance Exercises   267

Appendix D   Body Composition Assessments   273

D.1 Density of Water at Different Temperatures   273
D.2 Prediction Equations for Residual Volume (RV)   274
D.3 Standardized Sites for Skinfold Measurements   275
D.4 Skinfold Sites for Jackson's Generalized Skinfold Equations   280
D.5 Standardized Sites for Circumference Measurements   281
D.6 Standardized Sites for Bony Breadth Measurements   282

Appendix E   Energy Intake and Expenditure   283

E.1 Food Record and RDA Profile   283
E.2 Sample Computerized Analysis of Food Intake   285
E.3 Physical Activity Log   290
E.4 Compendium of Physical Activities   291

Appendix F   Flexibility and Low Back Care Exercises   303

F.1 Selected Flexibility Exercises   303
F.2 Exercise DO's and DON'Ts   308
F.3 Exercises for Low Back Care   311

Appendix G   Stress Assessment   312

G.1 Stress Inventory and Coping Strategies   312
G.2 Rathbone Manual Tension Test   316

Index   317

About the Author   323

Acknowledgments

I would like to acknowledge my editor, Elaine Mustain, for her critical and comprehensive review of this manuscript. This book reflects her expertise and careful attention to detail. Also, I am indebted to each of the following individuals for their unique contributions to the first, second, and third editions of this book:

Linda K. Gilkey and "Swede" Scholer, for taking the photographs; Jim Milani, Joseph Quatrochi, Lizbeth Soybel, and Angelo Collado, for serving as models for the photographs; Donna Lockner, for critically reviewing the nutrition information; Robert Robergs, Brent Ruby, and Peter Egan for doing the computer graphics; Carol-Ann Fernandez, Sandi Travis, and Kathi Kramer, for entering parts of manuscript on the word processor; Lorene Myers and Melinda Stegman, for proofreading previous editions of this book.

Your effort, cooperation, and expertise are truly appreciated.

Preface

Increased public awareness of the importance of physical activity for optimal health and longevity has led to an increased need for the leadership of highly qualified exercise scientists. Universities have responded to this need by offering graduate degree programs in exercise science. The third edition of *Advanced Fitness Assessment and Exercise Prescription* is intended for exercise science students enrolled in advanced professional courses dealing with physical fitness appraisal and exercise prescription.

A primary focus of this book is to provide exercise scientists with the knowledge and skills to assess the physical fitness of apparently healthy individuals. Since this text is not clinically oriented, there is limited information regarding the etiology and pathophysiology of cardiovascular disease, screening tests for pulmonary disorders, and the reading and interpretation of electrocardiograms. Exercise scientists working with coronary-prone individuals and cardiac patients are encouraged to consult clinically oriented books that provide detailed information concerning this population.

Advanced Fitness Assessment and Exercise Prescription provides a well-balanced approach to the assessment of physical fitness, addressing five components of total physical fitness:

- Cardiorespiratory endurance
- Muscular fitness
- Body weight and composition
- Flexibility
- Neuromuscular relaxation

This text is unique in its scope and in the depth of its content, organization, and approach to the subject matter. Introductory texts typically focus on field testing to evaluate physical fitness. Although this text includes some field tests, it emphasizes laboratory techniques for the assessment of physical fitness components. The scope and the depth of the information presented make this text an important resource for practitioners—especially those employed in health and fitness settings. This text is organized such that, for each physical fitness component, a chapter on assessment is followed by a chapter on exercise prescription. Key questions are presented at the beginning of each chapter, and key points and major concepts are summarized at the end of each chapter. You will find sources for purchasing equipment and supplies at the end of each chapter dealing with fitness assessment. This text synthesizes concepts, principles, and theories based on research in exercise physiology, kinesiology, and nutrition; and it applies appropriate tests and measurements to physical fitness testing and to the design of exercise programs. The net result is a direct and clear-cut approach to physical fitness assessment and exercise prescription.

You will note substantial changes and additions in the third edition of this text. Chapter 1 contains the U.S. Surgeon General's physical activity recommendations for health benefits. Chapter 2 covers preliminary health screening and risk classification, as well as guidelines for classification of blood pressure and hyperlipidemia in adults. Chapter 3 presents principles of physical fitness assessment and exercise prescription that are used to design all types of exercise programs. It also includes information about evaluation of field tests and prediction equations, exercise program adherence, and certification of exercise science professionals. Chapter 4 discusses guidelines for exercise testing based on the latest 1995 ACSM guidelines. This chapter also deals with graded exercise testing of children and older adults, as well as graded exercise tests using rowing and step ergometers. Chapter 5 compares aerobic exercise modes and provides an example of a multi-modal, cross-training program. Chapter 6 has been expanded to include sources of measurement error for muscular fitness tests, evaluation of muscle balance, and strength testing of children and older adults. Chapter 7 now contains guidelines for designing resistance training programs for athletes, experienced weightlifters, children, and older adults. Chapter 8 has been modified to include information about dual-energy x-ray absorptiometry and assessment of regional adiposity, as well as suitable skinfold and bioimpedance equations for measuring body fat of clients from diverse population subgroups. Chapter 9 includes guidelines for designing weight-loss and weight-gain programs, as well as exercise prescriptions for altering body composition. Chapter 10 presents goniometric test procedures and norms for evaluating flexibility, along with specific exercises for low back exercise programs.

An instructor's guide accompanies this text. It will assist instructors with the organization and preparation of the materials and assignments for their courses. This guide contains a sample course outline, instructions for class projects, guidelines for writing and presenting research abstracts, laboratory demonstrations and experiences, a checklist for evaluating practical laboratory skills, sample practice problems with solutions, and sample case studies.

These changes and additions to the text should provide a more comprehensive and advanced approach to physical fitness appraisal and exercise prescription than was available in the first two editions. I hope you will use the information in this book to improve your knowledge, skill, and professional competence as an exercise scientist.

CHAPTER 1

Physical Activity, Health, and Hypokinetic Diseases

Key Questions

- Is physical activity on the decline in the United States?
- What diseases are associated with a sedentary lifestyle, and what are the major risks for these diseases?
- What are the benefits of regular physical activity in terms of disease prevention, and how does it improve health?
- How much physical activity is needed for improved health benefits?
- What kinds of physical activities are suitable for typical people, and how often should they exercise?

One of the national health objectives for the year 2000 is to reduce to 15% the proportion of people aged 6 years and older who engage in no leisure-time physical activity (Public Health Service 1991). Epidemiological surveys of the U.S. population show that we are making progress toward this goal, with a modest decline (–2.3%) between 1986 and 1990 in the percentage of individuals classified as physically inactive (Casperson and Merritt 1995). Yet an estimated 60% of all American adults do not get the recommended amount of physical activity; 25% report no physical activity whatsoever; and nearly 50% of adolescents and young adults between the ages of 12 and 21 years are not physically active on a regular basis (U.S. Dept. of Health and Human Services 1996). As an exercise specialist, you have a challenging role to educate and motivate your clients to incorporate physical activity and regular exercise as an integral part of their lifestyles.

This chapter deals with physical activity trends, risk factors associated with hypokinetic diseases, the role of regular physical activity in disease prevention and health, and physical activity recommendations for improved health. For definitions of medical terminology used in this chapter, see appendix A.1.

PHYSICAL ACTIVITY, HEALTH, AND DISEASE: AN OVERVIEW

Modern technology has lessened the physical demands of everyday activities like cleaning the house, washing clothes and dishes, mowing the lawn, and traveling to work. What would have once required an hour of physical work now can be accomplished in just a few seconds by pushing a button or setting a dial. As a result, more time is available to pursue leisure activities. The unfortunate fact, however, is that many individuals pursue sedentary activities.

Although the human body is designed for movement and strenuous physical activity, exercise is not a part of the average lifestyle. One cannot expect the human body to function optimally and to remain healthy for extended periods if the body is abused or not used as intended. Thus, physical inactivity has led to a rise in hypokinetic diseases. The prefix *hypo* means "lack of," and *kinetic* refers to movement. Individuals who do not exercise regularly are at greater risk of developing hypokinetic diseases, such as coronary heart disease, hypertension, hypercholesterolemia, cancer, obesity, and musculoskeletal disorders (see figure 1.1).

For years, exercise scientists and health/fitness professionals have maintained that regular physical activity is the best defense against many diseases and disorders. The importance of regular physical activity in preventing disease and premature death and in maintaining a high quality of life has recently received recognition as a national health objective in the first U.S. Surgeon General's report on Physical Activity and Health (U.S. Dept. of Health and Human Services 1996). This report identifies physical inactivity as a serious, nationwide health problem; provides clear-cut scientific evidence linking physical activity to numerous health benefits; presents demographic data describing physical activity patterns and trends in the U.S. population; and makes physical activity recommendations for improved health (see page 3).

Modest health benefits can be realized by exercising enough to burn as few as 150 kilocalories (kcal) a day, or 1000 kcal a week. This amount of physical activity decreases the risk of coronary heart disease by 50% and the risk of hypertension, diabetes, and colon cancer by 30% (U.S. Dept. of Health and Human Services 1996). The Centers for Disease Control (CDC) and the American College of Sports Medicine (ACSM) have endorsed the following statement regarding physical activity (Pate et al. 1995):

Every U.S. adult should accumulate 30 minutes or more of moderate-intensity physical activity on most, preferably all, days of the week (see page 3).

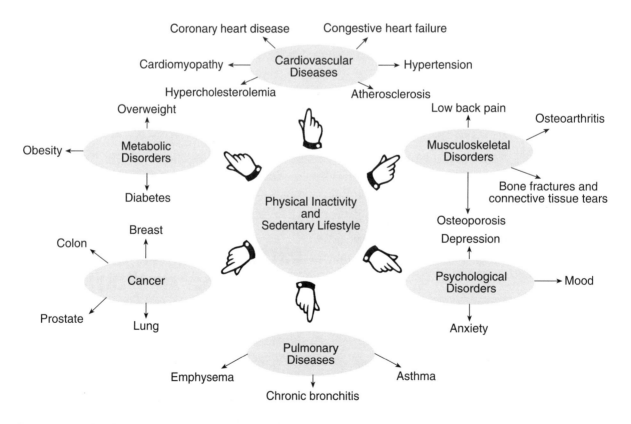

Figure 1.1   **Role of physical activity and exercise in disease prevention and rehabilitation.**

Health Benefits of Physical Activity

Reduced risk of

- dying prematurely
- dying prematurely from heart disease
- developing diabetes
- developing high blood pressure, and
- developing colon cancer

Reduction of

- blood pressure in people who already have high blood pressure, and
- feelings of depression and anxiety

Help in

- controlling body weight
- building and maintaining healthy bones, muscles, and joints
- developing strength and agility in older adults, so they are better able to move about without falling; and
- creating sense of psychological well-being

Data from U.S. Department of Health and Human Services, 1996, *Physical Activity and Health: A Report of the Surgeon General—At-a-Glance* (Washington, DC: Author).

Examples of Moderate Amounts of Physical Activity[*]

This list contains examples of moderate amounts of physical activity. More vigorous activities, such as stair walking and running, require less time (15 minutes). On the other hand, less vigorous activities, like washing and waxing the car, require more time (45 to 60 minutes).

Less Vigorous, More Time

Washing and waxing a car for 45-60 minutes

Washing windows or floors for 45-60 minutes

Playing volleyball for 45 minutes

Playing touch football for 30-45 minutes

Gardening for 30-45 minutes

Wheeling self in wheelchair for 30-40 minutes

Walking 1.75 miles (2.8 km) in 35 minutes (20-minute-per-mile pace)

Basketball (shooting baskets) for 30 minutes

Bicycling 5 miles (8.0 km) in 30 minutes

Dancing fast (social) for 30 minutes

Pushing a stroller 1.5 miles (2.4 km) in 30 minutes

Raking leaves for 30 minutes

Walking 2 miles (3.2 km) in 30 minutes (15-minute-per-mile pace)

Water aerobics for 30 minutes

More Vigorous, Less Time

Swimming laps for 20 minutes

Wheelchair basketball for 20 minutes

Playing basketball for 15-20 minutes

Bicycling 4 miles (6.4 km) in 15 minutes

Jumping rope for 15 minutes

Running 1.5 miles (2.4 km) in 15 minutes (10-minute-per-mile pace)

Shoveling snow for 15 minutes

Stair walking for 15 minutes

[*]A moderate amount of physical activity is roughly that which uses approximately 150 kilocalories of energy per day, or 1,000 kilocalories per week. Some activities can be performed at various intensities; the suggested durations correspond to expected intensity of effort.

Data from U.S. Dept. of Health and Human Services, 1996, *Physical Activity and Health: A Report of the Surgeon General—At-A-Glance* (Washington, DC: Author), 2.

The Exercise and Physical Activity Pyramid, developed by the Metropolitan Life Insurance Company (1995), illustrates a balanced plan of physical activity and exercise to promote a healthy lifestyle and improve physical fitness (see figure 1.2). You should encourage your clients to engage in physical activities around the home and workplace on a daily basis to establish a foundation (base of pyramid) for an active lifestyle. They should perform aerobic activities and flexibility exercises at least three to five days a week; they should do weight resistance exercises and recreational sport activities two to three days a week (middle levels of pyramid). High-intensity training and competitive sports (top of pyramid) require a solid fitness base to prevent injury, and offer relatively few health benefits. Most people should engage in these activities only sparingly. Later chapters contain more detailed exercise prescriptions for cardiovascular and musculoskeletal fitness

CARDIOVASCULAR DISEASE

In 1993 diseases of the heart and blood vessels claimed the lives of 954,138 individuals in the United States. It is estimated that cardiovascular disease (CVD) is responsible for more than 42% of all deaths, and that one-sixth of all people dying from CVD are younger than 65 years. More than 60 million, or one out of every four, Americans have some form of cardiovascular disease: hypertension (50.0 million), coronary heart disease (13.5 million), congestive heart failure (4.7 million), or stroke (3.8 million) (American Heart Association 1995). Other forms of CVD afflict millions more (see figure 1.1).

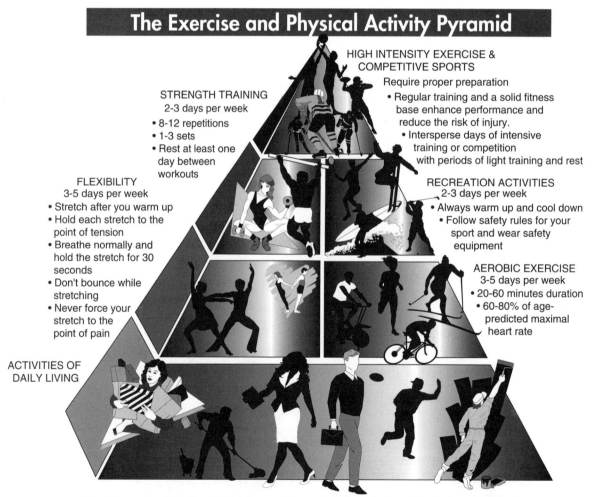

The Exercise and Physical Activity Pyramid

HIGH INTENSITY EXERCISE & COMPETITIVE SPORTS
Require proper preparation
• Regular training and a solid fitness base enhance performance and reduce the risk of injury.
• Intersperse days of intensive training or competition with periods of light training and rest

STRENGTH TRAINING
2-3 days per week
• 8-12 repetitions
• 1-3 sets
• Rest at least one day between workouts

FLEXIBILITY
3-5 days per week
• Stretch after you warm up
• Hold each stretch to the point of tension
• Breathe normally and hold the stretch for 30 seconds
• Don't bounce while stretching
• Never force your stretch to the point of pain

RECREATION ACTIVITIES
2-3 days per week
• Always warm up and cool down
• Follow safety rules for your sport and wear safety equipment

AEROBIC EXERCISE
3-5 days per week
• 20-60 minutes duration
• 60-80% of age-predicted maximal heart rate

ACTIVITIES OF DAILY LIVING

• Try to be active for at least 30 min everyday   • Daily physical activity is the base for fitness
• Activity can be continuous or in multiple segments of at least 10 min

Figure 1.2 Exercise and physical activity pyramid.
Adapted from "Exercise and Activity Pyramid" Metropolitan Life Insurance Company, 1995.

Coronary heart disease (CHD) accounts for more deaths annually than any other disease, with more than 489,000 people dying each year from CHD (American Heart Association 1995). Death rates for CHD are higher among Blacks than among Whites; but the Hispanic population has a lower prevalence of CHD than Whites (Public Health Service 1988).

Coronary heart disease is caused by a lack of blood supply to the heart muscle (myocardial ischemia) resulting from a progressive, degenerative disorder known as atherosclerosis. Atherosclerosis involves a buildup and deposition of fat and fibrous plaques in the intima, or inner lining, of the coronary arteries. These plaques restrict the blood flow to the myocardium and may produce angina pectoris, which is a temporary sensation of tightening and heavy pressure in the chest and shoulder region. A myocardial infarction, or heart attack, can occur if a blood clot, or thrombus, obstructs the coronary blood flow. In this case, blood flow through the coronary arteries is usually reduced by more than 80%. The portion of the myocardium supplied by the obstructed artery dies and eventually is replaced with scar tissue.

Although the death rate from heart attack in the United States declined almost 30% between 1983 and 1993, total deaths from CVD increased significantly in 1993. This is attributed to population growth, particularly middle-aged and older populations (American Heart Association 1995).

CHD Risk Factors

Epidemiological research indicates that many factors are associated with the risk of CHD. The greater the number and severity of risk factors, the greater the probability of CHD. The positive risk factors for CHD are as follows:

- Age
- Family history
- Hypercholesterolemia
- Hypertension
- Current cigarette smoking
- Diabetes mellitus
- Physical inactivity

Obesity and overweight are not independent risk factors, because they exert their effects through other risk factors (i.e., obese individuals tend to have hypertension, diabetes, sedentary lifestyle, and hypercholesterolemia). An increased level of high-density lipoprotein cholesterol (HDL-C > 60 mg · dl^{-1}) in the blood decreases CHD risk.

Physical Activity and CHD

As an exercise scientist, you must educate your clients about the benefits of physical activity and regular exercise for preventing CHD. Physically active people have lower incidences of myocardial infarction and mortality from CHD and tend to develop CHD at a later age compared to their sedentary counterparts (Berlin and Colditz 1990). Individuals who exercise regularly reduce their relative risk of developing CHD by a factor of 1.5 to 2.4 (American Heart Association 1995; Powell et al. 1987). Physical activity exerts its effect independently of smoking, hypertension, hypercholesterolemia, obesity, diabetes, or family history of CHD (Bouchard, Shephard, and Stephens 1994). Also, people who engage in regular exercise as part of their rehabilitation following a myocardial infarction have improved survival rates compared to individuals who do not exercise during their rehabilitation (O'Connor et al. 1989).

HYPERTENSION

Hypertension is a chronic, persistent elevation of blood pressure, affecting an estimated one out of every four adults in the United States. About 50 million Americans, age 6 years and older, have high blood pressure (American Heart Association 1995). Table 1.1 summarizes the risk factors associated with developing hypertension. Up to age 55, men are at greater risk of hypertension than women. After age 74, however, women are at greater risk than men. Also, Blacks and Hispanics have a greater prevalence of hypertension compared to Asians, American Indians, and Whites in the United States (American Heart Association 1995).

Physical Activity and Hypertension

Epidemiological studies report an inverse relationship between blood pressure and physical activity level in women and men (Hagberg 1990; Paffenbarger, Jung, Leung, and Hyde 1991; Reaven, Barrett-Connor, and Edelstein 1991). Regular physical activity (i.e., aerobic exercise performed at an intensity of 40 to 60% of maximal oxygen uptake, 3 to 5 times a week) reduces systolic and diastolic

Table 1.1   Summary of Factors Associated With Disease Risk

Factor	CHD	Diabetes	Hypertension	Hyperlipidemia	Low back pain	Obesity	Osteoporosis
Age	↑	↑	↑	↑	↑	↑	↑
Gender	M > F[a]	F > M	F > M[b]	F > M[b]	F = M	F > M	F > M[b]
Race	B, H > A, AI, W	AI, B, H > A, W	B, H > A, AI, W	B, H, W > A, AI		AI, B, H, W > A	A, W > AI, B
Family history	↑	↑	↑	↑			↑
SES	↓	↓	↓	↓	↓	↓	↑
Alcohol use			↑	↑			↑
Smoking	↑		↑	↑			↑
Nutrition							
Na intake			↑				
Ca intake							↓
Fat/cholesterol intake	↑			↑		↑	
CHO intake		↑					
Intake > Expenditure						↑	
Physical activity	↓	↓	↓	↓	↓	↓	↓
Exercise amenorrhea							↑
Flexibility					↓		
Muscular strength							↓
Skeletal frame size							↓
Other diseases							
Anorexia nervosa							↑
Diabetes	↑						
Hypertension	↑						
Hyperlipidemia	↑						
Obesity and overweight	↑	↑	↑	↑			

↑ = Direct relationship—as factor increases, risk increases; ↓ = indirect relationship—as factor increases, risk decreases.
[a] Males (M) at higher risk than females (F) up to age 55 years
[b] Menopausal females at higher risk than males
CHD = coronary heart disease; A = Asian; AI = American Indian; B = Black; H = Hispanic; W = White; Na = sodium; Ca = calcium; SES = socioeconomic status (reflects income and education levels).

blood pressure by about 10 mmHg in hypertensive individuals; moreover, these reductions in blood pressure in overweight and normal weight individuals are independent of weight loss (Hagberg 1990). Regular physical activity, however, does not lower blood pressure which is already normal (Fagard and Tipton 1994).

While endurance training lowers blood pressure in men and women with mild to moderate hypertension (Hagberg 1990), resistance training also lowers blood pressure in both adolescents and adults with hypertension (Hagberg et al. 1984; Harris and Holly 1987). However, Cononie et al. (1991) reported no change in blood pressure of older men and women (70 to 79 years) with normal or slightly elevated blood pressures in response to six months of resistance training.

HYPERCHOLESTEROLEMIA

Hypercholesterolemia is an elevation in blood cholesterol, particularly low-density lipoprotein cholesterol (LDL-C), and is associated with increased risk of developing CVD. Hypercholesterolemia also is referred to as hyperlipidemia, which is an increase in blood lipid levels. The average total cholesterol (TC) levels in the blood of men and women are 211 and 215 mg $\cdot$ dl^{-1}, respectively. Risk factors for hypercholesterolemia are identified in table 1.1.

In the body, cholesterol and triglycerides are transported as lipoproteins (a lipid bound to a protein carrier). Low-density lipoproteins (LDL) are larger molecules that precipitate in the plasma and are actively transported into the vascular walls. Excess LDL-cholesterol (LDL-C) stimulates the formation of plaque on the intima of the coronary arteries. This reduces the cross-sectional area and obstructs blood flow through the coronary arteries, eventually producing a myocardial infarction.

The high-density lipoproteins (HDL) are smaller molecules that remain suspended in the plasma and are metabolized by the liver. HDL serves a protective function by picking up excess cholesterol from the arterial walls and removing it from the body. HDL-cholesterol (HDL-C) values exceeding 45 mg $\cdot$ dl^{-1} are desirable, and women tend to have higher HDL-C compared to men.

Physical Activity and Lipid Profiles

Regular physical activity, especially habitual aerobic exercise, positively affects lipid metabolism and lipid profiles (Despres and Lamarche 1994). Cross-sectional comparisons of lipid profiles in physically active and sedentary women and men suggest that physical fitness is inversely related to TC and TC/HDL-C ratio (Despres and Lamarche 1994; Shoenhair and Wells 1995). Regular endurance exercise also lowers plasma triglycerides and sometimes reduces TC and LDL-C levels in individuals with initially high levels (Bouchard and Despres 1995). HDL-C increases in response to endurance training; however, this response is less dramatic in women than in men (Lokey and Tran 1989).

Although some researchers have reported improved lipid profiles following resistance training (Fripp and Hodgson 1987; Goldberg et al. 1984; Hurley et al. 1988), methodological flaws in the study design, such as no control group or only one baseline blood sample, suggest that more research is needed to justify this claim. In fact, some researchers have observed that resistance training does not improve lipid profiles in men at risk for CHD (Kokkinos et al. 1991) and in obese women (Manning et al. 1991) when body weight remains stable. These findings suggest that changes in lipid profiles in response to resistance training may be partially dependent on weight loss and the total training volume (Manning et al. 1991).

CIGARETTE SMOKING

Since 1965, smoking has declined 40% among U.S. adults. Yet 417,000 Americans died of smoking-related diseases in 1990 (American Heart Association 1995), and every day approximately 3,000 young people in the United States become smokers.

Cigarette smoking has been linked to lung cancer, pulmonary disorders, and CHD. Smokers have more than twice the risk of heart attack compared to nonsmokers. The nicotine contained in cigarette smoke produces an increase in heart rate and blood pressure, and inhibits the anticlotting mechanisms of the blood.

When individuals stop smoking, their risk of CHD declines rapidly regardless of how long or how much they have smoked. Ten years after quitting, the risk of death from CHD for individuals who had smoked a pack a day or less is almost the same as that of people who never smoked (American Heart Association 1995).

DIABETES MELLITUS

Approximately 13 million people in the United States have diabetes; 90 to 95% of these individuals have Type II, or noninsulin-dependent diabetes mellitus (NIDDM) (Kriska, Blair, and Pereira 1994). Type I, or insulin-dependent diabetes mellitus, usually occurs before the age of 30 years but can develop at any age. Table 1.1 presents risk factors for developing diabetes.

Research suggests that regular physical activity reduces one's risk of developing NIDDM through its association with weight loss and the effects of exercise on insulin sensitivity and glucose tolerance (Kriska et al. 1994; Wells 1996). Manson et al. (1991) reported that women who engaged in vigorous exercise at least once a week have a reduced risk of diabetes. The reduction in diabetes risk, however, appears to be associated with the frequency of exercise. The risk of diabetes decreased 23, 38, and 42%, respectively, in male physicians who exercised vigorously 1, 2 to 4, or 5 or more times a week (Manson et al. 1992). Vigorous exercise was defined as physical activity of sufficient duration to produce sweating. Specific guidelines for prescribing exercise programs for Type I and Type II diabetics are available elsewhere (Sherman and Albright 1990, 1992).

OBESITY AND OVERWEIGHT

Obesity can be defined as a body weight that exceeds the desirable level for a given age, sex, and skeletal frame by more than 20% (National Institutes of Health 1985), or as an excess of body fat at which health risks begin to increase (Public Health Service 1988). The National Health and Nutrition Examination Survey (NHANES III) reported that 61 million adults, or approximately one out of every three, are 20% or more above their desirable body weight (Kuczmarski et al. 1994), and the prevalence of obesity has increased 36% since the early 1960s (American Heart Association 1995). The prevalence of overweight among young Americans is also on the rise; more than one in every five children and adolescents are overweight (Troiano et al. 1995).

Table 1.1 summarizes factors associated with increased risk of obesity.

Excess body weight and fatness pose a threat to both the quality and length of one's life. Obese individuals have a shorter life expectancy and greater risks of CHD, hypercholesterolemia, hypertension, diabetes mellitus, certain cancers, chronic obstructive pulmonary disease, and osteoarthritis of the spine, hip, and knees (National Institutes of Health 1985). Although some studies have reported that obesity is not an independent risk factor for CHD, one epidemiological prospective study of cardiovascular disease in a general population of men and women (the Framingham Heart Study) showed that increased obesity was associated with increased risk, independent of other CHD risk factors (Hubert et al. 1983).

Obesity may be caused by improper diet, overeating, hormonal imbalances, genetic factors, and lack of physical activity. As an exercise specialist, you combat this problem by planning exercise programs and scientifically sound diets for your clients, in consultation with trained nutrition professionals. Restricting caloric intake and increasing caloric expenditure through exercise are effective ways of reducing body weight and fatness, while normalizing blood pressure and blood lipid profiles.

MUSCULOSKELETAL DISEASES AND DISORDERS

Diseases and disorders of the musculoskeletal system, such as osteoporosis, osteoarthritis, bone fractures, connective tissue tears, and low back syndrome, are other types of hypokinetic disease. A loss of bone mass due to aging and physical inactivity is characteristic of osteoporosis (see table 1.1 for osteoporosis risk factors). Approximately 25 million Americans have this disease, which increases the risk of bone fracture in both women and men. Adequate calcium intake and regular physical activity help counteract age-related bone loss. Epidemiological studies show that the incidence of bone fractures is lower in women with higher levels of physical activity. Although no data have demonstrated that exercise alone can prevent the loss of bone mass during and after menopause, the ACSM (1995) recommends increasing physical activity, especially weight-bearing exercise and resistance training exercise, to counteract bone loss due to aging. However, exercise should not be substituted for hormone replacement therapy at menopause.

Low back pain afflicts millions of people each year. More than 80% of all low back problems are produced by muscular weakness or imbalance caused by a lack of physical activity (see table 1.1). If the muscles are not strong enough to support the vertebral column in proper alignment, poor posture results and low back pain develops. Excessive weight, poor flexibility, and improper lifting habits also contribute to low back problems.

Because the origin of low back problems is often functional rather than structural, in many cases it can be corrected through an exercise program designed to develop strength and flexibility in the appropriate muscle groups. Also, people who remain physically active throughout life retain more bone, ligament, and tendon strength and are therefore less prone to bone fractures and connective tissue tears (Pollock, Wilmore, and Fox 1978).

Key Points

- Although physical inactivity is on the decline in the U.S., 60% of all Americans still do not get the recommended amount of physical activity needed for health benefits.

- Lack of regular physical activity and a sedentary lifestyle have led to a rise in hypokinetic diseases in the United States.

- The major hypokinetic diseases are cardiovascular diseases, diabetes, obesity, and musculoskeletal disorders.

- Cardiovascular diseases are responsible for 42% of all deaths in the U.S.

- The positive risk factors for coronary heart disease are the following: age, family history, hypercholesterolemia, hypertension, cigarette smoking, diabetes mellitus, and physical inactivity.

- The prevalence of obesity in the U.S. is on the rise; one out of every three adults and more than one out of every five adolescents and children are overweight.

- Osteoporosis and low back syndrome are musculoskeletal disorders afflicting millions of people in the U.S. each year.

- To benefit health and prevent disease, every U.S. adult should accumulate 30 minutes or more of moderate-intensity physical activity on most, preferably all, days of the week.

REFERENCES

American College of Sports Medicine. 1995. ACSM position stand on osteoporosis and exercise. *Medicine and Science in Sports and Exercise* 27: i-vii.

American Heart Association. 1995. *Heart and stroke facts: 1996 statistical supplement*. Dallas: Author.

Berlin, J.A., and Colditz, G.A. 1990. A meta-analysis of physical activity in the prevention of coronary heart disease. *American Journal of Epidemiology* 132: 612-628.

Bouchard, C., and Despres, J.P. 1995. Physical activity and health: Atherosclerotic, metabolic, and hypertensive diseases. *Research Quarterly for Exercise and Sport* 66: 268-275.

Bouchard, C., Shephard, R.J., and Stephens, T., eds. 1994. *Physical activity, fitness, and health. International proceedings and conference statement*. Champaign, IL: Human Kinetics.

Casperson, C.J., and Merritt, R.K. 1995. Physical activity trends among 26 states, 1986-1990. *Medicine and Science in Sports and Exercise* 27: 713-720.

Cononie, C.C., Graves, J.E., Pollock, M.L., Phillips, M.I., Sumners, C., and Hagberg, J.M. 1991. Effect of exercise training on blood pressure in 70- to 79-yr-old men and women. *Medicine and Science in Sports and Exercise* 23: 505-511.

Despres, J.P., and Lamarche, B. 1994. Low-intensity endurance training, plasma lipoproteins, and the risk of coronary heart disease. *Journal of Internal Medicine* 236: 7-22. DHHS Centers for Disease Control and Prevention. Atlanta: CDC.

Fagard, R.H., and Tipton, C.M. 1994. Physical activity, fitness, and hypertension. In C. Bouchard, R.J. Shephard, and T. Stephens, eds., *Physical activity, fitness, and health*, 633-655. Champaign, IL: Human Kinetics.

Fripp, R.R., and Hodgson, J.L. 1987. Effect of resistance training on plasma lipid and lipoprotein levels in male adolescents. *Journal of Pediatrics* 111: 926-931.

Goldberg, L.S., Elliot, L., Schultz, W., and Kloster, F.E. 1984. Changes in lipid and lipoprotein levels after weight training. *Journal of the American Medical Association* 252: 504-506.

Hagberg, J.M. 1990. Exercise, fitness, and hypertension. In C. Bouchard, R.J. Shephard, T. Stephens, J.R. Sutton, and B.D. McPherson, eds., *Exercise, fitness, and health: A consensus of current knowledge*, 455-466. Champaign, IL: Human Kinetics.

Hagberg, J.M., Ehsani, A.A., Goldring, D., Hernandez, A., Sinacore, D.R., and Holloszy, J.O. 1984. Effect of weight training on blood pressure and hemodynamics in hypertensive adolescents. *Journal of Pediatrics* 104: 147-151.

Harris, K.A., and Holly, R.G. 1987. Physiological response to circuit weight training in borderline, hypertensive subjects. *Medicine and Science in Sports and Exercise* 19: 246-252.

Hubert, H.B., Feinleib, M., McNamara, P.M., and Castelli, W.P. 1983. Obesity as an independent risk factor for cardiovascular disease: A 26 yr follow-up of participants in the Framingham Heart Study. *Circulation* 67: 968-977.

Hurley, B.F., Hagberg, J.M., Goldberg, A.P., Seals, D.R., Ehsani, A.A., Brennan, R.E., and Holloszy, J.O. 1988. Resistive training can reduce coronary risk factors without altering $\dot{V}O_2$max or percent body fat. *Medicine and Science in Sports and Exercise* 20: 150-154.

Kokkinos, P.F., Hurley, B.F., Smutok, M.A., Farmer, C., Reece, C., Shulman, R., Charabogos, C., Patterson, J., Will, S., Devane-Bell, J., and Goldberg, A.P. 1991. Strength training does not improve lipoprotein-lipid profiles in men at risk for CHD. *Medicine and Science in Sports and Exercise* 23: 1134-1139.

Kriska, A.M., Blair, S.N., and Pereira, M.A. 1994. The potential role of physical activity in the prevention of non-insulin dependent diabetes mellitus: The epidemiological evidence. In J.O. Holloszy, ed., *Exercise and Sport Sciences Reviews* 22: 121-143.

Kuczmarski, R.J., Flegal, K.M., Campbell, S.M., and Johnson, C.L. 1994. Increasing prevalence of overweight among U.S. adults: The National Health and Nutrition Examination Surveys, 1960 to 1991. *Journal of the American Medical Association* 272: 205-211.

Lokey, E.A., and Tran, Z.V. 1989. Effects of exercise training on serum lipids and lipoprotein concentrations in women: A meta-analysis. *International Journal of Sports Medicine* 10: 424-429.

Manning, J.M., Dooly-Manning, C.R., White, K., Kampa, I., Silas, S., Kessellhaut, M., and Ruoff, M. 1991. Effects of a resistance training program on lipoprotein-lipid levels in obese women. *Medicine and Science in Sports and Exercise* 23: 1222-1226.

Manson, J.E., Nathan, D.M., Krolewski, A.S., Stampfer, M.J., Willett, W.C., and Hennekens, C.H. 1992. A prospective study of exercise and incidence of diabetes among US male physicians. *Journal of the American Medical Association* 268: 63-67.

Manson, J.E., Rimm, E.B., Stampfer, M.J., Rosner, B., Hennekens, C.H., Speizer, F.E., Colditz, G.A., Willett, W.C., and Krolewski, A.S. 1991. Physical activity incidence of non-insulin dependent diabetes mellitus in women. *Lancet* 338: 774-778.

Metropolitan Life Insurance Company. 1995. *Your guide to physical activity for health.* New York: Author.

National Institutes of Health Consensus Development Panel. 1985. Health implications of obesity: National Institutes of Health consensus development conference statement. *Annals of Internal Medicine* 103: 1073-1077.

O'Connor, G., Buring, J., Yusuf, S., Goldhaber, S., Olmstead, E., Paffenbarger, R., and Hennekens, C. 1989. An overview of randomized trials of rehabilitation with exercise after myocardial infarction. *Circulation* 80: 234-244.

Paffenbarger, R.S., Jung, D.L., Leung, R.W., and Hyde, R.T. 1991. Physical activity and hypertension: An epidemiological view. *Annals of Medicine* 23: 319-327.

Pate, R.R., Pratt, M., Blair, S.N., Haskell, W.L., et al. 1995. Physical activity and public health: A recommendation from the Centers for Disease Control and Prevention and the American College of Sports Medicine. *Journal of the American Medical Association* 273: 402-407.

Pollock, M.L., Wilmore, J.H., and Fox, S.M. III. 1978. *Health and fitness through physical activity.* New York: John Wiley and Sons.

Powell, K.E., Thompson, P.D., Casperson, C.J., and Kendrick, J.S. 1987. Physical activity and the incidence of coronary heart disease. *Annual Review of Public Health* 8: 253-287.

Public Health Service. 1988. *The Surgeon General's report on nutrition and health.* DHHS [PHS] Publication No. 88-50210. Washington, DC: U.S. Government Printing Office.

Public Health Service. 1991. *Healthy People 2000.* DHHS [PHS] Publication No. 91-50212. Boston: Jones and Bartlett.

Reaven, P.D., Barrett-Connor, E., and Edelstein, S. 1991. Relation between leisure-time physical activity and blood pressure in older women. *Circulation* 83: 559-565.

Sherman, W.M., and Albright, A. 1990. Exercise and type I diabetes. *Gatorade Sports Science Institute Sports Science Exchange*, 3, no. 25. Burlington, IL: The Quaker Oats Company.

Sherman, W.M., and Albright, A. 1992. Exercise and type II diabetes. *Gatorade Sports Science Institute Sports Science Exchange*, 4, no. 37. Burlington, IL: The Quaker Oats Company.

Shoenhair, C.L., and Wells, C.L. 1995. Women, physical activity, and coronary heart disease: A review. *Medicine, Exercise, Nutrition and Health* 4: 200-206.

Troiano, R.P., Flegal, K.M., Kuczmarski, R.J., Campbell, S.M., and Johnson, C.L. 1995. Overweight prevalence and trends for children and adolescents. The National Health and Nutrition Examination Surveys. 1963-1991. *Archives of Pediatric and Adolescent Medicine* 149: 1085-1091.

U.S. Department of Health and Human Services. 1996. *Physical activity and health: A report of the Surgeon General at a Glance*. Atlanta, GA: U.S. Department of Health and Human Services, Centers for Disease Control and Prevention, National Center for Chronic Disease Prevention and Health Promotion.

Wells, C.L. 1996. Physical activity and women's health. In C. Corbin, and B. Pangrazi, eds., *Physical activity and fitness research digest*. Series 2, No. 5, 1-6. Washington, DC: President's Council on Physical Fitness and Sports.

CHAPTER 2

Preliminary Health Screening and Risk Classification

Key Questions

- What are the major components of the health evaluation, and how is this information used to screen clients for exercise testing and participation?
- What factors do I need to focus on when evaluating the client's medical history and lifestyle characteristics?
- How is the client's disease risk classified?
- Do all clients need a physical examination and medical clearance from their physician before taking an exercise test?
- What are the standards for classifying blood cholesterol levels?
- How is blood pressure measured and evaluated? Are automated blood pressure devices accurate?
- How is heart rate measured? Are heart rate monitors accurate?
- What is an ECG, and does every client need to have one before taking an exercise test?
- Is it safe to give a graded exercise test to all clients? When does a physician need to be present?
- What are the major components of the lifestyle evaluation, and how can this information be used?
- What are the purposes of informed consent?

Before assessing your client's physical fitness profile, you should classify the individual's health status and lifestyle. You will use information from the initial health and lifestyle evaluations to screen clients for physical fitness testing. You also will use this information to identify individuals with medical contraindications to exercise, with disease symptoms and risk factors, and with special needs.

This chapter discusses the components of a comprehensive health evaluation, coronary risk factor profile, medical history questionnaire, lifestyle evaluation, and informed consent. It also presents guidelines and standards for classifying blood cholesterol levels, blood pressures, and disease risk, along with techniques and procedures for measuring heart rate and blood pressure at rest and during exercise and conducting a resting 12-lead electrocardiogram (ECG).

HEALTH EVALUATION

The purpose of the health evaluation is to detect the presence of disease and to assess the initial disease risk classification of your clients. The components of a comprehensive health evaluation are listed in table 2.1. Minimally, for pretest health screening of clients for exercise testing and exercise program participation, you should

- administer the Physical Activity Readiness Questionnaire (PAR-Q),

- identify signs and symptoms of diseases,
- analyze the coronary risk profile, and
- classify the disease risk of your clients.

Physical Activity Readiness Questionnaire (PAR-Q)

The PAR-Q has seven questions designed to identify individuals who need medical clearance from their physicians prior to taking any physical fitness tests or starting an exercise program (see appendix A.2). If clients answer "yes" to any of these questions, they should be referred to their physicians to obtain medical clearance before engaging in physical activity. Also, older clients and those who are not used to regular physical activity should always check with their physicians before starting an exercise program.

Table 2.1   Components of a Comprehensive Health Evaluation

Component	Purpose
• PAR-Q	To determine client's readiness for physical activity
• Signs and symptoms of disease	To identify an individual in need of medical referral
• Coronary risk factor analysis	To determine the number of CHD risk factors for client
• Disease risk classification	To categorize client as apparently healthy, at increased risk, or with known disease
• Medical history	To review client's past and present personal and family health history, focusing on conditions requiring medical referral and clearance
• Physical examination	To detect signs and symptoms of disease
• Medical clearance	To obtain physician approval for exercise testing and participation
• Laboratory tests	To provide a more in-depth assessment of client's health status, particularly for someone with known disease
• Cholesterol and lipoprotein profile	To determine if client has hyperlipidemia; these values are also used in the coronary risk factor analysis
• Blood pressure assessment	To determine if client is hypertensive; these values are also used in the coronary risk factor analysis
• Resting heart rate and 12-lead ECG	To evaluate cardiac function and detect cardiac abnormalities that are contraindications to exercise
• Graded exercise test	To assess functional aerobic capacity and to detect cardiac abnormalities due to exercise stress

PROCEDURES FOR COMPREHENSIVE PRETEST HEALTH SCREENING

Here are step-by-step procedures you should follow when conducting a comprehensive health evaluation.

- Greet the client.
- Explain the purpose of the health evaluation and lifestyle evaluation.
- Obtain the client's informed consent for health screening.
- Administer and evaluate the PAR-Q; refer client to physician if necessary.
- Administer and evaluate client's medical history, focusing on signs, symptoms, and diseases; refer client to physician if necessary.
- Evaluate client's lifestyle profile.
- Evaluate and classify the client's cholesterol and lipoprotein levels if test results are available.
- Measure and classify the client's resting blood pressure and heart rate.
- Assess the client's coronary risk factors.
- Classify the client's disease risk.
- Evaluate the client's blood chemistry profile if test results are available.

If requested by the client's physician, you may include these additional items:

- Explain the purpose of and answer any questions about the 12-lead resting ECG and graded exercise test (GXT).
- Obtain the client's informed consent for these tests.
- Prepare the client and administer the 12-lead resting ECG.
- Have a physician interpret the results of the 12-lead resting ECG.
- Use the client's disease risk classification to determine whether a maximal or submaximal GXT should be administered and whether a physician needs to be present during this test.
- Assess the client's resting blood pressure and heart rate.
- Administer the GXT.
- Assess and classify the client's functional aerobic capacity.

Signs and Symptoms of Disease

As part of the pretest health screening, you should ask your clients if they have any of the following conditions (defined in appendix A.1):

Cardiovascular

Hypertension

Hypercholesterolemia

Heart murmurs

Myocardial infarction

Fainting/dizziness

Claudication

Chest pain

Palpitations

Ischemia

Tachycardia

Ankle edema

Stroke

Pulmonary

Asthma

Bronchitis

Emphysema

Nocturnal dyspnea

Coughing up blood

Exercise-induced asthma

Breathlessness during or after mild exertion

Metabolic

Diabetes

Obesity

Glucose intolerance

McArdle's syndrome

Hypoglycemia

Thyroid disease

Cirrhosis

Musculoskeletal

Osteoporosis

Osteoarthritis

Low back pain

Prosthesis

Muscular atrophy

Swollen joints

Orthopedic pain

Artificial joints

If so, refer them to their physicians to obtain a signed medical clearance prior to any exercise testing or participation. For definitions of the specific medical terms used, refer to appendix A.1.

Coronary Risk Factor Analysis

To assess your client's coronary risk profile, evaluate each item in table 2.2 carefully. Guidelines for classification of blood pressure and blood cholesterol levels in adults are presented in tables 2.3 and 2.4, respectively. If your client's high density lipoprotein cholesterol (HDL-C) exceeds 60 mg · dl^{-1}, subtract one from the total number of positive risk factors. Alternatively, you can use RISKO (see appendix A.3), a simple paper-and-pencil test developed by the American Heart Association (1994), or computer software programs to evaluate your client's CHD risk profile. This information is especially helpful in classifying the individual for exercise testing and in designing safe exercise programs.

Disease Risk Classification

Based on the results from the coronary risk factor analysis, you should classify individuals as apparently healthy, as being at increased risk, or as having known disease (see table 2.5). The ACSM (1995) defines apparently healthy as asymptomatic with no more than one major coronary risk factor (see table 2.2). Individuals who have signs or symptoms of cardiopulmonary or metabolic disease or who have two or more major coronary risk factors are at increased risk. Clients who have cardiac, pulmonary, or metabolic diseases are given a known disease classification.

Table 2.2   CHD Risk Factors

Positive risk factors	Criteria
1. Age	Men >45 yr; women >55 yr or premature menopause without estrogen replacement therapy
2. Family history	Myocardial infarction or sudden death before 55 yr of age for father or other first-degree male relative; or before 65 yr of age in mother or other first-degree, female relative
3. Cigarette smoking	Currently smoking
4. Hypertension	Blood pressure ≥140/90 mm Hg, measured on two separate occasions, or on antihypertensive medication
5. Hypercholesterolemia	TC >200 mg · dl^{-1} or HDL-C <35 mg · dl^{-1}
6. Diabetes mellitus	Persons with insulin-dependent diabetes who are >30 yr, or have had this disease for >15 yr; persons with noninsulin-dependent diabetes who are >35 yr
7. Physical inactivity	Persons defined by the combination of sedentary jobs involving sitting for a large part of the day and no regular exercise or active recreational pursuits

Negative risk factor*	
1. High HDL-C	Persons with serum HDL-C >60 mg · dl^{-1}

*If HDL-C is high, subtract one risk factor from the sum of the positive risk factors.

Adapted, by permission, from American College of Sports Medicine, 1995, *ACSM's Guidelines for Exercise Testing and Prescription* (Baltimore: Williams & Wilkins), 18.

Table 2.3   Classification of Blood Pressure for Adults 18 Years or Older[a]

Systolic BP (mm Hg)[b]	Category	Diastolic BP (mm Hg)
<130	Normal	<85
130-139	High normal	85-89
140-159	Stage I: Mild hypertension	90-99
160-179	Stage II: Moderate hypertension	100-109
180-209	Stage III: Severe hypertension	110-119
≥210	Stage IV: Very severe hypertension	≥120

[a]For individuals not taking antihypertensive drugs and not acutely ill. Based on average of two or more readings on two or more occasions.

[b]When systolic and diastolic pressures fall into different categories, use the higher category for classification.

Data from Joint National Committee (1993), "The Fifth Report of the Joint National Committee on Detection, Evaluation, and Treatment of High Blood Pressure," *Archives of Internal Medicine* 153: 161.

Table 2.4   Classification of Total Cholesterol, LDL-C, Triglycerides (mg · dl^{-1}), and HDL-C

Classification	TC	LDL-C	Triglycerides	Classification	HDL-C
Desirable	<200	<130	<200	Low	<35
Borderline high	200-239	130-159	200-400	Normal	35-60
High	≥240	≥160	400-1000	High	>60
Very high	—	—	>1000		

Data from National Cholesterol Education Program Committee (1993), "Summary of the Second Report of the National Cholesterol Education Program (NCEP) Expert Panel on Detection, Evaluation, and Treatment of High Blood Cholesterol in Adults (Adult Treatment Panel II)," *Journal of the American Medical Association* 269: 3017.

Table 2.5   Classification of Disease Risk

Classification	Criteria
Apparently healthy	Asymptomatic and apparently healthy individuals with no more than 1 major coronary risk factor
Increased risk	Individuals with signs or symptoms of cardiopulmonary or metabolic disease and/or 2 or more major coronary risk factors
Known disease	Individuals with known cardiac, pulmonary, or metabolic disease

Reproduced, by permission, from American College of Sports Medicine, 1995, *ACSM's Guidelines for Exercise Testing and Prescription* (Williams & Wilkins: Baltimore), 19.

Medical History Questionnaire

You should require your clients to complete a comprehensive medical history questionnaire that includes questions concerning personal and family health history (appendix A.4). Use the questionnaire to

- examine the client's record of personal illnesses, surgeries, and hospitalizations (Section A),

- assess previous medical diagnoses and signs and symptoms of disease that have occurred within the past year or are currently present (Section B), and

- analyze your client's family history of diabetes, heart disease, stroke, and hypertension (Section C).

Also, when reviewing the medical history, you should carefully focus on conditions that require medical referral (see page 15). If any of these conditions are noted, refer your client to a physician for a physical examination and medical clearance prior to exercise testing or starting an exercise program. It is also important to note the types of medication being used by the client. Drugs such as digitalis, beta-blockers, diuretics, vasodilators, bronchodilators, and insulin may alter the individual's heart rate, blood pressure, electrocardiogram, and exercise capacity. If your client reports a medical condition or drug that is unfamiliar to you, be certain to consult medical references or a physician to obtain more information before conducting any exercise tests or allowing the client to participate in an exercise program.

Physical Examination and Medical Clearance

Your prospective exercise program participants should obtain a physical examination and a signed medical clearance from a physician (appendix A.5), especially if they are

- men >40 years of age with two or more major coronary risk factors,

- women >50 years of age with two or more major coronary risk factors, or

- individuals of any age with known cardiovascular, pulmonary, or metabolic disease.

The physical examination should focus on signs and symptoms of CHD and include an evaluation of body weight, orthopedic problems, edema, acute illness, pulse rate, cardiac regularity, blood pressure (supine, sitting, and standing), and auscultation of the heart, lungs, and major arteries. The physical examination and medical history may reveal signs or symptoms of CHD, particularly if accompanied by shortness of breath, chest pains, leg cramps, or high blood pressure. Clients with these symptoms should obtain a signed medical clearance from their physician prior to exercise testing or exercise participation.

Laboratory Tests

Laboratory tests are also an important part of the health evaluation. Assess the blood lipid profile of all individuals, as well as fasting blood glucose levels, if indicated by family history or symptoms. For individuals with known coronary disease, additional tests may be indicated. These may include a resting 12-lead electrocardiogram, angiogram, echocardiogram, and a physician-monitored, graded exercise test. You also should obtain a chest x-ray, comprehensive blood chemistry, and a complete blood count (ACSM 1995). For clients with known pulmonary disease, ACSM (1995) recommends a chest x-ray, pulmonary function tests, and specialized pulmonary tests (e.g., blood gas analysis).

Cholesterol and Lipoprotein Profile

The National Cholesterol Education Program (NCEP) (1993) developed guidelines for classifying TC, LDL-C, and HDL-C levels (see table 2.4). A flow chart depicting the NCEP's recommendations for lipoprotein analysis and cholesterol treatment is presented in figure 2.1.

The NCEP recommends initially assessing the TC and HDL-C of the individual. If your client's TC is borderline high (200 to 239 mg · dl^{-1}) or high (≥240 mg · dl^{-1}), the HDL-C level is less than 35 mg · dl^{-1}, and the client has two or more risk factors for CHD, you should assess LDL-C following a nine- to twelve-hour fast. Refer clients to their physician for an extensive clinical evaluation and dietary therapy if they have high LDL-C (≥160 mg · dl^{-1}) or borderline high LDL-C (130 to 159 mg · dl^{-1}) and two or more risk factors.

In addition to TC and lipoproteins, you can assess triglycerides and the ratio of TC to HDL-C. Clients with triglyceride levels in excess of 200 mg · dl^{-1} or TC/HDL-C ratios greater than 5.0 are at higher risk.

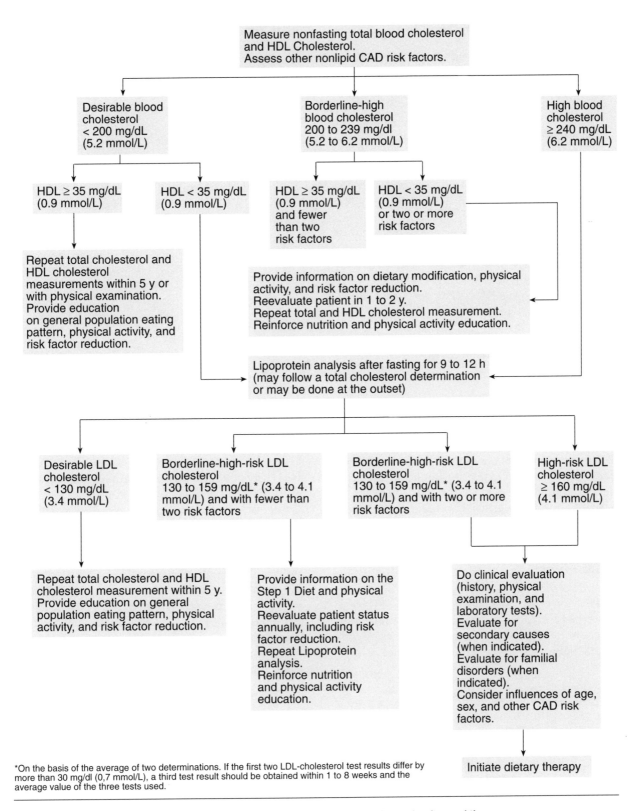

*On the basis of the average of two determinations. If the first two LDL-cholesterol test results differ by more than 30 mg/dl (0,7 mmol/L), a third test result should be obtained within 1 to 8 weeks and the average value of the three tests used.

Figure 2.1   National Cholesterol Education Program (1993)—guidelines for evaluation and therapy.

Diet and Physical Activity Therapy

The NCEP (1993) recommends a two-step dietary therapy to reduce serum cholesterol levels and to promote weight loss in individuals who are overweight. The Step I diet limits dietary intakes of saturated fat (8 to 10% of total calories), total fat (≤30% of total calories), and cholesterol (≤300 mg/day). The Step II diet is initiated if the Step I diet is found to be ineffective for reaching a healthy LDL-C level. The Step II diet limits saturated fat intake to ≤7% of the total calories and restricts dietary cholesterol to <200 mg/day.

Increased physical activity is an essential part of all dietary therapy, especially for overweight individuals who need to create a caloric deficit for weight loss. Weight reduction and exercise not only lower serum cholesterol levels but have these additional benefits for reducing risk of CHD (NCEP 1993):

- decrease in serum triglycerides
- elevation of HDL-C
- decrease in blood pressure
- reduction of risk for diabetes mellitus

As a last resort, some individuals may require drug therapy to alter their blood lipid profiles. Drug therapy, however, should not be substituted for dietary therapy (NCEP 1993). Drugs such as gemfibrozil, lovastatin, cholestyramine, and colestipol may lower LDL-C or raise HDL-C levels.

Blood Profile

Information obtained from a complete blood analysis can be used to assess your client's overall health status and readiness for exercise. Table 2.6 provides normal values for selected blood variables.

Blood Pressure Assessment

Blood pressure (BP) is a measure of the force or pressure exerted by the blood on the arteries. The highest pressure (systolic BP) reflects the pressure in the arteries during systole of the heart when myocardial contraction forces a large volume of blood into the arteries. Following systole, the arteries recoil and the pressure drops during diastole, or the filling phase of the heart. Diastolic BP is the lowest pressure in the artery during the cardiac

Table 2.6	Normal Values for Selected Blood Variables
Variable	**Ideal or typical values**
Triglycerides	<200 mg $\cdot$ dl^{-1}
Total cholesterol	<200 mg $\cdot$ dl^{-1}
LDL-cholesterol	<130 mg $\cdot$ dl^{-1}
HDL-cholesterol	>35 mg $\cdot$ dl^{-1}
TC/HDL-cholesterol	<3.5
Blood glucose	60-114 mg $\cdot$ dl^{-1}
Hemoglobin	13.5-17.5 g $\cdot$ dl^{-1} men 11.5-15.5 g $\cdot$ dl^{-1} women
Hematocrit	40-52% men 36-48% women
Potassium	3.5-5.5 meq $\cdot$ dl^{-1}
Blood urea nitrogen	4-24 mg $\cdot$ dl^{-1}
Creatinine	0.3-1.4 mg $\cdot$ dl^{-1}
Iron	40-190 μg $\cdot$ dL^{-1} men 35-180 μg $\cdot$ dL^{-1} women
Calcium	8.5-10.5 mg $\cdot$ dl^{-1}

cycle. Resting systolic BP usually varies between 110 and 140 mmHg, and diastolic BP between 60 and 80 mmHg. Usually a person is not classified as hypertensive unless the BP remains elevated (>140/90 mmHg) on two occasions (see table 2.3). The difference between the systolic and diastolic blood pressures is known as the pulse pressure. The pulse pressure creates a pulse wave that can be palpated at various sites in the body to determine pulse rate and to estimate blood pressure.

Effective treatments are available for hypertension. A sodium-restricted diet, weight reduction, restricted alcohol intake, and exercise may help to lower blood pressure in mild hypertensives. Many antihypertensive drugs are also available to lower blood pressure:

- Diuretics rid the body of excess salt and fluids.
- Beta-blockers reduce heart rate and cardiac output.
- Sympathetic nerve inhibitors prevent constriction of arterioles.
- Vasodilators induce relaxation in smooth muscles of arterial walls.
- Angiotensin converting enzyme (ACE) inhibitors disrupt the body's production of angiotensin, which constricts arterioles.

Procedures

The "gold standard" for assessing blood pressures is the direct measurement of intra-arterial BP. This method is invasive and requires catheterization. Therefore, in clinical or field settings, BP is typically measured indirectly by auscultation using a stethoscope and sphygmomanometer consisting of a BP cuff and either an anaeroid or mercury column manometer. A mercury column manometer is preferable because anaeroid manometers lose their calibration more easily. Technicians with impaired hearing can use an anesthesiologist's stethoscope, which magnifies sound. Alternatively, you can measure resting BP with automated devices The validity of these devices for measuring exercise blood pressures, however, has not yet been firmly established (Griffin, Robergs, and Heyward 1997). Also, you can obtain an estimate of resting BP using the palpation method described later. These estimates are generally within 10mmHg of auscultatory values (Reeves 1995).

To check the accuracy of an anaeroid manometer against a mercury unit, follow the procedures suggested by Reeves (1995):

- Disconnect the bulbs of both cuffs and reconnect the bulb and dial of the anaeroid unit to the cuff of the mercury unit.

- Roll the cuff up loosely, securing the Velcro strips, and hold the cuff steady while gradually inflating it.

- Hold the dial of the anaeroid manometer close to the mercury column and compare the two readings at several pressures throughout the range of the measurement scale (e.g., 40 to 220 mmHg). If the anaeroid and mercury manometer pressures differ by more than 2 to 3 mmHg, send the anaeroid manometer to the manufacturer for adjustment.

Measure resting BP in the supine and exercise (sitting or standing) positions prior to testing (ACSM 1995). The client should be wearing a short-sleeved or sleeveless garment and be seated in a quiet room. Take BP measurements rapidly, and completely deflate the cuffs for at least 30 seconds between consecutive readings. For more accurate results, obtain two or three determinations of pressure from each arm.

Proper cuff size is important, because a large cuff on a small arm causes low readings. Cuffs for average-sized adults are usually 12 to 14 cm (4.7 to 5.5 in) wide and 30 cm (11.8 in) in length. Smaller cuffs for children and larger cuffs for obese persons are also available. You should also use the larger cuff to measure BP of individuals with well-developed arm muscles.

To measure resting BP (seated position), use the following recommended procedures (Reeves 1995):

RESTING BLOOD PRESSURE MEASUREMENT

---

1. Seat the client in a quiet room for at least five minutes. The client's bare arm should be resting on a table so that the middle of the arm is at the level of the heart.

2. Estimate the client's arm circumference or measure it at the midpoint between the acromion process of the shoulder and the olecranon process of the elbow (see appendix D.5, description for measuring arm circumference) using an anthropometric tape measure. The bladder of the cuff should encircle 80% of an adult's arm and 100% of a child's arm.

3. Palpate the brachial artery pulse on the anteriomedial aspect of arm below the belly of the biceps brachii and 2 to 3 cm (1 inch) above the antecubital fossa. Wrap the deflated cuff firmly around the upper arm so that the midline of the cuff is over the brachial artery pulse. The lower edge of the cuff should be approximately 2.5 cm (1 inch) above the antecubital fossa. If the cuff is too loose, BP will be overestimated. Avoid placing the cuff over clothing, and if the shirt sleeve is rolled up, make certain that it is not occluding the circulation.

4. Position the manometer so that the center of the mercury column or dial is eye level and the cuff's tubing is not overlapping or obstructed.

5. Locate and palpate the radial pulse (see page 23 for anatomical description of this site), close the valve of the blood pressure unit completely by screwing it away from you, and rapidly inflate the cuff to 70 mmHg. Then slowly increase the pressure in 10 mmHg increments while palpating the radial pulse and note when the pulse disappears (estimate of systolic BP). Partially open the valve by unscrewing it toward you to slowly release the pressure at a rate of 2 to 3 mmHg per second, and note when the pulse reappears (estimate of diastolic BP). Fully open the valve to completely release the pressure in the cuff.

The estimate of systolic BP from the palpatory method is then used to determine how much the cuff needs to be inflated when measuring BP using the auscultatory technique. In this way, you can avoid over- or underinflating the cuff for clients with low or high blood pressures, respectively.

6.   Position the ear pieces of the stethoscope so that they are aligned with the auditory canals (i.e., angled anteriorily).

7.   Place the head (bell) of the stethoscope over the brachial pulse (about 1 cm or 0.4 in superior and medial to the antecubital fossa). Make certain that the entire head of the stethoscope is contacting the skin. To avoid extraneous noise, do not place any part of the head of the stethoscope underneath the cuff.

8.   Close the valve, and quickly and steadily inflate the cuff pressure to about 20 to 30 mmHg above the estimated systolic pressure previously determined by palpation.

9.   Partially open the valve to slowly release the pressure at a rate of 2 to 3 mmHg per second. Note when you hear the first sharp thud caused by the sudden rush of blood as the artery opens. This is known as the first Korotkoff sound and corresponds to the systolic pressure (Phase I).

10.   Continue reducing the pressure slowly (no more than 2 mmHg per second), noting when the metallic-tapping sound becomes muffled (Phase IV diastolic pressure) and when the sound disappears (Phase V diastolic pressure). Typically, the Phase V value is used as the index of diastolic pressure. However, both Phase IV and V diastolic pressures should be noted. During rhythmic exercise, the Phase V pressure tends to decrease due to reduction in peripheral resistance. In some cases, it may even drop to zero (Pollock, Wilmore, and Fox 1978).

11.   After noting the Phase V pressure, continue deflating the cuff for at least 10 mmHg, making certain that no additional sounds are heard. Then rapidly and completely deflate the cuff.

12.   Record all three BP values (Phase I, IV, and V) to the nearest 2 mmHg. Wait at least 30 seconds and repeat the measurement. Use the average of these two measurements.

It takes a great deal of practice to become proficient at measuring blood pressures. When you are first learning this method, it is highly recommended that you practice with a trained BP technician, using a dual- or multiple-head stethoscope so that you both can listen simultaneously and compare BP readings for the same trial.

Measuring BP during exercise is much more difficult than during rest. You should not attempt to measure exercise BP until you have demonstrated competency and confidence in your ability to measure resting BP. It is particularly difficult to obtain accurate BP measurements when the client is running on the treadmill, because of extraneous noise and movement of the arms while running. Sometimes you will not be able to determine diastolic BP due to the noise and vibration during exercise. Novice BP technicians should practice taking blood pressures during bicycle ergometer exercise first and then try measuring BP during treadmill exercise.

Measurement Error

Sources of error in measuring blood pressure are numerous (Reeves 1995). You need to be aware of the following sources of error and do as much as possible to control them:

- Inaccurate sphygmomanometer
- Improper cuff width or length
- Cuff not centered, too loose, or over clothing
- Arm unsupported, or elbow lower than heart level
- Poor auditory acuity of technician
- Improper rate of inflation or deflation of the cuff pressure
- Improper stethoscope placement or pressure
- Expectation bias and inexperience of the technician
- Slow reaction time of the technician
- Parallax error in reading the manometer
- Background noise
- Client holding treadmill handrails or cycle ergometer handlebars

Heart Rate Assessment

The client should rest 5 to 10 minutes in either a supine or seated position before you assess the resting heart rate. It is important that you measure resting heart rate carefully, because it is sometimes used in the calculation of target exercise heart rates for submaximal exercise tests as well as for exercise prescriptions. You can measure heart rate using auscultation, palpation, heart rate monitors, or ECG recordings.

Auscultation

When measuring resting heart rate by auscultation, place the bell of the stethoscope over the third intercostal space to the left of the sternum. Count the sounds from the heart for 30 or 60 seconds. The 30-second count is multiplied by 2 to convert it to beats per minute (bpm).

Palpation

When using the palpation technique for determining heart rate, palpate the pulse at one of the following sites:

- brachial artery—on the anteromedial aspect of the arm below the belly of the biceps brachii, approximately 2 to 3 cm (1 inch) above the antecubital fossa

- carotid artery—in the neck just lateral to the larynx

- radial artery—on the anterolateral aspect of the wrist directly in line with the base of the thumb

- temporal artery—along the hairline of the head at the temple

Heart Rate Monitors and ECG Recordings

Heart rate also can be measured using heart rate monitors or an ECG monitoring system. Generally, heart rate monitors are designed to detect either the pulse or the ECG electrical signal from the heart and provide a digital display of the heart rate. Pulse monitors use infrared sensors attached to the client's fingertip or earlobe to detect pulsations in blood flow during the cardiac cycle. Chest strap, wire, and wireless ECG-type monitors tend to be more accurate and reliable than pulse monitors, especially during vigorous exercise. However, the accuracy of wireless chest strap monitors may be affected by electrical equipment (such as some treadmills, stairclimbers, rowing machines, and video screens) generating radio or magnetic interference.

Most ECG monitoring systems provide a continuous digital display of the heart rate. This value is usually recorded at the top of the ECG strip recording. If your equipment does not provide a digital readout, you can use a heart rate ruler that converts the distance of two cardiac cycles to bpm. Alternatively, the heart rate can be counted by measuring the distance between four consecutive beats (R-R intervals) using a millimeter ruler. Convert the distance to beats per minute based on the paper speed of the recorder (usually $25 \text{ mm} \cdot \sec^{-1}$). For example, if the distance for 4 beats is 60 mm and the distance for 1 minute is 1500 mm (i.e., 25 mm x 60 seconds), the per minute heart rate is determined by setting up the following equation and solving for x:

4 beats / 60 mm = x(bpm) / 1500 mm

Cross-multiplying $60x = 6000$, then $x = 100$ bpm. You can use the sample ECG recordings in appendix A.6 to practice measuring heart rates using this method.

No matter which technique you use to measure heart rate, you should be aware that heart rate fluctuates easily due to temperature, anxiety, exercise, stress, eating, smoking, drinking coffee, time of day, and body position.

The average resting heart rate for adults is 60 to 80 bpm, with the average resting heart rate of women typically 7 to 10 bpm higher than that of men. Heart rates as low as 28 to 40 bpm have been reported for highly conditioned endurance athletes; whereas poorly trained, sedentary individuals may have heart rates that exceed 100 bpm. In a supine position, the resting heart rate is lower than in either a sitting or standing position.

Do not use resting heart rate as a measure of cardiorespiratory fitness. There is wide variability in resting heart rate within the population, and a low resting HR is not always indicative of cardiorespiratory fitness level. In some cases, a low resting heart rate indicates a diseased heart (McArdle, Katch, and Katch 1996). The following general guidelines may be used to classify resting heart rate:

<60 bpm = bradycardia (slow rate)
60–100 bpm = normal rate
>100 bpm = tachycardia (fast rate)

Twelve-Lead Electrocardiogram (ECG)

The ECG is a composite record of the electrical events in the heart during the cardiac cycle. As the heart depolarizes and repolarizes during contrac-tion, an electrical impulse spreads to the tissues surrounding the heart. Electrodes placed on opposite sides of the heart transmit the electrical potential to an ECG recorder.

In addition to obtaining baseline data, the resting ECG detects such contraindications to exercise testing as evidence of previous myocardial infarction, ischemic ST segment changes, conduction defects, and left ventricular hypertrophy. Reading and interpreting ECGs require a high degree of skill and practice. As an exercise technician, you can administer the resting 12-lead ECG, but a qualified physician should interpret the results. Only basic information about administering an ECG is included in this chapter. You should consult other references for more detailed information concerning the reading and interpretation of ECG abnormalities (Adamovich 1984; Conover 1992; Dubin 1980; Goldberger and Goldberger 1981; Goldman 1982).

ECG Basics

A typical normal ECG (figure 2.2) is composed of a P wave that represents depolarization of the atria. The P-R interval indicates the delay in the impulse at the atrioventricular (AV) node. Electrical currents generated during ventricular depolarization and contraction produce the QRS complex. The T wave and ST segment correspond to ventricular repolarization.

A lead is a pair of electrodes placed on the body and connected to an ECG recorder. An axis is an imaginary line connecting the two electrodes. A standard 12-lead ECG consists of three limb leads, three augmented unipolar leads, and six chest leads. Each of the 12 ECG leads records a different view of the heart's electrical activity.

Resting 12-Lead ECG

To measure the 12 leads, 10 electrodes are used. The electrodes for the three limb leads (I, II, and III) are placed on the right arm, left arm, and left leg. A ground electrode is placed on the right leg. This is electronically equivalent to placing the electrodes at the shoulders and the symphysis pubis. Limb lead I measures the voltage differential between the left and right arm electrodes. Limb leads II and III measure the voltage between the left leg and right (lead II) and left (lead III) arms. Figure 2.3 shows the three limb leads and three augmented unipolar leads.

The three augmented unipolar leads are aVF (feet), aVL (left), and aVR (right). The augmented unipolar lead compares the voltage across one of the limb

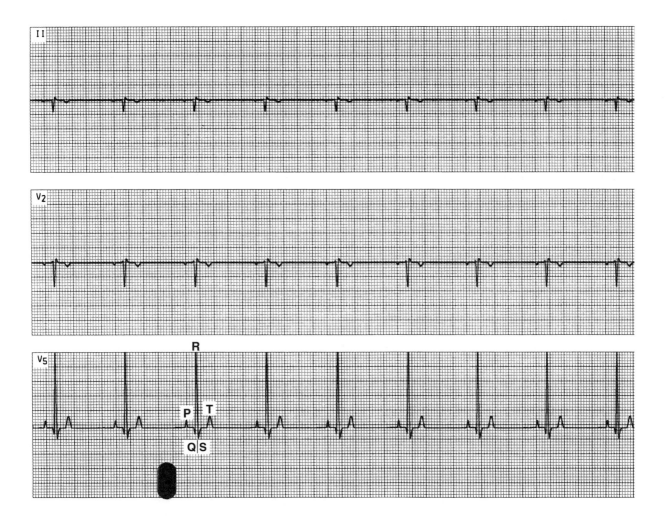

Figure 2.2 Typical normal ECG.

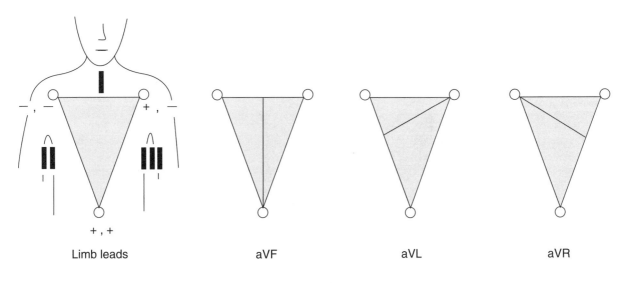

Figure 2.3 Three limb leads and three augmented unipolar leads.

electrodes with the average voltage across the two opposite electrodes. Lead aVL, for example, records the voltage across an electrode placed on the left arm and the average voltage across the other two limb electrodes (see figure 2.3).

The six chest electrodes (V_1 to V_6) measure the voltage across a specific area of the chest, with the average voltage across the other three limb leads. Figure 2.4 illustrates electrode placement for the chest leads, V_1 through V_6:

Anatomical Locations for Chest Electrodes

V_1—fourth intercostal space to the right of the sternal border

V_2—fourth intercostal space to the left of the sternal border

V_3—at the midpoint of a straight line between V2 and V4

V_4—fifth intercostal space along the midclavicular line

V_5—horizontal to V4 on the anterior axillary line

V_6—horizontal to V4 and V5 on the midaxillary line

During the resting ECG, the client should lie quietly in a supine position on a table. The electrode sites should be shaved, if hair is present, and cleaned with alcohol. Remove the superficial layer of skin at each site by rubbing it with fine grain emory paper or a gauze pad. Disposable electrodes contain electrode gel and adhesive disks. After applying the electrode, tap it firmly to test for noisy leads. You should always calibrate the ECG recorder prior to use by recording the standard 1-mV deflection per centimeter. Also, to standardize the time base for the ECG, set the paper speed to 25 mm per second.

Twelve-Lead Exercise ECG

To avoid poor ECG tracings, caused by moving limbs during exercise, the electrode configuration is modified slightly for an exercise 12-lead ECG. The right and left arm electrodes are placed below the right and left clavicles, respectively. The right and left leg electrodes are attached to the right and left sides of the trunk, below the rib cage on the anterior axillary line. The six chest electrodes are positioned as previously described (see figure 2.5).

Graded Exercise Test (GXT)

For some individuals, the client's physician may recommend that a graded exercise test be administered as part of the health evaluation to assess functional aerobic capacity. Coronary heart disease often is not detectable from the resting ECG, and abnormalities may not appear until the individual engages in relatively strenuous exercise.

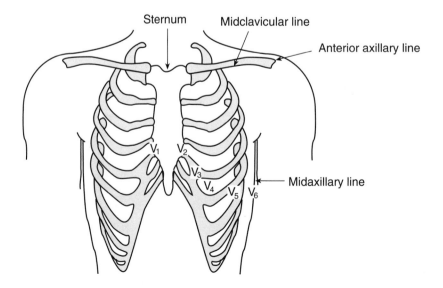

Figure 2.4   Electrode placement for chest leads, V_1 to V_6.

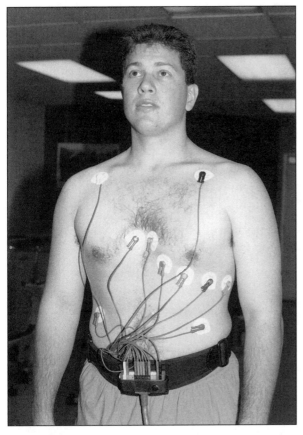

Figure 2.5   Electrode placement for 12-lead exercise ECG.

Use the client's risk classification to determine whether a maximal or submaximal exercise test should be administered and whether a physician needs to be present during the exercise testing (table 2.7). Also, you need to be familiar with medical conditions that are absolute and relative contraindications to exercise testing (see pg. 28) in an out-of-hospital setting. For definitions of the medical terms included in this list, refer to appendix A.1.

The ACSM (1995) recommends a maximal exercise test for healthy older men (>40 yr) and women (>50 yr) before beginning a vigorous (>60% of functional aerobic capacity) exercise program (see table 2.7). These maximal exercise tests should be administered with physician supervision. For apparently healthy individuals of any age, submaximal exercise testing can be done without physician supervision. However, the exercise tests should be conducted by exercise specialists, preferably who are ACSM-certified and who are well-trained and experienced in monitoring exercise tests and in handling emergencies (ACSM 1995). The results from these tests provide a basis for prescription of exercise for healthy and coronary-prone individuals, as well as for cardiopulmonary patients.

Table 2.7 ACSM Guidelines for Exercise Testing and Participation					
	Apparently healthy		**Increased risk[a]**		**Known disease[b]**
	Younger[c]	**Older**	**No symptoms**	**Symptoms**	
A. Medical exam and clinical exercise test recommended prior to:					
Moderate exercise (40-60% $\dot{V}O_2$max)	No[d]	No	No	Yes[e]	Yes
Vigorous exercise (>60% $\dot{V}O_2$max)	No	Yes	Yes	Yes	Yes
B. Physician supervision recommended during exercise test:[f]					
Submaximal testing	No	No	No	Yes	Yes
Maximal testing	No	Yes	Yes	Yes	Yes

[a] Persons with 2 or more risk factors or 1 or more signs or symptoms of cardiac, pulmonary, or metabolic diseases (see table 2.5)

[b] Persons with known cardiac, pulmonary, or metabolic disease

[c] Younger: ≤40 yr for men; ≤50 yr for women

[d] The "no" response means that an item is not necessary. The "no" response does not mean that the item should not be done.

[e] The "yes" response means that an item is recommended

[f] For physician supervision, this suggests that a physician is in close proximity and readily available should there be an emergent need.

Absolute and Relative Contraindications to Exercise Testing*

Absolute Contraindications

1. Recent significant change in resting ECG suggesting infarction or other acute cardiac events
2. Recent complicated myocardial infarction (unless client is stable and pain-free)
3. Unstable angina
4. Uncontrolled ventricular arrhythmia
5. Uncontrolled atrial arrhythmia that compromises cardiac function
6. Third-degree AV heart block without pacemaker
7. Acute congestive heart failure
8. Severe aortic stenosis
9. Suspected or known dissecting aneurysm
10. Active or suspected myocarditis or pericarditis
11. Thrombophlebitis or intracardia thrombi
12. Recent systemic or pulmonary embolism
13. Acute infections
14. Significant emotional distress (psychosis)

Relative Contraindications

1. Resting diastolic blood pressure >115 mmHg or resting systolic blood pressure >200 mmHg
2. Moderate valvular heart disease
3. Known electrolyte abnormalities (hypokalemia, hypomagnesemia)
4. Fixed-rate pacemaker (rarely used)
5. Frequent or complex ventricular ectopy
6. Ventricular aneurysm
7. Uncontrolled metabolic disease (e.g., diabetes, thyrotoxicosis, or myxedema)
8. Chronic infectious disease (e.g., mononucleosis, hepatitis, AIDS)
9. Neuromuscular, musculoskeletal, or rheumatoid disorders that are exacerbated by exercise
10. Advanced or complicated pregnancy

*For definitions of specific medical terms, refer to appendix A.1.

Reproduced, with permission, from American College of Sports Medicine, 1995, *ACSM's Guidelines for Exercise Testing and Prescription* (Baltimore: Williams & Wilkins), 42.

LIFESTYLE EVALUATION

Planning a well-rounded physical fitness program for an individual requires that you obtain information about the client's living habits. The lifestyle assessment provides useful information regarding the individual's risk factor profile. Factors such as smoking, lack of physical activity, and diets high in saturated fats or cholesterol increase the risk of CAD, atherosclerosis, and hypertension. These factors can be used to pinpoint patterns and habits that need modification and to assess the likelihood of the client's adherence to the exercise program. You can obtain the lifestyle profile by using the form in appendix A.7. You also may assess your client's psychological stress level as part of the lifestyle profile. A stress inventory (appendix G.1) is included for this purpose, and its use is discussed in chapter 11.

INFORMED CONSENT

Prior to conducting any physical fitness tests or exercise programs, you should see that each participant signs the informed consent (see appendix A.8). This form explains the purpose and nature of each physical fitness test, any inherent risks in the testing, and the expected benefits of the tests. The informed consent also ensures your clients that test results will remain confidential, and that their participation is strictly voluntary. If your client is underage (<18 years), a parent or guardian must also sign the informed consent. All consent forms should be approved by your institutional review board or legal counsel.

Key Points

- The purpose of the health evaluation is to detect disease and to assess disease risk.

- Important components of the health evaluation are a medical history, CHD risk factor analysis, physical examination, laboratory tests, and medical clearance.

- The resting evaluation of cardiorespiratory function includes heart rate, blood pressure, and a 12-lead ECG that is interpreted by a qualified physician.

- Resting blood pressure can be assessed using auscultation, palpation, or automated blood pressure devices.

- Heart rate may be taken using auscultation, palpation, heart rate monitors, or ECG recordings.

- The 12-lead ECG includes three limb leads (I, II, III), three augmented unipolar leads (aVF, aVR, aVL), and six chest leads (V_1 through V_6).

- A graded maximal exercise test is the best way to assess functional aerobic capacity.

- Unless contraindications to exercise are observed, a maximal exercise test is recommended for apparently healthy men more than 40 years old and apparently healthy women more than 50 years old before beginning a vigorous exercise program.

- The lifestyle evaluation includes information about the diet, tobacco and alcohol use, physical activity, and psychological stress levels of the individual.

- All clients are required to sign an informed consent prior to taking any physical fitness tests or participating in an exercise program.

SOURCES FOR EQUIPMENT

Product	Manufacturer's Address
Anaeroid or mercury sphygmomanometer and blood pressure cuffs	W.A. Baum Co. 620 Oak St. Copiague, NY 11726 (516) 226-3940
Electrocardiograph	Marquette Medical Systems 100 Marquette Dr. Jupiter, FL 33468 (800) 558-5102
Heart rate monitors	Creative Health Products 5148 Saddle Ridge Rd. Plymouth, MI 48170 (800) 742-4478

REFERENCES

Adomovich, D.R. 1984. *The heart.* East Moriches, NY: Sports Medicine Books.

American College of Sports Medicine. 1995. *ACSM's guidelines for exercise testing and prescription,* 5th ed. Baltimore, MD: Williams & Wilkins.

American Heart Association. 1994. *RISKO—A heart health appraisal.* Dallas, TX: Author.

Conover, M.B. 1992. *Understanding electrocardiography.* St. Louis: Mosby Year Book.

Dubin, D. 1980. *Rapid interpretation of EKGs.* Tampa, FL: Cover.

Goldberger, A.L., and Goldberger, E. 1981. *Clinical electrocardiography: A simplified approach.* St. Louis: C.V. Mosby.

Goldman, M.J. 1982. *Principles of clinical electrocardiography.* Cambridge, MD: Lange Medical.

Griffin, S., Robergs, R., and Heyward, V. 1997. Assessment of exercise blood pressure: A review. *Medicine and Science in Sports and Exercise* 29: 149-159

Joint National Committee on Detection, Evaluation, and Treatment of High Blood Pressure. 1993. The fifth report of the Joint National Committee on detection, evaluation, and treatment of high blood pressure (JNCV). *Archives of Internal Medicine* 153: 154-183.

McArdle, W.D., Katch, F.I., and Katch, V.L. 1996. *Exercise physiology: Energy, nutrition and human performance*, 4th ed. Baltimore: Williams & Wilkins.

National Cholesterol Education Program (NCEP). 1993. Summary of the second report of the National Cholesterol Education Program (NCEP) expert panel on detection, evaluation, and treatment of high blood cholesterol in adults (Adult Treatment Panel II). *Journal of the American Medical Association* 269: 3015-3023.

Pollock, M.L., Wilmore, J.H., and Fox, S.M. III. 1978. *Health and fitness through physical activity*. New York: John Wiley & Sons.

Reeves, R.A. 1995. Does this patient have hypertension? How to measure blood pressure. *Journal of the American Medical Association* 273: 1211-1218.

CHAPTER 3

Principles of Assessment, Prescription, and Exercise Program Adherence

Key Questions

- What are the essential components of a physical fitness profile?
- What are the purposes of physical fitness tests, and how can I use the results?
- Several physical fitness tests are available; how do I select the best one for my client?
- Are field tests as good as laboratory tests for measuring physical fitness?
- What is the best way to interpret test results for my client?
- What are the essential elements of an exercise prescription?
- Is one type of exercise better than others for improving each component of physical fitness?
- Does high-intensity exercise improve physical fitness faster than low-intensity exercise?
- Is it safe to exercise every day?
- When should I increase the frequency, intensity, and duration in an exercise prescription? Can these elements be increased simultaneously?
- Do older people benefit as much from exercise as younger people?
- How can I get my clients to stick with their exercise programs?
- Do I need to be professionally certified or licensed in order to work in this field?

Health/fitness professionals need to master the basic principles of physical fitness assessment and exercise prescription. Results from physical fitness tests are used to plan scientifically sound exercise programs, individualized to meet your client's needs, interests, and abilities. With your knowledge, leadership, and guidance, your clients can reduce their risk of disease and improve their health and physical fitness levels safely and effectively.

As an exercise specialist, you will have diverse responsibilities such as

- educating clients about the positive benefits of regular physical activity;

- conducting pretest health evaluations to screen clients for exercise participation (see chapter 2);

- selecting, administering, and interpreting tests designed to assess each component of physical fitness;

- designing individualized exercise programs;

- leading exercise classes;

- analyzing your clients' exercise performance and correcting performance errors;

- educating your clients about the "do's and don'ts" of exercise; and

- motivating your clients to improve their adherence to exercise.

Exercise specialists play many roles: educator, leader, technician, and artist. To be effective in these roles, you must integrate knowledge from many disciplines such as anatomy, physiology, chemistry, nutrition, education, and psychology, as well as refine your exercise testing, prescription, and leadership skills.

This chapter presents principles of exercise testing and prescription, along with information about exercise program adherence and the importance of professional certification for individuals in the field of exercise science.

COMPONENTS OF PHYSICAL FITNESS

Physical fitness is the ability to perform occupational, recreational, and daily activities without becoming unduly fatigued. As an exercise specialist, one of your primary responsibilities is to assess each of the following physical fitness components:

1. Cardiorespiratory endurance. Cardiorespiratory endurance is the ability of the heart, lungs, and circulatory system to supply oxygen and nutrients to working muscles efficiently. Exercise physiologists measure the maximum oxygen consumption ($\dot{V}O_2$max), or the rate of oxygen utilization of the muscles during aerobic exercise, in order to assess cardiorespiratory endurance and functional aero-

bic capacity. Physical fitness evaluations should include a test of cardiorespiratory function during rest and exercise. Graded exercise tests (GXT) are used for this purpose. Improved cardiorespiratory endurance is one of the most important benefits of aerobic exercise training programs. Chapters 4 and 5 present detailed information about graded exercise testing and aerobic exercise programs.

2. Musculoskeletal fitness. Musculoskeletal fitness refers to the ability of the skeletal and muscular systems to perform work. This requires muscular strength, muscular endurance, and bone strength. Muscular strength is the maximal force or tension level that can be produced by a muscle group; muscular endurance is the ability of a muscle to maintain submaximal force levels for extended periods; bone strength is directly related to the risk of bone fracture and is a function of the mineral content and density of the bone tissue. Resistance training is one of the most effective ways to improve the strength of muscles and bones and to develop muscular endurance. Chapters 6 and 7 provide detailed information about assessing musculoskeletal fitness and designing resistance training programs.

3. Body weight and body composition. Body weight refers to the size or mass of the individual. Body composition views the body weight in terms of the absolute and relative amounts of muscle, bone, and fat tissues. Aerobic exercise and resistance training are effective in altering body weight and composition. Chapters 8 and 9 discuss body composition assessment techniques and exercise programs for weight management.

4. Flexibility. Flexibility is the ability to move a joint or series of joints fluidly through the complete range of motion. Flexibility is limited by factors such as bony structure of the joint and the size and strength of muscles, ligaments, and other connective tissues. Daily stretching exercises can greatly improve flexibility. Chapter 10 gives more information about assessing flexibility and designing stretching programs.

5. Neuromuscular relaxation. Neuromuscular relaxation refers to the ability to reduce or eliminate unnecessary tension or contraction in a muscle group. Progressive relaxation exercise and Tai Chi are examples of effective techniques for decreasing stress and neuromuscular tension levels. Chapter 11 provides additional information about neuromuscular tension and stress assessment, as well as the use of regular physical activity as a stress management technique.

PURPOSES OF PHYSICAL FITNESS TESTING

As mentioned in chapter 2, it is imperative that you carefully screen your clients for exercise testing, classify their disease risk, identify any contraindications to exercise testing, and obtain their informed consent prior to conducting any physical fitness tests. You can use laboratory and field tests to assess each component of physical fitness and to develop physical fitness profiles for your clients. Results from these tests enable you to identify strengths and weaknesses and to set realistic and attainable goals for your clients. Data from specific tests (e.g., heart rates from a GXT) will help you make accurate and precise exercise prescriptions for each client. Also, you can use baseline and follow-up data to evaluate the progress of exercise program participants.

TESTING ORDER AND THE TESTING ENVIRONMENT

When you administer a complete battery of physical fitness tests in a single session, the ACSM (1995) recommends using the following test sequence to minimize the effects of previous tests on subsequent test performance:

- Resting blood pressure and heart rate
- Body composition
- Cardiorespiratory endurance
- Muscular fitness
- Flexibility

If your physical fitness test battery includes an evaluation of neuromuscular tension and stress levels, these tests should follow the evaluation of resting heart rate and blood pressure.

Often clients are apprehensive about taking physical fitness tests. Test anxiety may affect the validity and reliability of test results. Therefore, you should put your client at ease by establishing good rapport, projecting a sense of relaxed confidence, and creating a testing environment that is friendly, quiet, private, safe, and comfortable. Room temperature should be maintained at 70° to 74° F (21° to 23° C), and the relative humidity should be controlled whenever possible. For pretest health screening and interpretation of the client's test results, the room

should have comfortable chairs and a table for completing questionnaires and paperwork, as well as an examination table or bed for the resting evaluation of heart rate, blood pressure, and the 12-lead ECG. All equipment used for physical testing should be carefully calibrated and prepared before your client arrives for testing. This will ensure valid test data and efficient use of time.

TEST VALIDITY, RELIABILITY, AND OBJECTIVITY

To accurately assess your client's physical fitness status, you must select tests that are valid, reliable, and objective. These basic concepts must be fully understood in order to evaluate the relative worth of specific physical fitness tests and prediction equations.

Test Validity

With regard to physical fitness testing, *test validity* is the ability of a test to *accurately measure*, with minimal error, a specific physical fitness component. When the physical fitness component is *directly* measured, *reference* or *criterion measures* are obtained. However, some physical fitness components cannot be measured directly, requiring the use of *indirect* measures to estimate the value of the reference measure. For example, exercise physiologists consider the direct measurement of $\dot{V}O_2max$ (i.e., collection and analysis of expired gas samples) during maximal exercise to be the criterion measure of cardiorespiratory endurance. Direct measurement of $\dot{V}O_2max$, however, requires expensive equipment and considerable technical expertise. Therefore in the laboratory setting, $\dot{V}O_2max$ is usually estimated using formulas to convert the amount of work output during a GXT to oxygen consumption (see chapter 4). In field settings, prediction equations are used to estimate $\dot{V}O_2max$ from a combination of physiological, demographic, and performance predictor variables. Because field tests and conversion formulas indirectly measure the physical fitness component, these equations have *prediction errors*.

One way that researchers quantify the validity of physical fitness tests is by calculating the relationship between predicted scores (y') and criterion scores (y) using correlation coefficients ($r_{yy'}$). The value, $r_{yy'}$ is known as the *validity coefficient*. The magnitude of the validity coefficient cannot exceed 1.0. The closer the value is to 1.0, the stronger the validity of the test. Valid physical fitness field tests and prediction equations typically have validity coefficients in excess of $r_{y,y'} = 0.80$.

Test Reliability

Reliability is the ability of a test to yield *consistent* and *stable* scores across trials and over time. For example, the skinfold test is considered reliable because a trained skinfold technician obtains similar skinfold values when taking duplicate measurements on the same person. Researchers quantify reliability by calculating the relationship between trial 1 and trial 2 test scores or day 1 and day 2 test scores. This value, $r_{x1,x2}$, is known as the *reliability coefficient*. The magnitude of the reliability coefficient cannot exceed 1.0. In general, physical fitness tests have high reliability coefficients, typically exceeding $r_{x1,x2} = 0.90$.

It is important to know that test reliability affects test validity. Tests with poor reliability have poor validity because unreliable tests fail to produce consistent test scores. It is possible, though, for a test to have excellent reliability ($r_{x1,x2} > 0.90$) but poor validity. Even when a test yields stable and precise values across trials or between days, it may not validly measure a specific physical fitness component. For example, researchers reported high test-retest reliability ($r_{x1,x2} = 0.99$) for the sit-and-reach test, but also noted that this test has poor validity ($r_{y,y'} = 0.12$) as a measure of low back flexibility in women (Jackson and Langford 1989).

Test Objectivity

Objectivity is also known as *intertester reliability*. Objective tests yield similar test scores for a given individual when the same test is administered by different technicians. Objectivity is quantified by calculating the correlation between pairs of test scores measured on the same individuals by two different technicians. This value, $r_{1,2}$, is known as the *objectivity coefficient*. Like validity and reliability coefficients, the magnitude of the objectivity coefficient cannot exceed 1.0. Most physical fitness tests have high objectivity coefficients ($r_{1,2} > 0.90$), especially when technicians are highly trained, practice together, and carefully follow standardized testing procedures.

EVALUATING PREDICTION EQUATIONS

Although reference measures obtained in the laboratory setting provide the most valid assessment of each physical fitness component, these tests are expensive, time-consuming, and require considerable technical expertise. In field and clinical settings, you can obtain estimates of these reference measures by selecting valid field tests and prediction equations that have good predictive accuracy. Table 3.1 provides an overview of the types of tests used in laboratory and field settings to assess each physical fitness component.

To select the most appropriate tests for measuring your client's physical fitness, it is important to be able to evaluate the relative worth of the fitness tests and their prediction equations. To do this, you should ask the following questions:

1. What reference measure was used to develop the prediction equation?

As mentioned earlier, the reference or criterion measure of a specific physical fitness component is obtained by *directly* measuring the component. Reference measures are used as the "gold standard" to validate field tests and to develop prediction equations that accurately estimate the reference measure. For example, skinfold prediction equations are developed and cross-validated by comparing the estimated body density, calculated from the skinfold equation, to the reference measure of body density obtained from hydrodensitometry (underwater weighing). Similarly, the validity of the sit-and-reach test for measuring low back flexibility was tested by comparing sit-and-reach scores to range of motion values (reference measure) directly measured by x-ray or goniometric methods. Table 3.1 describes reference measures that experts commonly use to assess each physical fitness component. Field tests and prediction equations, developed using *indirect* methods instead of reference methods as a criterion, have questionable validity.

2. How large was the sample used to develop the prediction equation? What is the ratio of sample size to the number of predictor variables in the equation?

Large randomly-selected samples (N = 100 to 400 subjects) generally are needed to insure that data are representative of the population for whom the

Table 3.1   Direct (Reference) and Indirect (Field) Measures of Physical Fitness Components

Physical fitness component	Reference measure	Laboratory or reference method	Indirect measures or field tests	Prediction error (SEE)	Chapter
Cardiorespiratory endurance	Direct measurement of $\dot{V}O_2$max $(ml \cdot kg^{-1} \cdot min^{-1})$	Maximal GXT	Submaximal GXT, distance run/walk tests, step tests	<5.0 ml $\cdot$ kg^{-1} $\cdot$ min^{-1}	4
Body composition	Db (g $\cdot$ cc^{-1}), FFM (kg) or % BF	Hydrodensitometry or dual-energy x-ray absorptiometry	Bioimpedance, skinfold, anthropometry, near-infrared interactance	<0.0080 g $\cdot$ cc^{-1} Db <3.5 kg FFM men <2.8 kg FFM women $<3.5\%$ BF	8
Muscular strength	Maximal force (kg) or torque (Nm)	Isokinetic or 1-RM tests	Submaximal tests (2- to 10-RM value)	<2.0 kg	6
Bone strength	Bone mineral content and bone density	Dual-energy x-ray absorptiometry	Anthropometric measures of bony width	NR	8
Flexibility	ROM at joint (degrees)	X-ray or goniometry	Linear measures of ROM	$<6°$	10
NM relaxation	Electrical activity in resting muscles	Electromyography	Rathbone manual tension test	NR	11

Db = total body density; FFM = fat-free mass; % BF = relative body fat; SEE = standard error of estimate; GXT = graded exercise test; ROM = range of motion; RM = repetition maximum; NR = not reported; kg = kilogram; Nm = newton-meter; g = gram; cc = cubic centimeter; ml = milliliter; min = minute.

prediction equation was developed. Also, equations based on large samples tend to have more stable regression weights for each predictor variable in the equation.

In multiple regression, the correlation between the reference measure of the physical fitness component and the predictors in the equation is represented by the ***multiple correlation coefficient (R_{mc})***. The larger the R_{mc} (up to maximum value of 1.00), the stronger the relationship. The size of R_{mc} will be artificially inflated if there are too many predictors in the equation compared to the total number of subjects. Statisticians recommend that there should be a minimum of 10 to 20 subjects per predictor variable. For example, if an SKF prediction equation has three predictors (e.g., triceps SKF, calf SKF, and age), then the minimum sample size needs to be 30 to 60 subjects. Prediction equations that are based on small samples and/or that have a poor subject-to-predictor ratio are suspect and should not be used.

3. What was the size of the R_{mc} and the standard error of estimate (SEE) for the prediction equation?

In general, the R_{mc} for equations predicting physical fitness components exceeds 0.80. This means that at least 64% [$R^2 = (0.80)^2 \chi 100$] of variance in the reference measure can be accounted for by the predictors in the equation. As you can easily see, the larger the R_{mc}, the greater the amount of shared variance between the reference measure and predictor variables. When you evaluate the relative worth of a prediction equation, it is more important to note the size of the prediction error (SEE) than that of the R_{mc} because the magnitude of R_{mc} is greatly affected by sample size and variability of the data.

The SEE reflects the degree of deviation of individual data points (subjects' scores) around the line of best fit through the entire sample's data points. *The line of best fit is the regression line that depicts the linear relationship between the reference measure and the predictors.* The closer to the regression line individual data points fall, the smaller the SEE or prediction error (see figure 3.1). Table 3.1 presents standards for evaluating prediction errors of physical fitness prediction equations.

4. To whom is the prediction equation applicable?

To answer this question, you need to pay close attention to the physical characteristics of the sample used to derive the equation. Factors such as age, gender, race, fitness level, and body fat need to

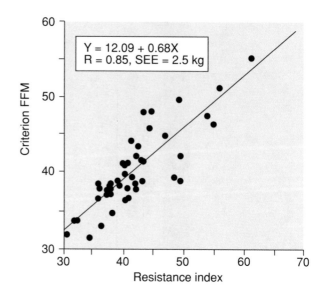

Figure 3.1   Line of best fit and SEE.

be examined carefully. Prediction equations are either ***population-specific*** or ***generalized***. Population-specific equations are intended only for individuals from a specific homogeneous group. For example, separate SKF equations have been developed for prepubescent boys and girls (see chapter 8). Population-specific equations are likely to systematically over- or underestimate the physical fitness component if they are applied to individuals who do not belong to that population subgroup.

On the other hand, there are generalized prediction equations which can be applied to individuals who differ greatly in physical characteristics. Generalized equations are developed using diverse, heterogeneous samples and account for differences in physical characteristics by including these variables as predictors in the equation. For example, the prediction equation for the Rockport walking test (see chapter 4) is a generalized equation because gender and age are predictors in this equation.

5. How were the variables measured by the researchers who developed the prediction equation?

It is important to know not only which variables are included in a prediction equation but how each of these predictors was measured by the researchers developing the equation. Although it is highly recommended that standardized procedures be used for all physical fitness testing, this is not always done. For example, the suprailiac skinfold used in the skinfold equations developed by Jackson, Pollock, and Ward (1980) is measured above the iliac crest at the *anterior axillary line*. In contrast, the *Anthropometric Standardization Reference Manual*

(Lohman, Roche, and Martorell 1988) recommends that the suprailiac skinfold be measured above the iliac crest at the *midaxillary line*. For most individuals, there will be a difference between skinfold thicknesses measured at these two sites. Thus, larger than expected prediction errors may result if physical fitness variables are not measured following the descriptions provided by the researchers who developed the equation.

6. Was the prediction equation cross-validated on another sample from the population?

An equation must be tested on other samples from the population before its validity or predictive accuracy can be determined. For example, the American College of Sports Medicine developed an equation to estimate energy expenditure ($\dot{V}O_2$) from work output during steady-state exercise on a bicycle ergometer (see chapter 4). This equation was cross-validated on independent samples of men and women by other researchers (Lang et al. 1992; Latin et al. 1993). In general, prediction equations that have not been cross-validated on the original study sample or on additional samples in other studies should not be used.

7. What was the size of the correlation ($r_{y,y'}$) between the reference measure (y) and predicted (y') scores (validity coefficient)? What was the size of the prediction error (SEE) when this equation was applied to the cross-validation sample?

As noted above, an equation with good predictive accuracy should yield a moderately high validity coefficient ($r_{y,y'}$ >0.80) and an acceptable SEE (see table 3.1). Keep in mind that the SEE represents the degree of deviation of individual scores from the regression line (see figure 3.1).

ADMINISTERING AND INTERPRETING PHYSICAL FITNESS TESTS

To obtain good test results, it is important to prepare your clients for physical fitness testing by giving them appropriate instructions at least one day before the scheduled exercise tests.

Pretest Instructions

Give the client directions to the testing facility, and make special arrangements if the facility requires a parking pass. Make sure the client has the following instructions in preparation for the test:

- Wear comfortable clothing, socks, and athletic shoes if available.
- Drink plenty of fluids during the 24-hour period before the test.
- Refrain from eating, smoking, and drinking alcohol or caffeine for three hours prior to the test.
- Do not engage in strenuous physical activity the day of the test.
- Get adequate sleep (6 to 8 hours) the night before the test.

Test Administration

Later chapters give detailed procedures for administering laboratory and field tests for each physical fitness component. Your technical skills and expertise in administering these tests are directly related to your mastery of standardized testing procedures and the amount of time that you spend practicing testing techniques. For example, to become a proficient skinfold technician, you probably should practice on at least 50 to 100 people (Jackson and Pollock 1985). You also need a great deal of practice to measure exercise blood pressures and heart rates accurately and to coordinate the timing of these measurements during a graded exercise test on the treadmill or bicycle ergometer. Remember that you cannot obtain valid test scores if you do not follow the standardized testing procedures.

Test Interpretation

After collecting the test data, you must analyze and interpret the results for your client. Computer software programs are available that display and compare the client's test results to normative data. Some graphs display the individual's physical fitness profile, so that you and your client can easily pinpoint strengths as well as physical fitness components in need of improvement.

To classify your client's physical fitness status, you should compare test scores to established norms. For this purpose, age-gender norms are provided for many of the cardiorespiratory fitness, muscular fitness, body composition, and flexibility tests included in this book. For some tests, percentile rankings are used to classify your client's performance. To illustrate the interpretation of a percentile ranking, let's use the example of a 35-year-old male client whose sit-and-reach score ranks in the 60th percentile. This ranking means that his score is better than 60% of all males of the same age taking this test.

Talking to Your Clients

When interpreting results for clients, use lay language rather than highly technical terms and jargon. Whenever possible, try to phrase poor results in positive terms. For example, if a female client's body fat level is classified as *obese*, do not embarrass and alarm her by saying: "Your underwater weighing test indicates that you are obese and need to lose at least 20 pounds to achieve a healthy body fat level in order to reduce your risk of diseases linked to obesity. You need to decrease your caloric intake and increase your caloric expenditure by dieting and exercising. The sooner you start a weight management program, the better."

Instead, you should use a more positive and less intimidating approach when interpreting this result. The following approach is more appropriate, especially for clients with low self-esteem or little motivation to initiate and adhere to an exercise program: "People with greater than 32% body fat are at risk for disease. If you wish, I will evaluate your daily calorie intake and suggest healthy foods you like to eat that are low in fat. Also, we can discuss ways to increase your physical activity level. I think we can find some activities that you will enjoy and have time for, so that you'll burn more calories each day. With these changes, you should be able to lower your body fat to a healthy level in a reasonable amount of time."

BASIC PRINCIPLES FOR EXERCISE PROGRAM DESIGN

A number of basic training principles apply to all types of exercise programs, whether they are designed to improve cardiorespiratory endurance, musculoskeletal fitness, body composition, or flexibility.

Specificity Training Principle

The specificity training principle states that the body's physiological and metabolic responses and adaptations to exercise training are specific to the type of exercise and the muscle groups involved. For example, physical activities requiring continuous, dynamic, and rhythmical contractions of large muscle groups are best suited for stimulating improvements in cardiorespiratory endurance; stretching exercises develop range of joint motion and flexibility; and resistance exercises are effective for improving muscular strength and muscular endurance. Furthermore, the gains in muscular fitness are specific to the exercised muscle groups, type and speed of contraction, and training intensity.

Overload Training Principle

To promote improvements in physical fitness components, the physiological systems of the body must be taxed using loads that are greater than those to which the individual is accustomed. Overload can be achieved by increasing the frequency, intensity or duration of aerobic exercise. Muscle groups can be effectively overloaded by increasing the number of repetitions, sets, or exercises in programs designed to improve muscular fitness and flexibility.

Principle of Progression

Throughout the training program, you must progressively increase the training volume, or overload, to stimulate further improvements. The progression needs to be gradual because "doing too much, too soon" may cause musculoskeletal injuries and is a major reason why some individuals drop out of exercise programs.

Principle of Initial Values

Individuals with low initial physical fitness levels will show greater relative (%) gains and a faster rate of improvement in response to exercise training compared to individuals with average or high fitness levels. For example, during the first month of an aerobic exercise program, the $\dot{V}O_2$max of a client with poor cardiorespiratory endurance capacity may improve 12% or more; a highly trained endurance athlete may improve only 1% or less.

Principle of Interindividual Variability

Individual responses to a training stimulus are quite variable and depend on factors such as age, initial fitness level, and health status. You therefore must design exercise programs with the specific needs, interests, and abilities of each client in mind, and develop personalized exercise prescriptions that take into account individual differences and preferences.

Principle of Diminishing Returns

Each person has a genetic ceiling that limits the possible extent of improvement due to exercise training. As individuals approach their genetic ceiling, the rate of improvement in physical fitness slows and eventually levels off.

Principle of Reversibility

The positive physiological effects and health benefits of regular physical activity and exercise are reversible. When individuals discontinue their exercise programs (detraining), exercise capacity diminishes quickly, and within a few months most of the training improvements are lost.

THE ART AND SCIENCE OF EXERCISE PRESCRIPTION

Traditionally, some exercise specialists have focused more on rigidly applying scientific principles of exercise prescription, with little or no attention to the *art* of exercise prescription. As an exercise programming artist, you need to be creative, flexible, and able to modify the exercise prescription based on your client's goals, behaviors, and responses to the exercise. Using both a scientific and artistic approach will enable you to personalize the exercise prescription, increasing the probability of your clients' making long-term commitments to include physical activity and exercise as an indispensable part of their lifestyles.

Basic Elements of the Exercise Prescription

Although prescriptions are individualized for each client, there are basic elements common to all exercise prescriptions. These basic elements include mode, intensity, duration, frequency, and progression.

Mode

As mentioned earlier, the specificity of training principle implies that certain types of exercise training are better suited than others to developing specific components of physical fitness. Table 3.2 presents types of training and examples of exercise modes that optimize improvements for each physical fitness component.

To promote changes in body composition, bone health, neuromuscular tension, and stress levels, many experts recommend using more than one type of exercise training. For body composition changes, you should prescribe a combination of aerobic exercise to reduce body fat and resistance exercise to build muscle and bone. Similarly, weight-bearing, aerobic activities and resistance training are both effective for building bone mass for improved bone health. Although many different kinds of physical activity can be used to reduce neuromuscular tension and stress levels (see chapter 11), some experts favor using exercise modes that require focusing on specific muscle groups during the activity to induce a state of relaxation (e.g., progressive relaxation techniques and Tai Chi).

Intensity

Exercise intensity dictates the specific physiological and metabolic changes in the body during exercise training. As mentioned previously, the initial exercise intensity in the exercise prescription depends on the client's program goals, age, capabilities, preferences, and fitness level and should stress, but not overtax, the cardiopulmonary and musculoskeletal systems (ACSM 1995). Later chapters provide detailed guidelines for selecting exercise intensities for the development of each physical fitness component, as well as for the progression of exercise intensity.

Duration

Duration and intensity of exercise are inversely related; the higher the intensity, the shorter the duration of the exercise. Exercise duration depends not only on the intensity of exercise but also on the client's health status, initial fitness level, functional capability, and program goals. For improved *health benefits*, the ACSM and Centers for Disease Control and Prevention (CDC) recommend that *every individual should accumulate 30 minutes or more of moderate physical activity on most, but preferably all, days of the week* (Pate et al. 1995). This amount of physical activity can be achieved in either one continuous bout of exercise or multiple bouts of shorter duration throughout the day (e.g., 10 minute bouts, 3

Table 3.2   Types of Training and Exercise Modes for Improving Physical Fitness Components

Physical fitness component	Type of training	Exercise modes
Cardiorespiratory endurance	Aerobic exercise	Walking, jogging, cycling, rowing, stairclimbing, simulated cross-country skiing, aerobic dance, and step aerobics
Muscular strength and muscular endurance Bone strength	Resistance exercise Weight-bearing aerobic exercise and resistance exercise	Free weights and exercise machines Walking, jogging, aerobic dance, step aerobics, stairclimbing, simulated cross-country skiing, free weights, and exercise machines
Body composition	Aerobic exercise and resistance exercise	Same modes listed for cardiorespiratory endurance and muscular strength
Flexibility	Stretching exercise	Static stretches and PNF stretches
Neuromuscular tension/stress	Relaxation exercises requiring mild physical exertion and concentration	Progressive relaxation exercise and Tai Chi

PNF = proprioceptive neuromuscular facilitation

times a day), depending on the client's functional capacity and time constraints.

As the client adapts to the exercise training, the duration of exercise may be slowly increased about every 2 to 3 weeks. For older and less fit individuals, the ACSM (1995) recommends increasing exercise duration, rather than intensity, in the initial stages of the exercise program. For most clients, the duration of aerobic, resistance, and flexibility exercise workouts should not exceed 60 minutes (ACSM 1995). This will lessen the chance of overuse injuries and exercise "burnout."

Frequency

Frequency typically refers to the total number of weekly exercise sessions. Research shows that exercising 3 days a week on alternate days is sufficient to improve various components of physical fitness. However, frequency is related to the duration and intensity of exercise and varies depending on the client's program goals and preferences, time constraints, and functional capacity. Sedentary clients with poor initial fitness levels may exercise more than once a day. When improved health is the primary goal of the exercise program, the ACSM and CDC recommend *daily* physical activity of moderate intensity. Therefore, when you prescribe daily physical activity for an apparently healthy client, it is important to vary the type of exercise (i.e., aerobic, resistance, and flexibility exercises) or exercise mode (e.g., walking, cycling, and weightlifting) to lessen the risk of overuse injuries to the bones, joints, and muscles.

Progression of Exercise

Throughout the exercise program, physiological and metabolic changes enable the individual to perform more work. For continued improvements, the cardiopulmonary and musculoskeletal systems must be progressively overloaded by periodically increasing the frequency, intensity, and duration of exercise.

When applying the principle of progression to an exercise prescription, you should increase the frequency, intensity, and duration of exercise *gradually*, and you should do so *one element at a time*. A simultaneous increase in frequency, intensity, and duration, or in any combination of these elements, may overtax the individual's physiological systems, thereby increasing the risk of exercise-related injuries and exercise burnout. Generally, for older and less fit clients, it is better to increase exercise duration, instead of exercise intensity, especially during the initial stage of their exercise prescriptions.

Stages of Progression in the Exercise Program

Most individualized exercise programs include *initial conditioning, improvement, and maintenance* stages. The *initial conditioning stage* typically lasts 4 weeks and serves as a primer to familiarize the client with exercise training. During this stage, you should prescribe stretching exercises, light calisthenics, and low-intensity aerobic or resistance exercises. Have your clients *progress slowly by increasing exercise duration first*, followed by small increases in exercise intensity. The initial stage of the exercise program may be skipped for some physically active individuals, provided that their initial fitness level is good-to-excellent and they are accustomed to the exercise modes prescribed for their programs.

The *improvement stage* of the exercise program typically lasts 4 to 5 months, and the rate of progression is more rapid compared to the initial conditioning stage. During this stage the frequency, intensity, and duration systematically and slowly progress, increasing *one element at a time*, until the client's fitness goal is reached.

The *maintenance stage* of the exercise program is designed to maintain the level of fitness achieved by the client at the end of the improvement stage. This stage usually begins 6 months after the exercise program begins and should be continued on a regular, long-term basis. The amount of exercise required to maintain the client's physical fitness level is less than that needed to improve specific fitness components. Thus, the frequency of a specific mode of exercise used to develop any given fitness component can be decreased and replaced with other types of physical activities. By the end of the improvement stage, for example, a client may be jogging 5 days a week. For maintenance, jogging may be reduced to 2 or 3 days a week, and different aerobic activities (e.g., rollerblading and stairclimbing) or other types of exercise and sport activities (e.g., weightlifting or tennis) may be substituted. Including a variety of enjoyable physical activities during this stage helps to counteract boredom and to maintain the client's interest level.

EXERCISE PROGRAM ADHERENCE

Exercise professionals are faced with the challenge of convincing individuals to start exercising and getting them to make a lifelong commitment to a physically active lifestyle. Three out of every five adults (60%) in the United States do not get the recommended amount of physical activity, and 25% of the adult population reports no physical activity at all (U.S. Dept. of Health and Human Services 1996). Exercise specialists play an important role in educating the public about *why* regular physical activity is absolutely essential for good health and *how* to exercise safely and effectively.

Of those individuals starting an exercise program, half will drop out within six months (Dishman 1982). As an exercise specialist, you must help the client develop a positive attitude toward physical activity and make a firm commitment to the exercise program. To increase adherence, you need to be aware of factors related to attrition.

Adherence to an exercise program is related to biological, psychological, behavioral, social, and environmental factors. Predictors of exercise program adherence are listed on this page. The most critical factors characterizing the exercise program dropout are as follows (Martin and Dubbert 1985):

- Overweight
- Low self motivation
- Anxiety about exercise
- No spousal support
- Inconvenient exercise facility
- Exercise intensity that is too high
- No social support during and after exercise

As the exercise specialist, you should focus particularly on those factors which are under your control such as setting individualized goals for the client, providing social support and reinforcement, and prescribing low-to-moderate exercise intensities.

To motivate your clients to exercise on a regular basis, prescribe physical activity that is enjoyable and fun. In an aerobic exercise program, for example, the participant does not need to do the same thing, such as walking or jogging, during every exercise session. Other aerobic activities, such as swimming, cross-country skiing, and step aerobics may be substituted as long as the client exercises at the prescribed training intensity.

Some individuals need the added motivation of exercising with a partner or with a formal group. Whether your clients choose to exercise alone or with others, have them select a regular time and place to exercise, because consistency is a critical factor for instilling the exercise habit.

You can use behavior modification techniques to increase program retention. Sometimes it can be effective to give rewards such as T-shirts, certifi-

Factors Related to Exercise Program Adherence

Biological Factors

Relative body fat
Overweight

Psychological Factors

Self motivation
Self efficacy
Attainment of exercise
  goals
Depression/anxiety/
  introversion

Social Factors

Family support
Family problems
Exercise/job conflicts
Income and education
  levels

Behavioral Factors

Smoking
Leisure time
Credit rating
Type A behavior prone

Program Factors

Social support (group
  vs. individual
  exercise)
Location and conve-
  nience of exercise
  facility
Exercise leadership and
  supervision
Initial exercise intensity
Variety of exercise
  modes
Program costs

cates, emblems, and pins to recognize the attainment of specific goals, such as walking a total of 50 miles (80.5 km) in one month. Help your client set both short-term and long-term goals that are attainable. For this purpose, you can periodically re-evaluate your client's fitness levels to assess improvement. You can state goals in performance or physiological terms. An example of a short-term performance goal is to complete a 3-mile (4.8 km) fun run in less than 33 minutes. A long-term physiological goal might be to increase maximum oxygen uptake ($\dot{V}O_2$max) by 15% in four months. As the exercise specialist, you must help each individual set realistic goals.

The key to increasing exercise program adherence lies in the leadership, education, and motivation which you provide. First, you must be a positive role model. You also must be knowledgeable, able to educate clients about exercise and fitness, and able to provide motivation and encourage social support (see next page for strategies you may use to increase exercise adherence).

CERTIFICATION AND LICENSURE

Exercise specialists need to have extensive knowledge and technical skills in order to be effective. Historically, individuals working in exercise settings, such as health/fitness clubs, were not necessarily

STRATEGIES TO INCREASE EXERCISE PROGRAM ADHERENCE

Program Strategies

- Offer both group and individual activities
- Select times and locations that are convenient for program participants
- Offer a variety of exercise and fitness activities
- Monitor the progress of program participants
- Set realistic short-term and long-term goals for each participant
- Educate participants about exercise, physical fitness, and health benefits
- Provide incentives for exercise
- Encourage social support

Behavioral Strategies for Exercise Leaders

- Be a positive role model and actively participate in exercise sessions
- Show interest in participants (e.g., follow-up phone calls when participant has several unexplained absences)
- Exhibit enthusiasm
- Develop good rapport with each program participant (e.g., learn their names)
- Reward accomplishments of participants
- Motivate and encourage participants to make a long-term commitment to exercise
- Attend to orthopedic and musculoskeletal problems of participants

required to have specialized education and training in exercise science. Often, the only prerequisites for employment as a health/fitness instructor or exercise leader were personal experience with exercise and a lean or muscular body. Over the past 15 years, however, professional organizations such as the American College of Sports Medicine have increased public awareness about all aspects of exercise and fitness, including the importance of dealing with highly trained and qualified exercise professionals.

Professional certification and licensure are two ways to ensure the competency of professionals in the field of exercise science. Although many professional organizations offer certification programs for exercise professionals, Louisiana was the first state in the United States to pass a law requiring licensure of all clinical exercise physiologists (Herbert 1995). This requirement places clinical exercise physiologists on par with other health professionals (e.g., nurses, nutritionists, physical therapists, and occupational therapists) who are required to have licenses to practice in many states. In the future, it is highly probable that other states will pass legislation requiring licensure of exercise professionals.

A number of professional organizations (e.g., the American College of Sports of Medicine, the National Strength and Conditioning Association, and the YMCA of the USA) offer certification workshops and examinations for health/fitness instructors, exercise leaders, personal trainers, and health/fitness directors working with healthy populations. Clinical-track workshops and certifications are also available for exercise specialists, exercise technologists, and program directors who are working with higher-risk individuals enrolled in exercise rehabilitation programs. Some of these professional certifications require an undergraduate or graduate degree in exercise science or a closely allied field, as well as experience working in health/fitness or clinical settings. Your career goals will dictate which type of professional certification is best for you.

There are many advantages to obtaining either state licensure or professional certification. You will have a better chance of finding a job in the health/fitness field, because many employers now hire only professionally certified health/fitness instructors. Certification by reputable, professional organizations upgrades the quality of the typical person working in the field and ensures employers and their clientele that employees have mastered the knowledge and skills needed to be competent exercise science professionals. Hence, the likelihood of lawsuits resulting from negligence or incompetence may be lessened. Also, certification and licensure help to validate exercise specialists as health professionals who are equally deserving of the respect afforded to professionals in other allied health professions.

Key Points

- The essential components of physical fitness are cardiorespiratory endurance, musculoskeletal fitness, body composition, flexibility, and neuromuscular relaxation.

- Valid, reliable, and objective laboratory and field tests have been developed to assess each fitness component.

- Test validity refers to the ability of a physical fitness test to accurately measure a specific fitness component.

- Test reliability is the ability of a test to yield consistent and stable scores across trials and over time.

- Objective tests give similar test scores when different technicians administer the test to the same client.

- To obtain valid and reliable test results, standardized testing procedures must be followed, and technical skills are needed.

- Established norms for most tests are available and are used to classify physical fitness status based on the client's test scores.

- When interpreting test results to clients, be positive and use simple, nontechnical terms.

- To design an effective exercise program, training principles must be understood and applied. These principles include: specificity, overload, progression, initial values, individual variability, diminishing returns, and reversibility.

- The basic elements of an exercise prescription are mode, intensity, duration, and frequency.

- Each exercise prescription should be individualized to meet the needs, interests, and abilities of the client.

- The three stages of an exercise program are initial conditioning, improvement, and maintenance.

- Throughout the improvement stage of an exercise program, the frequency, intensity, and duration of exercise are increased, one at a time.

- Exercise adherence is related to biological, psychological, behavioral, social, environmental, and program factors.

- Professional certification and licensure are two ways to ensure competence of professionals working in the exercise science field.

REFERENCES

American College of Sports Medicine. 1995. *ACSM's guidelines for exercise testing and prescription.* Baltimore, MD: Williams & Wilkins.

Dishman, R.K. 1982. Compliance/adherence in health-related exercise. *Health Psychology* 1:237-267.

Herbert, D.L. 1995. First state licenses exercise physiologists. *Fitness Management* October, 26-27.

Jackson, A.S., and Pollock, M.L. 1985. Practical assessment of body composition. *The Physician and Sportsmedicine* 13: 76-90.

Jackson, A.S., Pollock, M.L., and Ward, A. 1980. Generalized equations for predicting body density of women. *Medicine and Science in Sports and Exercise* 12: 175-182.

Jackson, A.W., and Langford, N.J. 1989. The criterion-related validity of the sit-and-reach test: Replication and extension of previous findings. *Research Quarterly for Exercise and Sport* 60: 384-387.

Lang, P.B., Latin, R.W., Berg, K.E., and Mellion, M.B. 1992. The accuracy of the ACSM cycle ergometry equation. *Medicine and Science in Sports and Exercise* 24: 272-276.

Latin, R.W., Berg, K.E., Smith, P., Tolle, R., and Woodby-Brown, S. 1993. Validation of a cycle ergometry equation for predicting steady-rate VO_2. *Medicine and Science in Sports and Exercise* 25: 970-974.

Lohman, T.G., Roche, A.F., and Martorell, R., eds. 1988. *Anthropometric standardization reference manual.* Champaign, IL: Human Kinetics.

Martin, J.E., and Dubbert, P.M. 1985. Adherence to exercise. In R.L. Terjung, ed., *Exercise and sport sciences reviews* 13: 137-167. New York: Academic Press.

Pate, R.R., Pratt, M., Blair, S.N., Haskell, W.L., et al. 1995. Physical activity and public health: A recommendation from the Centers for Disease Control and Prevention and the American College of Sports Medicine. *Journal of the American Medical Association* 273: 402-407.

U.S. Department of Health and Human Services. 1996. *Physical activity and health: A report of the Surgeon General.* Atlanta, GA: U.S. Department of Health and Human Services, Centers for Disease Control and Prevention, National Center for Chronic Disease Prevention and Health Promotion.

CHAPTER 4

Assessing Cardiorespiratory Fitness

Key Questions

- How is cardiorespiratory fitness ($\dot{V}O_2$max) assessed?
- What is a graded exercise test?
- How is $\dot{V}O_2$ estimated from graded exercise test and field test data?
- Should all clients be given a maximal graded exercise test? What factors should be considered in determining whether to give your client a maximal or submaximal exercise test?
- How accurate are submaximal exercise tests and field tests in assessing cardiorespiratory fitness?
- What exercise modes are suitable for graded exercise testing?
- What are the standardized testing procedures for graded exercise testing?
- What are the criteria for terminating a graded exercise test?
- Is it safe to give children and older adults a graded exercise test?

One of the most important components of physical fitness is cardiorespiratory endurance. Cardiorespiratory endurance is the ability to perform dynamic exercise involving large muscle groups at moderate to high intensity for prolonged periods (ACSM 1995). Every physical fitness evaluation should include an assessment of cardiorespiratory function during both rest and exercise. Exercise physiologists consider directly measured maximum oxygen uptake ($\dot{V}O_2$max) or peak $\dot{V}O_2$ to be the most valid measure of functional capacity of the cardiorespiratory system.

The *$\dot{V}O_2$max*, or rate of oxygen uptake during maximal aerobic exercise, reflects

1. the capacity of the heart, lungs, and blood to transport oxygen to the working muscles, and

2. the utilization of oxygen by the muscles during exercise.

Maximal and submaximal $\dot{V}O_2$ is expressed in absolute or relative terms. Absolute $\dot{V}O_2$ is measured in liters per minute ($L \cdot min^{-1}$) or milliliters per minute ($ml \cdot min^{-1}$) and provides a measure of energy cost for non-weight-bearing activities such as leg or arm cycle ergometry. Absolute $\dot{V}O_2$ is directly related to body size; thus men typically have a larger absolute $\dot{V}O_2$max than women.

To compare individuals who differ in body size, $\dot{V}O_2$ is expressed relative to body weight, i.e., $ml \cdot kg^{-1} \cdot min^{-1}$. Relative $\dot{V}O_2$ is used to estimate the energy cost of weight-bearing activities such as walking, running, aerobic dancing, stairclimbing, and bench stepping. Sometimes $\dot{V}O_2$ is expressed relative to the individual's fat-free mass (see chapter 8), that is, ml · kg FFM^{-1}· min^{-1}. For example, your client's improvement in relative $\dot{V}O_2$max following a 16-week aerobic exercise program may reflect both improved capacity of the cardiorespiratory system (increase in absolute $\dot{V}O_2$max) and weight loss (increase in relative $\dot{V}O_2$ expressed as ml · kg^{-1} · min^{-1} due to a decrease in body weight). Thus, expressing $\dot{V}O_2$max relative to fat-free mass, instead of body weight, provides you with an estimate of cardiorespiratory endurance that is independent of changes in body weight.

This chapter presents guidelines for graded exercise testing, as well as for maximal and submaximal exercise test protocols and procedures. The chapter also addresses graded exercise testing for children and older adults, and includes a discussion of cardiorespiratory field tests. All of the test protocols included in this chapter are summarized in appendix B.1.

EXERCISE EVALUATION

Exercise scientists and physicians use exercise tests to evaluate functional aerobic capacity ($\dot{V}O_2$max) objectively. The $\dot{V}O_2$max, determined from graded maximal or submaximal exercise tests, is used to classify the cardiorespiratory fitness level of your client (see table 4.1). You can use baseline and follow-up data to evaluate the progress of exercise program participants and to set realistic goals for your clients. You can use the heart rate and oxygen

uptake data from the graded exercise test to make accurate, precise exercise prescriptions.

As discussed in chapter 2, before beginning a vigorous (>60% $\dot{V}O_2$max) exercise program, the American College of Sports Medicine (ACSM) recommends a graded maximal exercise test (GXT) for

- apparently healthy men older than 40 years,
- apparently healthy women older than 50 years,
- higher risk individuals with or without symptoms of CHD, regardless of age, and
- all individuals with known cardiac, pulmonary, or metabolic disease, regardless of age.

However, you may use submaximal exercise tests for healthy individuals of any age, as well as clients with increased risk factors but no symptoms of CHD, if they are starting a moderate (40% to 60% $\dot{V}O_2$max) exercise program (ACSM 1995). For medical conditions that are absolute and relative contraindications to exercise testing in an out-of-hospital setting, see chapter 2, page 28.

Guidelines for Exercise Testing

You may use a maximal or submaximal graded exercise test (GXT) to assess the cardiorespiratory fitness of the individual. The selection of a maximal or submaximal GXT depends on

- your client's age and risk stratification (apparently healthy, increased risk, or known disease),

Table 4.1	Cardiorespiratory Fitness Classification				
	Maximal oxygen uptake (ml · kg^{-1} · min^{-1})				
Age (yr)	Poor	Fair	Good	Excellent	Superior
Women					
20-29	≤31	32-34	35-37	38-41	42+
30-39	≤29	30-32	33-35	36-39	40+
40-49	≤27	28-30	31-32	33-36	37+
50-59	≤24	25-27	28-29	30-32	33+
60+	≤23	24-25	26-27	28-31	32+
Men					
20-29	≤37	38-41	42-44	45-48	49+
30-39	≤35	36-39	40-42	43-47	48+
40-49	≤33	34-37	38-40	41-44	45+
50-59	≤30	31-34	35-37	38-41	42+
60+	≤26	27-30	31-34	35-38	39+

The Physical Fitness Specialist Certification Manual, The Cooper Institute for Aerobics Research, Dallas, TX, revised 1997.

- your reasons for administering the test (physical fitness testing or clinical testing), and

- the availability of appropriate equipment and qualified personnel.

In clinical and research settings, $\dot{V}O_2$max is typically measured directly and requires expensive equipment and experienced personnel. Although $\dot{V}O_2$max can be predicted from maximal exercise intensity with a fair degree of accuracy, submaximal tests also provide a reasonable estimate of your client's cardiorespiratory fitness level and are less costly, time-consuming, and risky. Submaximal exercise testing, however, is considered to be less sensitive as a diagnostic tool for CHD.

In either case, the exercise test should be a multistage, graded test. This means that the individual exercises at gradually increasing submaximal work loads. Many commonly used exercise test protocols require that each work load be performed for 3 minutes. The graded exercise test measures maximum aerobic capacity ($\dot{V}O_2$max) when the oxygen uptake plateaus, that is, it does not increase by more than 150 ml · min^{-1} with a further increase in work load. Other criteria (ACSM 1995) used to indicate the attainment of $\dot{V}O_2$max are

- failure of the heart rate to increase with increases in exercise intensity,

- venous lactate concentration exceeding 8 mM/L,

- respiratory exchange ratio greater than 1.15, and

- RPE greater than 17 using the original Borg scale (6-20).

Many poorly conditioned individuals are unable to attain $\dot{V}O_2$max. If the test is terminated prior to reaching $\dot{V}O_2$max, the graded exercise test is a measure of the functional aerobic capacity ($\dot{V}O_2$ peak) rather than maximum aerobic capacity. For CHD screening and classification purposes, bringing a person to at least 85% of the age-predicted maximum heart rate is desirable, because some ECG abnormalities do not appear until the heart rate reaches this level of intensity (Pollock et al. 1978).

Evidence suggests that maximal exercise tests are no more dangerous than submaximal tests (Pollock et al. 1978; Rochmis and Blackburn 1971; Shephard 1977), provided you carefully follow guidelines for exercise tolerance testing and monitor the physiological responses of the exercise participant continuously. Shephard (1977) predicted one fatality in

every 10 to 20 years for a population of five million middle-aged Canadians who undergo maximal exercise testing. For high-risk patients, he estimated 1 fibrillation per 5000 submaximal exercise tests and 1 fibrillation per 3000 maximal exercise tests.

General Procedures for Cardiorespiratory Fitness Testing

At least one day before the exercise test, you should give your client pretest instructions (see chapter 3, page 37). Prior to graded exercise testing, the client should read and sign the informed consent and complete the physical activity readiness questionnaire (PAR-Q & YOU, see appendix A.2).

Step-by-step procedures, as recommended by the ACSM (1995), for administering a GXT are listed below.

PROCEDURES FOR ADMINISTERING A GXT

- Measure the client's resting HR and BP (see chapter 2 for these procedures).

- Begin the GXT with a 2- to 3-minute warm-up to familiarize clients with the exercise equipment and prepare them for the first stage of the exercise test.

- During the test, monitor HR, BP, and ratings of perceived exertion (RPE) at regular intervals. Measure exercise HR near the end of each minute of each exercise stage. Assess exercise BP and RPE near the end of each exercise stage. Throughout the exercise test, continuously monitor the client's physical appearance and symptoms.

- Discontinue the GXT when the test termination criteria are reached, if the client requests to stop the test, or if any of the indications for stopping an exercise test are apparent (see page 51).

- Have the client cool down by exercising at a low work rate that does not exceed the intensity of the first stage of the exercise test (e.g., walking on the treadmill at 2 mph (53.6 m·min^{-1}) and 0% grade or cycling on the bicycle ergometer at 50 to 60 rpm and zero resistance). Active recovery reduces the risk of hypotension from venous pooling in the extremities.

- During recovery, continue measuring postexercise HR, BP, and RPE for at least 4 minutes, or longer if there are any abnormal responses. The HR and BP during active recovery should be stable, but may be higher than pre-exercise levels. Continue monitoring the client's physical appearance during recovery.

- If your client has signs of discomfort, or if an emergency occurs, use a passive cool-down with the client in a sitting or supine position.

Pretest, exercise, and recovery HRs can be measured using the palpation or auscultation techniques (see chapter 2) if a heart rate monitor or ECG recorder is unavailable. Because of extraneous noise and vibration during exercise, it may be difficult to obtain accurate measurements of BP, especially when your client is running on the treadmill. To become proficient at taking exercise BP, you need to practice as much as possible.

To obtain *ratings of perceived exertion* (RPE) during exercise testing, you can use either the original (6 to 20) or revised (0 to 10) RPE scale (see table 4.2). These scales allow clients to rate their degree of exertion *subjectively* during exercise and are highly related to exercise heart rates and $\dot{V}O_2$. Both RPE scales take into account the linear rise in HR and

$\dot{V}O_2$ during exercise. The revised scale also reflects nonlinear changes in blood lactate and ventilation during exercise. Ratings of 10 on the revised scale and 19 on the original scale usually correspond with the maximal level of exercise. RPEs are useful in determining the endpoints of the GXT, particularly for patients who are taking beta-blockers or other medications that may alter the heart rate response to exercise. You can teach your clients how to use the RPE scale to monitor relative intensities during aerobic exercise programs.

Test Termination

In a maximal or submaximal graded exercise test, the exercise usually continues until the client voluntarily terminates the test or reaches a predetermined endpoint. As an exercise technician, however, you must be acutely aware of all indicators for stopping a test. If you notice any of the signs or symptoms listed on page 51, you should stop the exercise test prior to the client's reaching $\dot{V}O_2$max (for maximal GXT) or the predetermined endpoint (for submaximal GXT).

Table 4.2   Ratings of Perceived Exertion (RPE) Scales

Category scale	Category-ratio scale
6 No exertion at all	0 Nothing at all
7 Extremely light	0.5 Extremely weak (just noticeable)
8	1 Very weak
9 Very light	2 Weak (light)
10	3 Moderate
11 Light	4
12	5 Strong (heavy)
13 Somewhat hard	6
14	7 Very strong
15 Hard	8
16	9
17 Very hard	10 Extremely strong (almost max)
18	
19 Extremely hard	
20 Maximal exertion	

Reprinted, by permission, from G. Borg, 1982, *Psychophysical judgment and the process of perception*, H.G. Geissler and P. Petzold, Berlin: VEB Deutscher Verlag der Wissenschaften, 25-34.

General Indications for Stopping an Exercise Test in Apparently Healthy Adults*

1. Onset of angina or angina-like symptoms

2. Significant drop (20 mmHg) in systolic blood pressure or a failure of the systolic blood pressure to rise with an increase in exercise intensity

3. Excessive rise in blood pressure: systolic pressure >260 mmHg or diastolic pressure >115 mmHg

4. Signs of poor perfusion: lightheadedness, confusion, ataxia, pallor, cyanosis, nausea, or cold and clammy skin

5. Failure of heart rate to increase with increased exercise intensity

6. Noticeable change in heart rhythm

7. Subject requests to stop

8. Physical or verbal manifestations of severe fatigue

9. Failure of the testing equipment

*Assumes that testing is nondiagnostic and is being performed without direct physician involvement or electrocardiographic monitoring. For definitive and specific termination criteria for clinical testing, see next column.

Reproduced, with permission, from American College of Sports Medicine, 1995, *ACSM's Guidelines for Exercise Testing and Prescription* (Baltimore: Williams & Wilkins), 78.

General Procedures for Clinical Exercise Testing

You can use a maximal GXT for diagnostic and functional testing in order to determine safe levels of exercise for clients with or without heart disease. For clinical testing, measure both the BP and 12-lead ECG (see chapter 2 for these procedures) in the supine and exercise postures prior to exercise testing. During exercise, monitor the 12-lead ECG every minute and record it during the last minute of each exercise stage. Monitor the exercise BP and RPE at regular intervals, as previously described for physical fitness testing. In addition, whenever symptoms or ECG changes occur during exercise, record the 12-lead ECG, HR, BP, and RPE (ACSM 1995). *If you notice any of the signs or symptoms listed at the top of this page, stop the exercise test immediately.* ST-segment elevation with a horizontal or downward slope is indicative of severe CHD or coronary spasm. Horizontal or downsloping ST-segment depression (>2 mm) reflects myocardial ischemia. The onset, duration, and magnitude of the ST-segment depression is related to the severity of the ischemia. Failure of systolic BP to rise or a significant drop in systolic BP (20 mmHg) during the exercise test are indicators of CHD or heart failure (Hanson 1988).

Absolute and Relative Indications* for Termination of a Clinical GXT

Absolute Indications

1. Acute myocardial infarction or suspicion of a myocardial infarction

2. Onset of moderate-to-severe angina

3. Drop in systolic blood pressure with increasing workload, accompanied by signs or symptoms or drop below standing resting pressure

4. Serious arrhythmias (e.g., second- or third-degree AV block, atrial fibrillation with fast ventricular response or sustained ventricular tachycardia or increasing premature ventricular contractions.)

5. Signs of poor perfusion, including pallor, cyanosis, or cold and clammy skin

6. Unusual or severe shortness of breath

7. Central nervous system symptoms, including ataxia, vertigo, visual or gait problems, or confusion

8. Technical inability to monitor the ECG

9. Patient's request

Relative Indications

1. Pronounced ECG changes from baseline [>2mm of horizontal or downsloping ST-segment depression, or >2mm of ST-segment elevation (except in aVR)]

2. Any chest pain that is increasing

3. Physical or verbal manifestations of severe fatigue or shortness of breath

4. Wheezing

5. Leg cramps or intermittent claudication (grade 3 on 4-point scale)

6. Hypertensive response (Systolic BP >260 mmHg; Diastolic BP >115 mmHg)

7. Less serious arrhythmias such as supraventricular tachycardia

8. Exercise-induced bundle branch block that cannot be distinguished from ventricular tachycardia

*For definitions of specific terms, refer to appendix A.1.

Reprinted, by permission, from American College of Sports Medicine,1995, *ACSM's Guidelines for Exercise Testing and Prescription* (Baltimore: Williams & Wilkins), 97.

Immediately following exercise, record a 10-second ECG while the client is upright. Then monitor the ECG for at least 6 to 8 minutes with the client in a supine position (passive recovery). However, if your client is having difficulty breathing, he or she should sit down. Even though an active cool-down may decrease hypotension, it is not recommended following a GXT that is given for diagnostic purposes because active cool-down may increase the magnitude of ST-segment depression.

MAXIMAL EXERCISE TEST PROTOCOLS

Many maximal exercise test protocols have been devised to assess aerobic capacity. As the exercise technician, you must be able to select an exercise mode and test protocol that is suitable for your clients given their age, gender, and health and fitness status. Commonly used modes of exercise are treadmill walking, running, and stationary cycling. Arm ergometry is useful for paraplegics and patients who have limited use of the lower extremities. Bench stepping is not highly recommended but could be useful in field situations when large groups need to be tested. Whichever mode of exercise you choose, be sure to follow the general principles of exercise testing below.

GENERAL PRINCIPLES OF EXERCISE TESTING

1. Typically, you will use either a treadmill or stationary bicycle ergometer for graded exercise testing (GXT). Be sure to calibrate all equipment before use.

2. Begin the GXT with a 2- to 3-minute warm-up to orient the client to the equipment and prepare the client for the first stage of the GXT.

3. The initial exercise intensity should be considerably lower than the anticipated maximal capacity.

4. Exercise intensity should be increased gradually throughout the stages of the test. Work increments may be 2 METs or greater for apparently healthy individuals and as small as 0.5 MET in patients with disease.

5. Closely observe contraindications for testing and indications for stopping the exercise test. When in any doubt about the safety of or benefits of testing, do not perform the test at that time.

6. Monitor the heart rate at least two times, but preferably each minute, during each stage of the GXT. Measure heart rate near the end of each minute. If the heart rate does not reach steady state (two heart rates within ± 5-6 bpm), extend the work stage an additional minute or until the heart rate stabilizes.

7. Measure blood pressure and RPE once, at the latter portions of each stage of the GXT.

8. Continually monitor client appearance and symptoms.

9. For submaximal GXTs, terminate the test when the client's heart rate reaches 70% HRR (heart rate range) or 85% HR max, unless the protocol specifies a different termination criterion. Also stop the test immediately if there is an emergency situation, if the client fails to conform to the exercise protocol, or if the client experiences signs of discomfort.

10. The test should include a cool-down period of at least 4 minutes, or longer if you observe abnormal responses in heart rate and blood pressure. Monitor heart rate and blood pressure during recovery. For active recovery, the work load should be no more than that used during the first stage of the GXT. Use a passive recovery in emergency situations or when clients experience signs of discomfort and cannot perform an active cool-down.

11. Estimate exercise tolerance in METs for the treadmill or ergometer protocol used; or make a direct assessment if you're measuring oxygen uptake during the GXT.

12. The testing area should be quiet and private. The room temperature should be 21° to 23° C (70° to 72° F) and the humidity 60% or less if possible.

The exercise test may be continuous or discontinuous. A continuous $\dot{V}O_2$max test is performed with no rest between work increments. For discontinuous tests, the subject is given a 5- to 10-minute rest interval between work loads. On average, discontinuous tests take five times longer to administer than continuous tests.

McArdle, Katch, and Pechar (1973) compared the $\dot{V}O_2$max scores as measured by six commonly used continuous and discontinuous treadmill and bicycle ergometer tests. They noted that the $\dot{V}O_2$max scores for the bike ergometer tests were approximately 6 to 11% lower than values for the treadmill tests. Many subjects identified local discomfort and fatigue in the thigh muscles as the major factors limiting further work on both the continuous and discontinuous bicycle ergometer tests. For the treadmill tests, subjects indicated windedness and general fatigue as the limiting factors and complained of localized fatigue and discomfort in the calf muscles and lower back.

Treadmill Maximal Exercise Tests

The exercise is performed on a motor-driven treadmill with variable speed and incline (see figure 4.1).

Speed varies up to 25 mph (670 m · min^{-1}), and incline is measured in units of elevation per 100 horizontal units and is expressed as a percentage. The work load on the treadmill is raised by increasing the speed or incline or both. Work load is usually expressed in miles per hour and percent grade.

It is difficult and expensive to measure the oxygen consumption during exercise. Therefore, the ACSM (1995) has developed equations (table 4.3) to estimate the metabolic cost of exercise ($\dot{V}O_2$). These equations provide a valid estimate of $\dot{V}O_2$ only for steady-state exercise. When used to estimate the maximum rate of energy expenditure ($\dot{V}O_2$max), the measured $\dot{V}O_2$ will be less than the estimated $\dot{V}O_2$ if a steady state is not reached. Also, since maximal exercise involves both aerobic and anaerobic components, the $\dot{V}O_2$max will be overestimated since the contribution of the anaerobic component is not known.

The ACSM metabolic equations in table 4.3 are useful in clinical settings for estimating the rate of energy expenditure for treadmill walking or running . The total energy expenditure, in ml · kg^{-1} · min^{-1}, is a function of three components: *horizontal, vertical,* and *resting* energy expenditures. See page 55 for an example of how to take these three factors into account when figuring $\dot{V}O_2$.

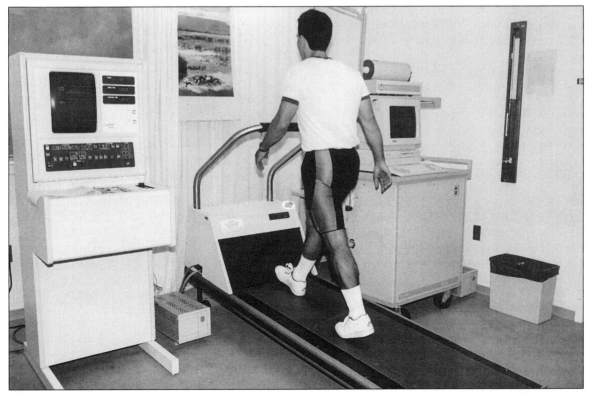

Figure 4.1   Treadmill.

Table 4.3 Summary of Metabolic Calculations

$\dot{V}O_2$ mode (units)	= Resting component (R)	+ Horizontal component (H)	+ Vertical component (V)	Comments
Walking ($ml \cdot kg^{-1} \cdot min^{-1}$)	= $3.5\ ml \cdot kg^{-1} \cdot min^{-1}$	+ speed ($m \cdot min^{-1}$) × 0.1	+ grade (decimal) × $m \cdot min^{-1}$ × 1.8	1. For speeds of 50-100 $m \cdot min^{-1}$ (1.9-3.7 mph) 2. 1 mph = 26.8 $m \cdot min^{-1}$
Running ($ml \cdot kg^{-1} \cdot min^{-1}$)	= $3.5\ ml \cdot kg^{-1} \cdot min^{-1}$	+ speed ($m \cdot min^{-1}$) × 0.2	+ grade (decimal) × $m \cdot min^{-1}$ × 0.9	1. For speeds > 134 $m \cdot min^{-1}$ (>5.0 mph) 2. If truly jogging (not walking), this equation can also be used for speeds of 80-134 $m \cdot min^{-1}$ (3-5 mph)
Leg ergometer ($ml \cdot min^{-1}$)	= $3.5\ ml \cdot kg^{-1} \cdot min^{-1}$ × kg BW	+ None	+ $kgm \cdot min^{-1}$ × 2	1. For work rates between 300-1200 $kgm \cdot min^{-1}$ 2. $kgm \cdot min^{-1}$ = kg × m/rev × rev/min 3. Multiply resting component by BW (kg) to convert to $ml \cdot min^{-1}$ 4. Monarch and Bodyguard = 6 m/rev, Tunturi = 3 m/rev
Arm ergometer ($ml \cdot min^{-1}$)	= $3.5\ ml \cdot kg^{-1} \cdot min^{-1}$ × kg BW	+ None	+ $kgm \cdot min^{-1}$ × 3	1. For work rates between 150-750 $kgm \cdot min^{-1}$ 2. $kgm \cdot min^{-1}$ = kg × m/rev × rev/min 3. Multiply resting component by BW (kg) to convert to $ml \cdot min^{-1}$
Stepping ($ml \cdot kg^{-1} \cdot min^{-1}$)	= Included in H and V components	+ Steps/min × 0.35	+ m/step × steps/min × 1.33 × 1.8	1. 1.33 includes both positive component of going up (1.0) + negative component of going down (0.33) 2. Stepping height in meters 3. 1 inch = .0254 m

Reproduced, with permission, from American College of Sports Medicine, 1995, ACSM's Guidelines for Exercise Testing and Prescription (Baltimore: Williams & Wilkins), 278-281.

TO INSURE VALID ESTIMATION . . .

Before using any of the ACSM metabolic equations to estimate $\dot{V}O_2$, make certain that all units of measure match those in the equation (see facing page).

- Convert body weight in pounds to kilograms (1 kg = 2.2 lb). For example, 170 lb/2.2 = 77.3 kg.
- Convert treadmill speed in mph to m · min⁻¹ (1 mph = 26.8 m · min⁻¹). For example, 5.0 mph × 26.8 = 134.0 m · min⁻¹.
- Convert treadmill grade from percent to decimal form by dividing by 100. For example, 12% / 100 = 0.12.
- Convert METs to ml · kg⁻¹ · min⁻¹ by multiplying (1 MET = 3.5 ml · kg⁻¹ · min⁻¹). For example, 6 METs × 3.5 = 21.0 ml · kg⁻¹ · min⁻¹.
- Convert watts to kgm · min⁻¹ (1 watt = 6 kgm · min⁻¹) by multiplying. For example, 150 watts × 6 = 900 kgm · min⁻¹.
- For non-weight-bearing exercise modes, like arm and leg cycle ergometry, convert ml · kg⁻¹ · min⁻¹ to ml · min⁻¹ by multiplying by the body weight in kg. For example, 30 ml · kg⁻¹ · min⁻¹ × 70 kg = 2100 ml · min⁻¹.
- For weight-bearing exercise modes, like walking, running, and bench stepping, convert ml · min⁻¹ to ml · kg⁻¹ · min⁻¹ by dividing body weight in kg. For example, 2400 ml · min⁻¹/ 60 kg = 40 ml · kg⁻¹ · min⁻¹.
- Convert step height in inches to meters (1 in = 0.0254 m) by multiplying. For example, 8 in × 0.0254 = 0.2032 m.

FOR EXAMPLE . . .

To calculate the $\dot{V}O_2$ for a 70 kg subject who is walking on the treadmill at a speed of 3.5 mph and a grade of 10%, follow these steps:

ACSM Walking Equation

$\dot{V}O_2$ = Resting Component + Horizontal Component + Vertical Component

(ml · kg⁻¹ · min⁻¹) = 3.5 + speed (m · min⁻¹) × 0.1 + grade (decimal) × speed (m · min⁻¹) × 1.8

1. Convert the speed in mph to m · min⁻¹; 1 mph = 26.8 m · min⁻¹.

   3.5 mph × 26.8 = 93.8 m · min⁻¹

2. Calculate the horizontal component (H).

   H = speed (m · min⁻¹) × 0.1

   = 93.8 m · min⁻¹ × 0.1

   = 9.38 ml · kg⁻¹ · min⁻¹

3. Calculate the vertical component (V). Convert % grade into decimal by dividing by 100.

   V = grade (decimal) × speed × 1.8

   = 0.10 × (93.8 m · min⁻¹) × 1.8

   = 16.88 ml · kg⁻¹ · min⁻¹

4. Calculate the total $\dot{V}O_2$ in ml · kg⁻¹ · min⁻¹ by adding the horizontal, vertical, and resting (R) components (R = 1 MET = 3.5 ml · kg⁻¹ · min⁻¹).

   $\dot{V}O_2$ = H + V + R

   = (9.38 + 16.88 + 3.5) ml · kg⁻¹ · min⁻¹

   = 29.76 ml · kg⁻¹·min⁻¹

5. Calculate the rate of energy expenditure (E) in METs, by converting $\dot{V}O_2$ to METs.

   E = $\dot{V}O_2$ /1 MET or 3.5 ml · kg⁻¹ · min⁻¹

   = 29.76 ml · kg⁻¹ · min⁻¹/3.5

   = 8.5 METs

The $\dot{V}O_2$ estimated from the ACSM walking equation (see table 4.3) is reasonably accurate for walking speeds between 50 to 100 m · min^{-1} (1.9 to 3.7 mph). However, since the equation is more accurate for walking up a grade than on the level, $\dot{V}O_2$ may be underestimated as much as 15 to 20% when walking on the level (ACSM 1995). For the ACSM running/jogging equations, the $\dot{V}O_2$ estimates are relatively accurate for speeds exceeding 134 m · min^{-1} (5 mph) and speeds as low as 80 m · min^{-1} (3 mph) providing the client is jogging and not walking (ACSM 1995).

Figure 4.2 illustrates commonly used treadmill exercise test protocols. These protocols conform to the general guidelines for maximal exercise testing. Some of the protocols are designed for a specific population, such as well-conditioned athletes or high-risk cardiac patients. The exercise intensity for each stage of the various treadmill test protocols can be expressed in METs. The MET estimations for each stage of some commonly used treadmill protocols are listed in table 4.4

Population-specific and generalized equations have been developed to estimate $\dot{V}O_2$max from exercise time for some treadmill protocols (see table 4.5). These equations may provide a more accurate estimation of $\dot{V}O_2$max than the ACSM metabolic equations.

It is important for exercise technicians to keep in mind that the initial work load for some of the protocols designed for highly trained athletes is too intense (exceeding 2 to 3.5 METs) for the average individual. The Balke and Bruce protocols are well suited for normal risk individuals, and the Bruce protocol is easily adapted for high-risk individuals using an initial work load of 1.7 mph (45.6 m · min^{-1}) at 0 to 5% grade.

Balke Treadmill Protocol

To administer the Balke and Ware (1959) exercise test protocol (see figure 4.2), set the treadmill speed at 3.4 mph (91.1 m · min^{-1}) and the initial grade of the treadmill at 0% during the first minute of exercise. Maintain a constant speed on the treadmill throughout the entire exercise test. At the start of the second minute of exercise, increase the grade to 2%. Thereafter, at the beginning of every additional minute of exercise, increase the grade by only 1%.

Use the prediction equation for the Balke protocol in table 4.5 to estimate your client's $\dot{V}O_2$max from exercise time. Alternatively, you can use a nomogram (see figure 4.3), developed for the Balke treadmill protocol, to calculate the $\dot{V}O_2$max of your client. To use this nomogram, locate the time corresponding to the last complete minute of exercise during the protocol along the vertical axis labeled "Balke Time," and draw a horizontal line from the time axis to the oxygen uptake axis. Be certain to plot the exercise time of women and men in the appropriate column when using this nomogram.

Bruce Treadmill Protocol

The Bruce, Kusumi, and Hosmer (1973) exercise test is a multistaged treadmill protocol (see figure 4.2). The work load is increased by changing both the treadmill speed and percent grade. During the first stage (minutes 1 to 3) of the test, the normal individual walks at a 1.7-mph pace at 10% grade. At the start of the second stage (minutes 4 to 6), increase the grade by 2% and the speed to 2.5 mph (67 m · min^{-1}). In each subsequent stage of the test, increase the grade 2% and the speed by either 0.8 or 0.9 mph (21.44 or 24.12 m · min^{-1}) until the subject is exhausted. Prediction equations for this protocol have been developed to estimate the $\dot{V}O_2$max of active and sedentary women and men, cardiac patients, and elderly individuals (see table 4.5). As an alternative, you may use the nomogram (see figure 4.4), developed for the Bruce protocol. Plot the client's exercise time for this protocol along the vertical axis labeled "Bruce Time," and draw a horizontal line from the time axis to the oxygen uptake. Again, be certain to use the column appropriate for men or women.

Modified Bruce Protocol

The modified Bruce protocol (see figure 4.2) is more suitable than the Bruce protocol for high-risk and elderly individuals. With the exception of the first two stages, this protocol is similar to the standard Bruce protocol. Stage 1 starts at 0% grade and a 1.7 mph walking pace. For stage 2, the grade is increased to 5%. McInnis and Balady (1994) compared physiological responses to the standard and modified Bruce protocols in patients with CHD; they reported similar heart rate and blood pressure responses at matched exercise stages despite the additional 6 minutes of low-intensity exercise performed using the modified Bruce protocol.

Note that the prediction equations for the Bruce protocol (see table 4.5) can only be used for the standard, not the modified, Bruce protocol. To estimate $\dot{V}O_2$ for the modified Bruce protocol, use the ACSM metabolic equation for walking (see table 4.3).

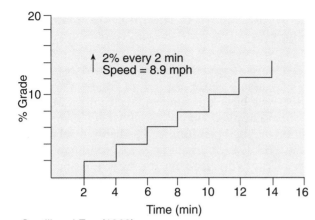

Costill and Fox (1969)
For: highly trained
Warmup: 10-min walk or run
Initial work load: 8.9 mph, 0%, 2 min

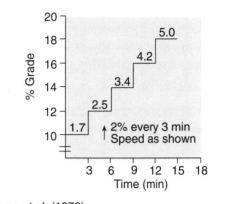

Bruce et al. (1973)
For: normal and high risk
Initial work load: 1.7 mph, 10% 3 min = normal
                   1.7 mph, 0-5% 3 min = high risk

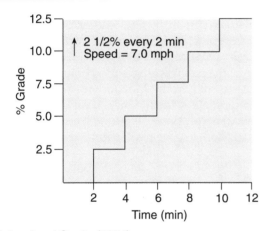

Maksud and Coutts (1971)
For: highly trained
Warmup: 10-min walking 3.5 mph, 0%
Initial work load: 7 mph, 0%, 2 min

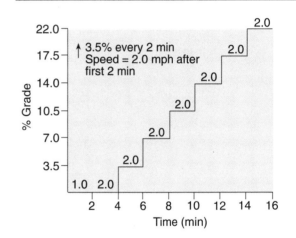

Naughton et al. (1964)
For: cardiac and high risk
Initial work load: 1.0 mph, 0%, 2 min

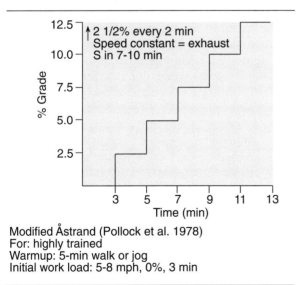

Modified Åstrand (Pollock et al. 1978)
For: highly trained
Warmup: 5-min walk or jog
Initial work load: 5-8 mph, 0%, 3 min

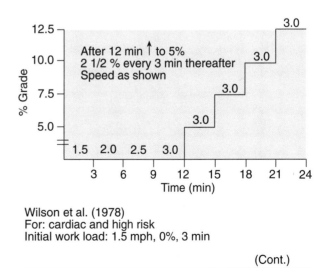

Wilson et al. (1978)
For: cardiac and high risk
Initial work load: 1.5 mph, 0%, 3 min

(Cont.)

Figure 4.2   Treadmill exercise test protocols.

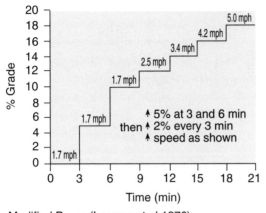

Modified Bruce (Lerman et al. 1976)
For: normal and high risk
Initial workload: 1.7 mph, 0%, 3 min

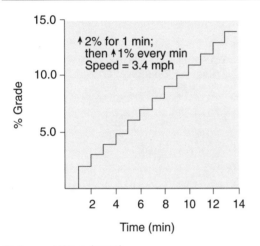

Balke and Ware (1959)
For: normal risk
Initial work load: 3.4 mph. 0%, 1 min

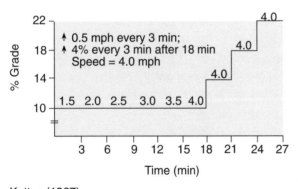

Kattus (1967)
For: cardiac and high risk
Initial work load: 1.5 mph, 10%, 3min

Figure 4.2 *(Continued).*

Bicycle Ergometer Maximal Exercise Tests

The bicycle ergometer is a widely used instrument for assessing cardiorespiratory fitness. On a friction-type bicycle ergometer (see figure 4.5), resistance is applied against the flywheel using a belt and weighted pendulums. The handwheel adjusts the work load by tightening or loosening the brake belt. The work load on the bicycle ergometer is raised by increasing the resistance on the flywheel. The power output (P) is usually expressed in kilogram-meters per minute ($kgm \cdot min^{-1}$) or watts (W) ($1\ watt = 6\ kgm \cdot min^{-1}$) and is easily measured using the equation:

Power = Force × Distance / Time

where force equals the resistance or tension setting on the ergometer (kilograms) and distance is the distance traveled by the flywheel rim for each revolution of the pedal times number of revolutions per minute (rpm). On the Monark and Bodyguard bicycle ergometers, the flywheel travels 6 meters (m) per pedal revolution. Therefore, if a resistance of 2 kg is applied and the pedaling rate is 60 rpm, then

Power = 2 kg × 6 m × 60 rpm
= 720 kgm · min⁻¹ or 120 W

To calculate the distance traveled by the flywheel of cycle ergometers with varying sized flywheels, measure the circumference (in meters) of the resistance track on the flywheel and multiply the circumference by the number of flywheel revolutions during one complete revolution (360 degrees) of the pedal (Gledhill and Jamnik 1995).

When standardizing the work performed on a friction-type bicycle ergometer, the client should maintain a constant pedaling rate. Some cycle ergometers have a speedometer that displays the individual's pedaling rate. Check this dial frequently to make certain that your client is maintaining a constant pedaling frequency throughout the test. If a speedometer is not available, use a metronome to establish your client's pedaling cadence. Controlling the pedaling rate on an electrically braked bicycle ergometer is unnecessary. An electromagnetic braking force adjusts the resistance for slower or faster pedaling rates, thereby keeping the power output constant. This type of bicycle ergometer, however, is difficult to calibrate.

Table 4.4 MET Estimates for Each Stage of Commonly Used Treadmill Protocols

Stage[a]	Bruce	Modified Bruce[b]	Balke	Naughton
1	4.6	2.3	3.6	1.8
2	7.0	3.5	4.5	3.5
3	10.2	4.6	5.0	4.5
4	12.1	7.0	5.5	5.4
5	14.9	10.2	5.9	6.4
6	17.0	12.1	6.4	7.4
7	19.3	14.9	6.9	8.3

[a] Percentage grade and speed for each stage are illustrated in figure 4.2.
[b] Stage 1 = 0% grade, 1.7 mph; Stage 2 = 5% grade, 1.7 mph.

Table 4.5 Population-Specific and Generalized Equations for Treadmill Protocols

Protocol	Population	Reference	Equation
Balke	Active and sedentary men	Pollock et al. 1976	$\dot{V}O_2max = 1.444(Time) + 14.99$ $r = 0.92$, SEE = 2.50 ml $\cdot$ kg^{-1} $\cdot$ min^{-1}
	Active and sedentary women[a]	Pollock et al. 1982	$\dot{V}O_2max = 1.38(Time) + 5.22$ $r = 0.94$, SEE = 2.20 ml $\cdot$ kg^{-1} $\cdot$ min^{-1}
Bruce[b]	Active and sedentary men; male cardiac patients	Foster et al. 1984	$\dot{V}O_2max = 14.76 - 1.379(Time) + 0.451(Time^2) - 0.012(Time^3)$ $r = 0.98$, SEE = 3.35 ml $\cdot$ kg^{-1} $\cdot$ min^{-1}
	Active and sedentary women	Pollock et al. 1982	$\dot{V}O_2max = 4.38(Time) - 3.90$ $r = 0.91$, SEE = 2.7 ml $\cdot$ kg^{-1} $\cdot$ min^{-1}
	Cardiac patients and elderly[c]	McConnell and Clark, 1987	$\dot{V}O_2max = 2.282(Time) + 8.545$ $r = 0.82$, SEE = 4.9 ml $\cdot$ kg^{-1} $\cdot$ min^{-1}
Naughton	Male cardiac patients	Foster et al. 1983	$\dot{V}O_2max = 1.61(Time) + 3.60$ $r = 0.97$, SEE = 2.60 ml $\cdot$ kg^{-1} $\cdot$ min^{-1}

[a] For women, the Balke protocol was modified: Speed 3.0 mph, initial work load 0% grade for 3 min, increasing 2.5% every 3 min thereafter.
[b] For use with the standard Bruce protocol, *not* modified Bruce protocol.
[c] This equation is used only for treadmill walking while holding the handrails.

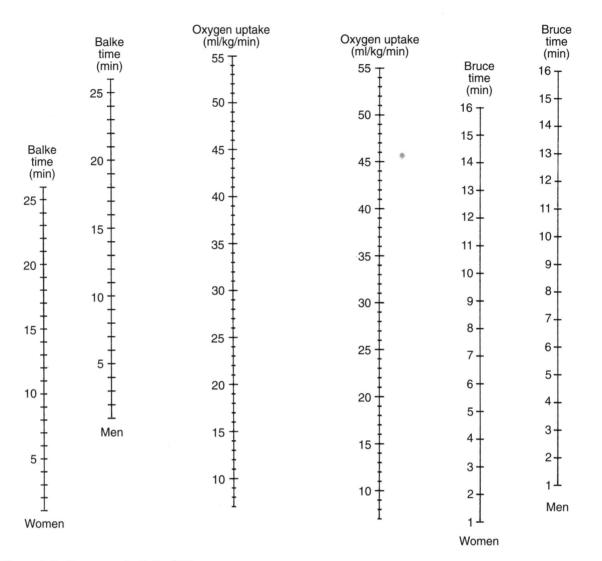

Figure 4.3   Nomogram for Balke GXT.
Reprinted, by permission, from N. Ng: Metcalc, 1995, Human Kinetics, Champaign, 30.

Figure 4.4   Nomogram for Standard Bruce GXT.
Reprinted, by permission, from N. Ng: Metcalc, 1995, Human Kinetics, Champaign, 32.

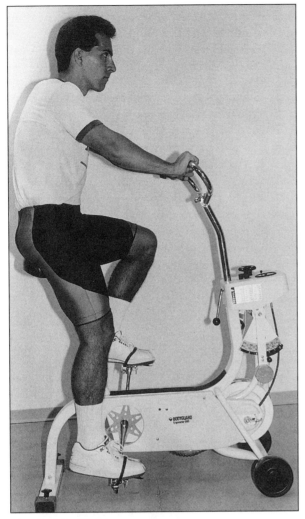

Figure 4.5 Bicycle ergometer.

TESTING WITH BICYCLE ERGOMETERS

The following guidelines are suggested for use of bicycle ergometers (Sinning 1975):

1. Calibrate the bicycle often by hanging known weights from the belt of the flywheel and reading the dial on the handwheel.

2. Always release the tension on the belt between tests.

3. Establish pedaling frequency prior to setting the work load.

4. Check the load setting frequently during the test, because it may change as the belt warms up.

5. Set the metronome so that one revolution is completed for every two beats (e.g., set the metronome at 120 for a test requiring a pedaling frequency of 60 rpm).

6. Adjust the height of the seat so the knee is slightly flexed (about 5°) at maximal leg extension with the ball of the foot on the pedal.

7. Have the client assume an upright, seated posture with hands properly positioned on the handlebars.

Most cycle ergometer test protocols for untrained cyclists use a pedaling rate of 50 or 60 rpm, and power outputs are increased by 150 to 300 kgm · min^{-1} (25 to 50 W) in each stage of the test. However, you can use higher pedaling rates (≥80 rpm) for trained cyclists. A pedaling rate of 60 rpm produces the highest $\dot{V}O_2$max when compared with rates of 50, 70, or 80 rpm (Hermansen and Saltin 1969). Figure 4.6 illustrates some widely used discontinuous and continuous maximal exercise test protocols for the bicycle ergometer.

To calculate the energy expenditure for bicycle ergometer exercise, use the ACSM equations provided in table 4.3. The total energy expenditure, in ml · min^{-1}, is a function of two components. The resistive or *vertical component (V)* is the energy expended per minute to overcome the resistance (kg) applied to the flywheel while pedaling at a constant frequency. The *resting component (R)* is the amount of oxygen consumed per minute by the client at rest and is dependent on body weight. The resting component is calculated by multiplying the resting metabolic equivalent (1 MET or 3.5 ml · kg^{-1} · min^{-1}) by the client's body weight (BW) in kilograms. For an example of such a calculation, see ACSM Leg Ergometry Equations on page 62.

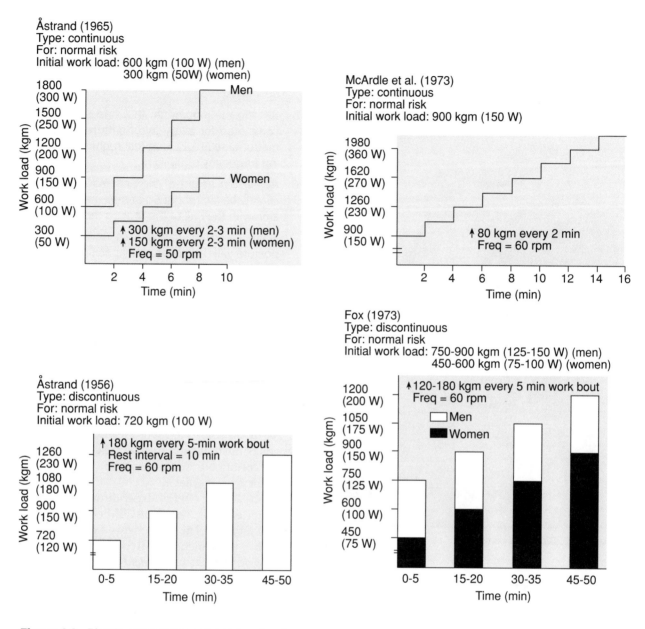

Figure 4.6 Bicycle ergometer exercise test protocols.

ACSM LEG ERGOMETRY EQUATION

To calculate the energy expenditure of a 62-kg (136-lb) woman cycling at a work rate of 450 kgm · min⁻¹, follow these steps:

1. Calculate the resistive component (V).

$$V = kgm \cdot min^{-1} \times 2$$
$$= 450 \; kgm \cdot min^{-1} \times 2$$
$$= 900 \; ml \cdot min^{-1}$$

2. Calculate the absolute $\dot{V}O_2$ by adding the resting component, corrected for body weight.

$\dot{V}O_2$ = V + (1 MET × BW)

= 900 ml · min^{-1} + [3.5 ml · kg^{-1} · min^{-1} × 62 kg]

= 900 ml · min^{-1} + 217 ml · min^{-1}

= 1117 ml · min^{-1}

3. Convert the absolute $\dot{V}O_2$ to relative $\dot{V}O_2$ by dividing by body weight.

relative $\dot{V}O_2$ = absolute $\dot{V}O_2$/BW

= 1117 ml · min^{-1}/62 kg

= 18 ml · kg^{-1} · min^{-1}

4. Express the relative energy expenditure in METs by dividing by 3.5 ml · kg^{-1} · min^{-1}.

METs = 18 ml · kg^{-1} · min^{-1}/3.5 ml · kg^{-1} · min^{-1}

= 5.14 METs

Although the ACSM cycle ergometry equation may provide a reasonable estimate of oxygen cost during submaximal, steady-state, cycle ergometer exercise for some individuals, this equation underestimates actual oxygen cost by as much as 263 to 290 ml · min^{-1}, respectively, in women and men (Lang et al. 1992; Latin and Berg 1994). These researchers suggest using revised equations for estimating the oxygen cost of cycle ergometer exercise (see below).

REVISED ACSM LEG ERGOMETRY EQUATIONS

Males (for 180 to 900 kgm · min^{-1} work loads)

$\dot{V}O_2$ = (kgm · min^{-1} × 1.9) + 260 ml · min^{-1} + (3.5 × BW in kg)

Females (for 0 to 750 kgm · min^{-1} work loads)

$\dot{V}O_2$ = (kgm · min^{-1} × 1.6) + 205 ml · min^{-1} + (3.5 × BW in kg)

These revised ACSM equations have been cross-validated for independent samples of young men and women (age = 26 years), as well as deconditioned, obese women, 23 to 60 years of age. Compared to the ACSM equations, the revised equations have smaller prediction errors and higher correlations for power outputs ≤900 kgm · min^{-1} for men and ≤720 kgm · min^{-1} for women (Andersen and Wadden 1995; Latin and Berg 1994). You should consider using these revised equations to estimate your client's energy cost of cycle ergometer exercise at moderate power outputs.

Keep in mind that these metabolic equations, as well as the ACSM equations, are accurate in estimating $\dot{V}O_2$ only if the client attains a steady state during the maximal GXT. If, for example, the client is able to complete only one minute of exercise during the last stage of the maximal test protocol, the power output from the previous stage (in which the client reached steady state) should be used to estimate $\dot{V}O_2$max rather than the power output corresponding to the last stage.

Åstrand Bicycle Ergometer Maximal Test Protocol

For the Åstrand (1965) continuous test protocol (see figure 4.6), the initial power output is 300 kgm · min^{-1} (50 W) for women and 600 kgm · min^{-1} (100 W) for men. Because the pedaling rate is 50 rpm, the resistance is 1 kg for women (1 kg × 6 m × 50 rpm = 300 kgm · min^{-1}) and 2 kg for men (2 kg × 6 m × 50 rpm = 600 kgm · min^{-1}). Have your client exercise at this initial work load for 2 minutes. Then increase the power output every 2 to 3 minutes in increments of 150 kgm · min^{-1} (25 W) and 300 kgm · min^{-1} (50 W) for women and men, respectively. Continue the test until the client is exhausted or can no longer maintain the pedaling rate of 50 rpm. Use either the ACSM metabolic equation for leg ergometry or the revised ACSM cycle ergometer equations (Latin et al. 1993, 1994) to estimate $\dot{V}O_2$ from your client's power output during the last stage of the GXT.

Fox Bicycle Ergometer Maximal Test Protocol

The Fox (1973) protocol is a discontinuous test consisting of a series of 5-minute exercise bouts with 10-minute rest intervals. The starting work load is between 750 kgm · min⁻¹ (125 W) and 900 kgm · min⁻¹ (150 W) for men and 450 kgm · min⁻¹ (75 W) and 600 kgm · min⁻¹ (100 W) for women. The progressive increments in work depend on the client's heart rate response and usually are between 120 and 180 kgm · min⁻¹ (20 and 30 W). The client exercises until exhausted or until no longer able to pedal for at least 3 minutes at a power output that is 60 to 90 kgm · min⁻¹ (10 to 15 W) higher than the previous work load. You can use the metabolic equations to convert the power output from the last stage of this protocol to $\dot{V}O_2$max.

Bench Stepping Maximal Exercise Tests

The least desirable mode of exercise for maximum exercise testing is bench stepping. During bench stepping, the individual is performing both positive (up phase) and negative (down phase) work. Approximately one-quarter to one-third less energy is expended during negative work (Morehouse 1972). This factor, coupled with adjusting the step height and stepping rate for differences in body weight, makes standardization of the work extremely difficult. Most step test protocols increase the intensity of the work by gradually increasing the height of the bench or the stepping rate. The work (W) performed can be calculated using the equation, W = F × D, where F is body weight in kilograms and D is bench height times number of steps per minute. For example, a 50-kg (110 lb) woman stepping at a rate of 22 steps · min⁻¹ on a 30-cm (0.30-m or 11.8-in) bench is performing 330 kgm · min⁻¹ of work (50 kg × 0.30 m × 22 steps · min⁻¹).

The following equations can be used to adjust the step height and stepping rate for differences in body weight to achieve a given work rate (Morehouse 1972):

Step height (cm) = work (kg cm · min⁻¹)/[body weight (kg) × stepping rate]

Stepping rate (steps · min⁻¹) = work (kg cm · min⁻¹)/ [body weight (kg) × step height (cm)]

For example, if you devise a graded step test protocol that requires a client weighing 60 kg (132 lb) to exercise at a work rate of 300 kgm · min⁻¹, and the stepping rate is set at 18 steps · min⁻¹, you need to determine the appropriate step height that corresponds to the work rate:

Step height = 300 kgm · min⁻¹/(60 kg × 18 steps · min⁻¹)

= 0.28 m or 28 cm

Alternatively, you may choose to keep the step height constant and vary the stepping cadence for each stage of the graded exercise test. For example, if the step height is set at 30 cm (0.30 m), and the protocol requires that a client weighing 60 kg (132 lb) exercise at a work rate of 450 kgm · min⁻¹, you need to calculate the corresponding stepping rate for this client:

Stepping rate = 450 kgm · min⁻¹ / (60 kg × 0.30 m)

= 25 steps · min⁻¹

You can calculate the energy expenditure in METs using the ACSM metabolic equation for stepping exercise (see table 4.3). For an example of such calculations, see ACSM Stepping Equation below.

ACSM STEPPING EQUATION

To calculate the energy expenditure for bench stepping using a 16-inch step height at a cadence of 24 steps · min⁻¹, follow these steps:

$\dot{V}O_2$ = horizontal component + vertical component

$\dot{V}O_2$ in ml · kg⁻¹ · min⁻¹ = (steps · min⁻¹ × 0.35) + (m/step × steps · min⁻¹ × 1.33 × 1.8)

1. Calculate the horizontal component (H).
   H = stepping rate × 0.35
   = 24 steps · min⁻¹ × 0.35
   = 8.4 ml · kg⁻¹ · min⁻¹

2. Convert the bench height to meters (1 in = 2.54 cm or 0.0254 m).
   ht = 16 in × 0.0254 m
   = 0.4064 m

3. Calculate the vertical component (V).
   V = bench height × stepping rate × 1.33 × 1.8
   = 0.4064 m × 24 steps · min⁻¹ × 1.33 × 1.8
   = 23.35 ml · kg⁻¹ · min⁻¹

4. Add the H and V to calculate relative $\dot{V}O_2$.
   $\dot{V}O_2$ = 8.4 ml · kg⁻¹ · min⁻¹ + 23.35 ml · kg⁻¹ · min⁻¹
   = 31.75 ml · kg⁻¹ · min⁻¹

5. Convert the $\dot{V}O_2$ to METs by dividing by 3.5 ml · kg⁻¹ · min⁻¹.
   METs = 31.75 ml · kg⁻¹ · min⁻¹/3.5 ml · kg⁻¹ · min⁻¹
   = 9.07 METs

Nagle, Balke, and Naughton Maximal Step Test Protocol

Nagle, Balke, and Naughton (1965) devised a graded step test for assessing work capacity. Have your client step at a rate of 30 steps/min on an automatically adjustable bench (2 to 50 cm or 0.8 to 19.6 in). Set the initial bench height at 2 cm, and increase the height 2 cm every minute of exercise. Use a metronome to establish the stepping cadence (4 beats per stepping cycle). To establish a cadence of 30 steps/min, for example, set the metronome at 120 (30 × 4). Terminate the test when the subject is fatigued or can no longer maintain the stepping cadence. Use the ACSM metabolic equation for stepping exercise to calculate the energy expenditure ($\dot{V}O_2$max) corresponding to the step height and stepping cadence during the last work stage of this protocol.

SUBMAXIMAL EXERCISE TEST PROTOCOLS

It is desirable to directly determine the functional aerobic capacity of the individual for diagnosing CHD, classifying the cardiorespiratory fitness level, and prescribing an aerobic exercise program. However, it is not always practical to do so. The actual measurement of $\dot{V}O_2$max requires expensive laboratory equipment, a considerable amount of time to administer, and a high level of motivation on the part of the client.

Alternatively, you can use submaximal exercise tests to predict or estimate the $\dot{V}O_2$max of the individual. Many of these tests are similar to the maximal exercise tests described previously, except that they are terminated at some predetermined heart rate intensity. You will monitor the heart rate, BP, and RPE during the submaximal exercise test. The treadmill, bicycle ergometer, or bench stepping exercises are commonly used for submaximal exercise testing.

Assumptions of Submaximal Exercise Tests

Submaximal exercise tests assume a steady-state HR at each exercise intensity, as well as a linear relationship between heart rate, oxygen uptake, and work intensity. While this is true for light-to-moderate work loads, the relationship between oxygen uptake and work becomes curvilinear at heavier work loads.

Another assumption of submaximal testing is that the mechanical efficiency during cycling or treadmill exercise is constant for all individuals. However, a client with poor mechanical efficiency while cycling has a higher submaximal heart rate at a given work load, and the actual $\dot{V}O_2$max is therefore underestimated (McArdle, Katch, and Katch 1996). As a result, $\dot{V}O_2$max predicted by submaximal exercise tests tends to be overestimated for highly trained individuals and underestimated for untrained, sedentary individuals.

Submaximal tests also assume that the maximum heart rate (HR max) for clients of a given age is similar. The HR max, however, has been shown to vary as much as ± 11 bpm, even after controlling for variability due to age and training status (Londeree and Moeschberger 1984). For submaximal tests, the HR max is estimated from age. The equation, HR max = 220 – age, yields a low estimate of the maximum heart rate, while the equation, HR max = 210 – (0.5 × age), gives a high estimate of maximum heart rate (ACSM 1995). The HR max of approximately 5 to 7% of men and women is more than 15 bpm less than their age-predicted HR max, while 9 to 13% have HR max values that exceed their age-predicted HR max by more than 15 bpm (Whaley et al. 1992). Due to individual variability in HR max, as well as the inaccuracy of using age-predicted HR max, you may expect considerable error (±10 to 15%) in estimating your client's $\dot{V}O_2$max—especially when submaximal data are extrapolated to an age-predicted HR max.

Treadmill Submaximal Exercise Tests

Treadmill submaximal tests provide an estimate of functional aerobic capacity ($\dot{V}O_2$max) and assume a linear increase in heart rate with successive increments in work load. Compared to clients with low cardiorespiratory fitness levels, the well-conditioned individual presumably is able to perform a greater quantity of work at a given submaximal heart rate.

You can use the treadmill maximal test protocols (figure 4.2) to identify the slope of the individual's heart rate response to exercise. The $\dot{V}O_2$max can be predicted from either one (single-stage model) or two (multistage model) submaximal heart rates. Mahar et al. (1985) reported that the accuracy of the single-stage model is similar to that of the multistage model.

Multistage Model

To estimate $\dot{V}O_2$max using the multistage model, use the heart rate and work load data from two or more submaximal stages of the treadmill test. Be sure your client reaches steady-state heart rates between 115 to 150 bpm (Golding, Meyers, and Sinning 1989). Determine the slope (b) by calculating the ratio of the difference between the two submaximal (SM) work loads (expressed as $\dot{V}O_2$) and the corresponding change in submaximal heart rates:

$$b = (SM_2 - SM_1)/(HR_2 - HR_1)$$

Calculate the $\dot{V}O_2$ for each work load using the ACSM metabolic equation (table 4.3), and use the following equation to predict $\dot{V}O_2$max:

$$\dot{V}O_2\text{max} = SM_2 + b\,(HR\,max - HR_2)$$

If the actual maximal heart rate is not known, estimate it using the formula, 220 – age. The following example illustrates the use of the multistage model for estimating $\dot{V}O_2$max for a submaximal treadmill test given to a 38-year-old male.

Protocol: Bruce

Submaximal data, Stage 2[a]:

$\dot{V}O_2$[b] = 24.5 ml · kg^{-1} · min^{-1} (SM$_2$)

HR = 145 bpm (HR$_2$)

Submaximal data, Stage 1[a]:

$\dot{V}O_2$[b] = 16.1 ml · kg^{-1} · min^{-1} (SM$_1$)

HR = 130 bpm (HR$_1$)

Maximum HR:

220 – age = 182 bpm

Slope (b): $(SM_2 - SM_1) / (HR_2 - HR_1)$

$b = (24.5 - 16.1) / (145 - 130)$

$b = 8.4/15$

$b = 0.56$

$\dot{V}O_2$max: $SM_2 + b(HR\,max - HR_2)$

$= 24.5 + 0.56(182 - 145)$

$= 24.5 + 20.72$

$\dot{V}O_2$max = 45.22

---

[a] Stages 1 and 2 refer to the last two stages of the GXT completed by the client, and not the first and second stage of the test protocol. For example, if the client completes three stages of the submaximal exercise test protocol, use data from stages 2 and 3 to estimate $\dot{V}O_2$.

[b] Calculate $\dot{V}O_2$ using ACSM metabolic equations (see table 4.3). $\dot{V}O_2$ can be expressed in L · min^{-1}, ml · kg^{-1} · min^{-1}, or METs.

Single-Stage Model

To estimate $\dot{V}O_2$max using the single-stage model, use one submaximal heart rate and one work load. The steady-state submaximal heart rate during a single-stage GXT should reach 130 to 150 bpm. Formulas for men and women have been developed (Shephard 1972).

Men

$$\dot{V}O_2\text{max} = SM_{\dot{V}O_2} \times [(HR\,max - 61)/(HR_{SM} - 61)]$$

Women

$$\dot{V}O_2\text{max} = SM_{\dot{V}O_2} \times [(HR\,max - 72)/(HR_{SM} - 72)]$$

Calculate $SM_{\dot{V}O_2}$ using the ACSM metabolic equations (see table 4.3). Estimate HR max (if not known) using the formula, 220 – age; HR_{SM} is the submaximal heart rate.

The following example illustrates the use of the single-stage model for estimating $\dot{V}O_2$max for a treadmill submaximal test given to a 45-year-old female.

Protocol: Balke

Submaximal data, Stage 3:

$\dot{V}O_2$ = 5.0 METs ($SM_{\dot{V}O_2}$)

HR = 148 bpm (HR_{SM})

Maximum HR:

220 – age = 175 bpm

$\dot{V}O_2$max: $= SM_{\dot{V}O_2} \times [(HR\,max - 72)/(HR_{SM} - 72)]$

$= 5 \times [(175 - 72)/(148 - 72)]$

$= 5 \times [103/76]$

$= 6.8$ METs

Single-Stage Treadmill Walking Test

Ebbeling et al. (1991) developed a single-stage treadmill walking test suitable for estimating $\dot{V}O_2$max of low risk, healthy adults who are 20 to 59 years of age. For this protocol, walking speed is individualized and ranges from 2.0 to 4.5 mph (53.6 to 120.6 m · min^{-1}) depending on your client's age, gender, and fitness level. Establish a walking pace during a 4-minute warm-up at 0% grade. The warm-up work bout should produce a HR within 50 to 70% of the individual's age-predicted HR max. The test consists of brisk walking at the selected pace for an additional 4 minutes at 5% grade. Record the steady-state HR at this work load and use it in the following equation to estimate $\dot{V}O_2$max:

$\dot{V}O_2max$ (ml · kg^{-1} · min^{-1})
= 15.1 + 21.8 (speed mph) – 0.327 (HR bpm)
– 0.263 (speed × age yr) + 0.00504 (HR × age)
+ 5.48 (gender: where female = 0; male = 1)

Single-Stage Treadmill Walking or Jogging Test

You can also estimate your client's $\dot{V}O_2max$ from a single 6-minute treadmill walk (50% $\dot{V}O_2max$) or run (70% $\dot{V}O_2max$) and steady-state HR from the last 2 minutes of exercise (Latin and Elias 1993). For the walking protocol, set the treadmill speed at 3.0 mph (80.4 m · min^{-1}) for women and 3.5 mph (93.8 m · min^{-1}) for men, and raise the grade to a level requiring 50 or 60% $\dot{V}O_2max$. For the running protocol, have the client run at a speed requiring about 70 to 80% $\dot{V}O_2max$ at 0% grade. Estimate the energy expenditure ($\dot{V}O_2$) of the exercise work load using the ACSM walking or running equations (see table 4.3). Plot the client's energy expenditure in L · min^{-1} and the steady-state exercise HR in the corresponding columns of the Åstrand-Rhyming nomogram (see figure 4.7). Connect these points with a ruler and read the estimated $\dot{V}O_2max$ at the point where the line intersects the $\dot{V}O_2max$ column.

Single-Stage Treadmill Jogging Test

You can estimate the $\dot{V}O_2max$ of younger adults (18 to 28 years) using a single-stage treadmill jogging test (George et al. 1993). For this test, select a comfortable jogging pace ranging from 4.3 to 7.5 mph (115.2 to 201 m · min^{-1}), but not more than 6.5 mph (174.2 m · min^{-1}) for women or 7.5 mph (201 m · min^{-1}) for men. Have the client jog at a constant speed for about 3 minutes. The steady-state exercise HR should not exceed 180 bpm. Estimate $\dot{V}O_2max$ using the following equation:

$\dot{V}O_2max$ (ml · kg^{-1} · min^{-1}) = 54.07 – 0.1938 (BW in kg)
+ 4.47 (speed in mph) – 0.1453 (HR in bpm)
+ 7.062 (gender: where male = 1; female = 0)

Bicycle Ergometer Submaximal Exercise Tests

Bicycle ergometer multistage, submaximal tests can be used to predict $\dot{V}O_2max$. These tests are either continuous or discontinuous and are based on the assumption that heart rate and oxygen uptake are linear functions of work rate. The heart rate response to submaximal work loads is used to predict $\dot{V}O_2max$.

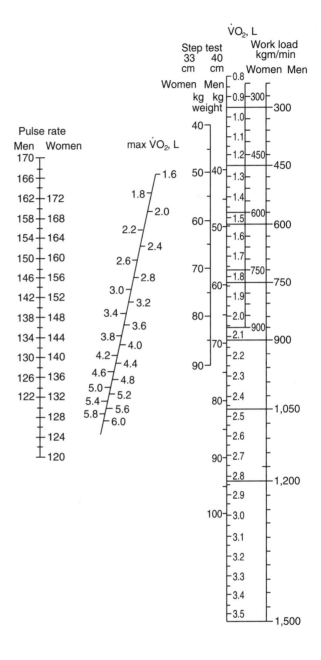

Figure 4.7 Modified Åstrand-Ryhming nomogram.
Reprinted, by permission, from I. Åstrand, "Aerobic capacity in men and women with special reference to age," *Acta Physiologica Scandinavica* 49 (Suppl. 169): 51.

YMCA Bicycle Ergometer Submaximal Exercise Test Protocol

Golding, Myers, and Sinning (1989) developed a bicycle ergometer submaximal protocol for women and men. This protocol uses three or four consecutive 3-minute work loads on the bicycle ergometer designed to raise the HR to between 110 and 150 bpm. The pedal rate is 50 rpm, and the initial work load is 150 kgm · min^{-1} (25 W). Use the heart rate during the last minute of the initial work load to determine subsequent work loads (see figure 4.8). If the HR is less than 80 bpm, set the second work load at 750 kgm · min^{-1}. If HR is 80 to 89 bpm or 90 to 100 bpm, the respective work loads are 600 or 450 kgm · min^{-1} for the second stage of the protocol. If the HR at the end of the first work load exceeds 100 bpm, set the second work load at 300 kgm · min^{-1}.

Set the third and fourth work loads accordingly (see figure 4.8). Measure the heart rate during the last 30 seconds of minutes 2 and 3 at each work load. If these heart rates differ by more than 5 bpm, extend the work load an additional minute until the HR stabilizes. If the client's steady-state HR reaches or exceeds 150 bpm during the third work load, terminate the test.

Calculate the energy expenditure ($\dot{V}O_2$) for the last two work loads using the ACSM metabolic equations (see table 4.3) or the revised ACSM equations (see page 63). To estimate $\dot{V}O_2$max from these data, use the equations for the multistage model to calculate the slope of the line depicting the heart rate response to the last two work loads. Alternatively, you can graph these data to estimate $\dot{V}O_2$max (see figure 4.9). To do this, plot the $\dot{V}O_2$ for each work load and corresponding heart rates. Connect these two data points with a straight edge, extending the line so that it intersects the predicted maximum heart rate line. To extrapolate $\dot{V}O_2$max, drop a perpendicular line from the point of intersection to the x-axis of the graph. If this is done carefully, the graphing method and multistage method will yield similar estimates of $\dot{V}O_2$max.

ACSM Bicycle Ergometer Submaximal Exercise Test Protocol

The American College of Sports Medicine (1991) developed a cycle ergometer submaximal exercise test protocol based on the individual's body weight and activity status (table 4.6). To select the most appropriate protocol (A, B or C), determine the subject's body weight classification and activity

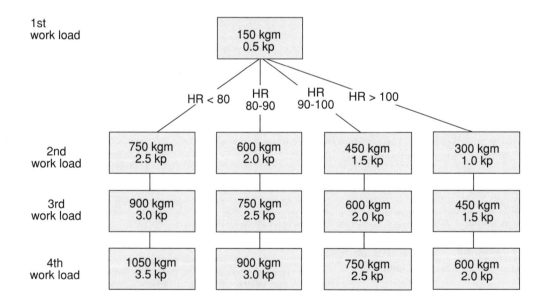

Directions:

1. Set the first work load at 150 kgm/min (0.5 kp)
2. If the HR in the third min is
   • less than (<) 80, set the second load at 750 kgm (2.5 kp);
   • 80-89, set the second load at at 600 kgm (2.0 kp);
   • 90-100, set the second load at 450 kgm (1.5 kp);
   • greater than (>) 100, set the second load at 300 kgm (1.0 kp)
3. Set the third and fourth (if required) loads according to the loads in the columns below the second loads.

Figure 4.8 YMCA bicycle ergometer protocol.
Reprinted from *Y's Way to Physical Fitness, 3rd edition* with permission of the YMCA of the USA, 101 N. Wacker Drive, Chicago, IL 60606.

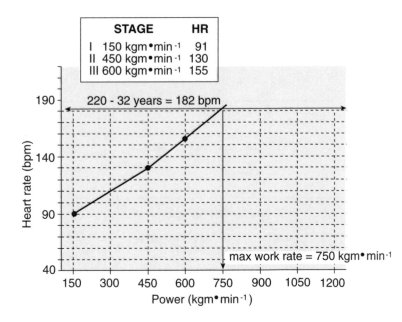

Figure 4.9   Plotting HR vs submaximal work rates to estimate maximal work capacity and $\dot{V}O_2$max.

status. Very active individuals are defined as those who have regularly participated in vigorous activities at least 20 minutes, three times per week, during the past three months.

Each protocol consists of four work loads, each lasting 2 minutes. Measure the heart rate during the last 15 seconds of each work load, and stop the test when the client's HR reaches 65 to 70% of the heart rate range (Karvonen method) or 85% of the age-predicted maximal heart rate (ACSM 1996). Using the graphing method, estimate the $\dot{V}O_2$max by plotting the HR response to the last two workloads and extending the line to the age-predicted HR max (see figure 4.9). Alternatively, you can use the multistage model equations to estimate $\dot{V}O_2$max.

In the ACSM (1991) *Guidelines for Exercise Testing and Prescription* (4th edition), the termination point for this protocol was only 65 to 70% of the age-predicted HR max, compared to the current recommendation of 85% HR max (ACSM 1996). Greiwe et al. (1995) tested the reliability and validity of the ACSM protocol in estimating $\dot{V}O_2$max using the 65 to 70% HR max termination criterion. They reported that this protocol significantly overestimated $\dot{V}O_2$max by 25% for women and men 21 to 54 years of age. Also, there were large intraindividual differences in the $\dot{V}O_2$max estimated from submaximal HR data from two separate submaximal trials, indicating poor reliability for this protocol and termination criterion. Because of the low termination criterion and the short, 2-minute stages for this protocol, the authors noted that subjects were un-

able to reach those exercise intensities that would tend to decrease intraindividual variability in submaximal HR. Thus, there were large errors in estimating $\dot{V}O_2$max from the submaximal HR data. Using the revised termination criterion (85% age-predicted HR max or 65 to 70% $\dot{V}O_2$max) may overcome this problem. However, more validation studies are needed to test this hypothesis.

Åstrand-Ryhming Bicycle Ergometer Submaximal Exercise Test Protocol

The Åstrand-Ryhming protocol (1954) is a single-stage test that uses a nomogram to predict $\dot{V}O_2$max from heart rate response to one 6-minute submaximal work load. A power output is selected that produces a heart rate between 130 and 150 bpm. The initial work load is usually 450 to 600 kgm · min[-1] (75 to 100 W) for women and 600 to 900 kgm · min[-1] (100 to 150 W) for men. An initial work load of 300 kgm · min[-1] (50 W) may be used for poorly conditioned or older individuals. Alternatively, you can use a nomogram (see figure 4.10) to estimate the initial work load for men by plotting the client's body weight and heart rate response after one minute of cycling at 600 kgm · min[-1] (100 W) (Terry et al. 1977). No such nomogram has been developed for women.

During the test, measure the heart rate every minute and record the average heart rate during the 5th and 6th minute. If the difference between these two heart rates exceeds 5 bpm, extend the work bout until a steady-state heart rate is achieved. If the

Table 4.6   ACSM Bicycle Ergometer Submaximal Test Protocols

Stages (2 min each)	Test protocols[a]		
	A	B	C
1	25[b] (150)	25 (150)	50 (300)
2	50 (300)	50 (300)	100 (600)
3	75 (450)	100 (600)	150 (900)
4	100 (600)	150 (900)	200 (1200)

BW in kg (lb)	Selection Criteria	
	Very Active[c]	
	No	Yes
<73 (≤160)	A	A
74-90 (161-199)	A	B
>91 (≥200)	B	C

[a]Terminate test protocol when HR reaches 70% HRR or 85% HR max.

[b]Work load in watts (kgm · min⁻¹)

[c]Very active = aerobic exercise 20 minutes, 3 days per week.

Reprinted, by permission, from American College of Sports Medicine, 1996, *ACSM Health/Fitness Instructor Certification Study Packet* (Baltimore: Williams & Wilkins), 16.

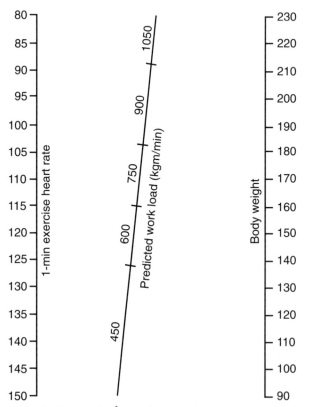

Figure 4.10   Nomogram for work load selection for Åstrand-Ryhming test.
Reprinted, by permission, from J.W. Terry et al., 1977, "A work load selection procedure for the Åstrand-Ryhming test," *Journal of Sports Medicine and Physical Fitness* 17: 363.

heart rate is less than 130 bpm at the end of the exercise bout, increase the work load by 300 kgm · min^{-1} (50 W) and have the client exercise an additional 6 minutes.

To estimate $\dot{V}O_2$max for this protocol, use the modified Åstrand-Ryhming nomogram (figure 4.7). This nomogram estimates $\dot{V}O_2$max (in L · min^{-1}) from submaximal treadmill, bicycle ergometer, and step test data. For each test mode, the submaximal heart rate is plotted with oxygen cost of treadmill exercise ($\dot{V}O_2$ in L · min^{-1}), power output (kgm · min^{-1}) for bicycle ergometer exercise, or body weight (kg) for stepping exercise. The correlation between measured $\dot{V}O_2$max and the $\dot{V}O_2$max estimated from this nomogram is r = 0.74; the prediction error is ±10 and ±15%, respectively, for well-trained and untrained individuals (Åstrand and Rodahl 1977).

For clients younger or older than 25 years, you must use age-correction factors to adjust the $\dot{V}O_2$max predicted from the nomogram for the effect of age. For example, if the estimated $\dot{V}O_2$max from the nomogram is 3.2 L · min^{-1} for a 45-year-old client, the adjusted $\dot{V}O_2$max is 2.5 L · min^{-1} (3.2 × 0.78 = 2.5 L · min^{-1}).

Age-Correction Factors for Åstrand-Ryhming Nomogram

Age	Correction factor
15	1.10
25	1.00
35	0.87
40	0.83
45	0.78
50	0.75
55	0.71
60	0.68
65	0.65

Fox Single-Stage Bicycle Ergometer Test Protocol

You can modify the maximal exercise test protocol (see figure 4.6) designed by Fox (1973) to predict $\dot{V}O_2$max (ml · min^{-1}). Have your client perform a single work load (e.g., 900 kgm · min^{-1} or 150 W) for 5 minutes. The standard error of estimate for this test is ±246 ml · min^{-1}, and the standard error of prediction is ±7.8%. The correlation between actual and predicted $\dot{V}O_2$max is r = 0.76. To estimate $\dot{V}O_2$max, measure the heart rate at the end of the fifth minute of exercise (HR$_5$) and use the following equation:

$$\dot{V}O_2max\ (ml \cdot min^{-1}) = 6300 - 19.26\ (HR_5)$$

Bench Stepping Submaximal Exercise Tests

Although there are many step tests to evaluate cardiorespiratory fitness, few provide equations for predicting $\dot{V}O_2$max. Only step test protocols with prediction equations are included in this section.

Åstrand-Ryhming Step Test Protocol

As mentioned previously, you can use the Åstrand-Ryhming nomogram (see figure 4.7) to predict $\dot{V}O_2$max from postexercise heart rate and body weight during bench stepping. For this protocol, the client steps at a rate of 22.5 steps · min^{-1} for 5 minutes. The bench height is 33 cm (13 in) for women and 40 cm (15.75 in) for men. Measure the postexercise heart rate by counting the number of beats between 15 and 30 seconds immediately after exercise (convert this 15-second count to beats per minute by multiplying by 4). Correct the predicted $\dot{V}O_2$max from the nomogram if your client is older or younger than 25 years (see age-correction factors at left).

Queen's College Step Test Protocol

McArdle et al. (1972) devised a step test to predict $\dot{V}O_2$max in which the client steps at a rate of 22 steps per minute (females) or 24 steps per minute (males) for 3 minutes. The bench height is 16.25 in. (41.3 cm) Have your client remain standing after the exercise. Wait 5 seconds, and then take a 15-second heart-rate count (either the client or the technician may count). Convert the count to beats per minute by multiplying by 4. If you are administering this test simultaneously to more than one client, you should teach your clients how to measure their own pulse rates (see page 74). To estimate $\dot{V}O_2$max in ml · kg^{-1} · min^{-1}, use the equations listed in table 4.7. The standard error of prediction for these equations is ±16%.

Additional Modes for Submaximal Exercise Testing

If you are working in the context of a health or fitness club, you may have access to stairclimbers and rowing ergometers. You can use some of these exercise machines for submaximal exercise testing of your clients.

Table 4.7   Prediction Equations for Cardiorespiratory Field Tests

Field test	Equation[a]	Source
Distance		
Run/Walk		
1.0-mi steady-state jog	$\dot{V}O_2max = 100.5 - 0.1636(BW\ kg) - 1.438(Time\ min) - 0.1928(HR\ bpm) + 8.344(Gender)^b$	George et al. 1993
1.0-mi run/walk (8-17 yr)	$\dot{V}O_2max = 108.94 - 8.41(Time\ min) + 0.34(Time\ min)^2 + 0.21(Age \times Gender)^b - 0.84(BMI)^c$	Cureton et al. 1995
1.5-mi run/walk	$\dot{V}O_2max = 88.02 - 0.1656(BW\ kg) - 2.76(Time\ min) + 3.716(Gender)^b$	George et al. 1993
12-min run	$\dot{V}O_2max = (Distance\ meters - 504.9)/44.73$	Cooper 1968
15-min run	$\dot{V}O_2max = 0.0178(Distance\ meters) + 9.6$	Balke 1963
1.0-mi walk	$\dot{V}O_2max = 132.853 - 0.0769(BW\ lb) - 0.3877(Age\ yr) + 6.315(Gender)^b - 3.2649(Time\ min) - 0.1565(HR\ bpm)$	Kline et al. 1987
Step tests		
Åstrand	Men: $\dot{V}O_2max\ (L \cdot min^{-1}) = 3.744[(BW\ kg + 5)/(HR - 62)]$ Women: $\dot{V}O_2max\ (L \cdot min^{-1}) = 3.750[(BW\ kg - 3)/(HR - 65)]$	Marley and Linnerud 1976
Queen's College	Men: $\dot{V}O_2max = 111.33 - (0.42\ HR\ bpm)$ Women: $\dot{V}O_2max = 65.81 - (0.1847\ HR\ bpm)$	McArdle et al. 1972

[a] All equations estimate $\dot{V}O_2max$ in $ml \cdot kg^{-1} \cdot min^{-1}$, unless otherwise specified.
[b] For gender, substitute 1 for male and 0 for female.
[c] BMI = body mass index or BW (in kg)/HT² (in meters).

Stairclimbing Submaximal Test Protocols

In light of the recent resurgence in bench stepping exercise and growing interest in step aerobic training, you may choose to use a simulated stairclimbing machine to estimate the aerobic capacity of some clients. The Stairmaster 4000 PT and 6000 PT are two step ergometers commonly used in health and fitness settings. The Stairmaster 4000 PT has step pedals which go up and down, whereas the 6000 PT model has a revolving staircase. Howley, Colacino, and Swensen (1992) reported that the HR response to increasing submaximal work loads (4.7 and 10 METs) was linear on the Stairmaster 4000 PT step ergometer. Also, compared to treadmill exercise, the HRs measured during stepping were systematically higher (7 to 11 bpm) at each submaximal intensity. However, the MET values read from the step ergometer were about 20% higher than the measured MET values. To obtain more accurate MET values for each submaximal intensity, use the following equation:

Actual METs = 0.556 + 0.745 (Stairmaster 4000 PT MET value)

To estimate $\dot{V}O_2max$, measure the steady-state HR and calculate the corrected MET value for each of two submaximal exercise intensities (e.g., 4 and 7 METs). Each stage of the test should last 3 to 6 minutes in order to achieve steady state. Then use either the multistage model formulas (see page 66) or the graphing method (see figure 4.9) to predict $\dot{V}O_2max$.

During the test, clients may hold the handrail lightly for balance, but should not support their body weight. If they support their body weight, $\dot{V}O_2max$ will be overestimated (Howley et al. 1992). Also, compared to treadmill testing, your clients' estimated $\dot{V}O_2max$ may be lower because stairclimbing produces systematically higher HRs at any given submaximal exercise intensity.

Rowing Ergometer Submaximal Test Protocols

Submaximal exercise protocols have been developed for the Concept II rowing ergometer and can be used to estimate your client's $\dot{V}O_2max$. The Hagerman (1993) protocol is designed for noncompetitive or unskilled rowers. Before beginning the test, set the fan blades in the fully closed position

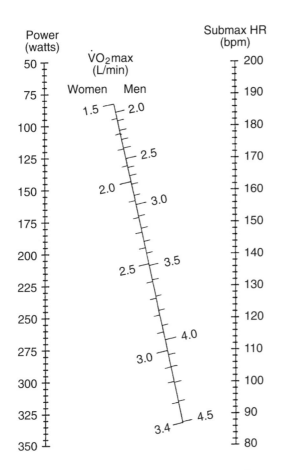

Figure 4.11 Concept II nomogram for estimating $\dot{V}O_2$max in noncompetitive and unskilled male and female rowers.
From "Concept II Rowing Ergometer Nomogram for prediction of Maximal Oxygen Consumption" by Dr. Fritz Hagerman, Ohio University, Athens, OH. The nomogram is not appropriate for use with non-Concept II ergometers and is designed to be used by noncompetitive or unskilled rowers participating in aerobic conditioning programs. Adapted by permission of CONCEPT II, INC, RR 1, BOX 1100, Morrisville, VT, (800) 245-5676.

exercise bout, rowing at an intensity of 80 to 90% HR max while maintaining constant 500 meter split times throughout the exercise bout. Measure your client's HR every 30 seconds, and average the 5-, 5 1/2-, and 6-minute HRs. Also, record the distance covered at the end of minutes 4 and 6.

Use the Lakomy nomogram (see figure 4.12) to estimate your client's $\dot{V}O_2$max from the distance covered during the last 2 minutes (subtract the 4-minute distance from the 6-minute distance) and the average exercise heart rate $[(HR_5 + HR_{5\,1/2} + HR_6)/3]$. This nomogram is based on an HR max of 191 bpm. Therefore, you need to apply correction factors for clients whose HR max is greater or less than 191 bpm. Also, to estimate your client's HR max for use with this nomogram, Lakomy and Lakomy (1993) recommend using the formula, HR max = 211 – age, instead of the standard formula, HR max = 220 – age. This adjustment accounts for the fact that the HR max for rowing exercise is 8 to 10 bpm lower than the standard, age-predicted HR max.

Maximal Heart Rate Correction Factors

HR max	Factor
205	1.11
200	1.07
195	1.03
190	0.99
185	0.95
180	0.92
175	0.88
170	0.85

FIELD TESTS

The maximal and submaximal exercise tests using the treadmill or bicycle ergometer are not well suited for measuring the cardiorespiratory fitness of large groups in a field situation. Thus, a number of performance tests, such as distance runs, have been devised to predict $\dot{V}O_2$max (see table 4.7). These tests are practical, inexpensive, less time-consuming, easy to administer to large groups, and can be used to classify the cardiorespiratory fitness level of healthy men (≤40 years) and women (≤50 years). You cannot use field tests to detect CHD because heart rate, ECG, and BP are usually not monitored during the performance. Most field tests used to assess cardiorespiratory endurance involve walking, running,

and select the small axle sprocket. For this test, select a submaximal exercise intensity (the HR should not exceed 170 bpm) that can be sustained for 5 to 10 minutes. Measure the exercise HR at the end of each minute. Continue the rowing exercise until the client achieves a steady-state HR. Use the Hagerman nomogram (see figure 4.11) to estimate $\dot{V}O_2$max from the submaximal power output (watts) and the steady-state HR during the last minute of exercise.

The Lakomy (1993) protocol is designed for both noncompetitive and skilled male rowers using the Concept II rowing ergometer. Prior to testing, set the fan blades in the fully closed position and select the large axle sprocket. This protocol begins with a 6-minute warm-up, rowing at an intensity of 50 to 60% HR max. The warm-up is followed by a 2-minute recovery period and a 6-minute submaximal

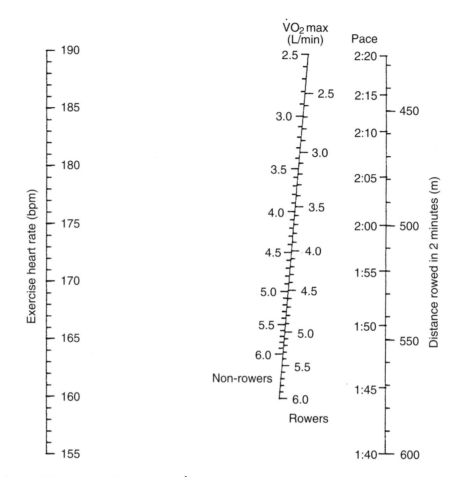

Figure 4.12 Concept II nomogram for estimating $\dot{V}O_2$max in noncompetitive and skilled male rowers.
From "Estimation of Maximum Oxygen Uptake from Submaximal Exercise on a Concept II Rowing Ergometer" by H.K.A. Lakomy and J. Lakomy, 1993, *Journal of Sports Sciences* 11, p. 230. Adapted by permission of E. & F.N. Spon (an imprint of Chapman & Hall).

swimming, cycling, or bench stepping, and require that clients be able to accurately measure their postexercise HR. Pollock, Broida, and Kendrick (1972) found that with practice, men could learn to measure their own pulse rates accurately. The correlation between manual and electronic measurements of pulse rate ranged between r = 0.91 to 0.94. Similar results (r = 0.95) were reported for college women for pulse rates measured manually and electronically (Witten 1973). Prior to administering field tests that require the measurement of heart rate, you should teach your clients how to measure their pulse rates using the palpation technique described below.

HOW TO MEASURE YOUR PULSE RATE

- Use your middle and index fingers to locate the radial pulse on the outside of your wrist just below the base of your thumb. Do not use your thumb to feel the pulse, because it has a pulse of its own and may produce an inaccurate count.

- If you cannot feel the radial pulse, try locating the carotid pulse by placing your fingers lightly on the front of your neck, just to the side of your voice box. Do not apply heavy pressure, because this will cause your heart rate to slow down.

- Use a stopwatch or the second hand of your wristwatch and count the number of pulse beats for either a 6-, 10-, or 15-second period.

- Convert the pulse count to beats per minute using the following multipliers: 6-second count times 10, 10-second count times 6, and 15-second count times 4.

- Remember this value and record it on your score card.

Distance Run Tests

The most commonly used distance runs involve distances of 1.0 or 1.5 miles (1600-2400 meters) to evaluate aerobic capacity. Distance run tests are based on the assumption that the more fit individual will be able to run a given distance in less time or run a greater distance in a given period of time. Using factor analysis, Disch, Frankiewicz, and Jackson (1975) noted that runs greater than 1.0 mile tended to load exclusively on the endurance factor rather than the speed factor.

You should be aware that the relationship between distance runs and $\dot{V}O_2$max has not been firmly established. Although performance on a distance run can be accurately measured, it may not be an accurate index of $\dot{V}O_2$max or a substitute for the direct measurement of $\dot{V}O_2$max. Endurance running performance may be influenced by other factors such as motivation, percent fat (Cureton et al. 1978; Katch et al. 1973), running efficiency (pacing ability), and lactate threshold (Costill and Fox 1969; Costill, Thomason, and Roberts 1973).

The correlations between distance run tests and $\dot{V}O_2$max tend to vary considerably (r = 0.27 to 0.90) depending on the subjects, sample size, and testing procedures (Burke 1976; Doolittle and Bigbee 1968; Falls, Ismail, and MacLeod 1966; George et al. 1993; Jackson and Coleman 1976, Metz and Alexander 1970; Ribisl and Kachadorian 1969; Rikli, Petray, and Baumgartner 1992; Vodak and Wilmore 1975; Zwiren et al. 1991). Generally, the longer the run, the higher the correlation with $\dot{V}O_2$max. Based on this observation, it is recommended that you select a test with a distance of at least 1.0 mile (1600 meters) or a duration of at least 9 minutes.

The most widely used distance run tests are the 9- or 12-minute runs and the 1.0- or 1.5-mile runs. Some physical fitness test batteries for children and adolescents recommend using either the 9-minute or 1.0-mile run tests.

Nine- or Twelve-Minute Run Tests

To administer the 9- or 12-minute run tests, use a 400-meter track or flat course with measured distances so that the number of laps completed can be easily counted and multiplied by the course distance. Place markers to divide the course into quarters or eighths of a mile, so that the exact distance covered in 9 or 12 minutes can be determined quickly. Instruct your clients to run as far as possible. Walking is allowed, but the objective of these tests is to cover as much distance as possible in either 9 or 12 minutes. At the end of the test, calculate the total distance covered in meters and use the appropri-

ate equation in table 4.7 to estimate the client's $\dot{V}O_2$max.

One and One-Half Mile Run/Walk Test

Conduct the 1.5-mile run/walk test on a 400-meter track or flat measured area. To measure the course, use an odometer or measuring wheel. For the 1.5-mile run, instruct your clients to cover the specified distance in the fastest possible time. Walking is allowed, but the objective is to cover the distance in the shortest possible time. Call out the elapsed time (in minutes and seconds) as the client crosses the finish line.

To use the $\dot{V}O_2$max prediction equation for the 1.5-mile run/walk test (see table 4.7), convert the seconds to minutes by dividing the seconds by 60. For example, if a client's time for the test is 12:30, the run time is converted to 12.5 minutes (30/60 seconds = 0.5 minute). This prediction equation estimates your client's $\dot{V}O_2$max from run time (in minutes), body weight (in kg), and gender.

One-Mile Jogging Test

One limitation of distance run tests is that individuals are encouraged to run as fast as possible and give a maximal effort, thereby increasing the risk of cardiovascular and orthopedic injuries. The potential risk is even greater for untrained individuals who do not run or jog regularly and have difficulty selecting a proper jogging pace. To address this problem, George et al. (1993) developed a submaximal, 1-mile track jogging test for 18- to 29-year old women and men that requires only moderate, steady-state exertion.

For this test, instruct your clients to select a comfortable, moderate jogging pace and to measure their postexercise heart rate immediately following the test. The elapsed time for 1 mile should be at least 8 minutes for males and 9 minutes for females, and the postexercise HR (15-second count $\times$ 4) should not exceed 180 bpm. To help establish a suitable pace, precede the timed, 1-mile test with a 2- to 3-minute warm-up jog. Use either an indoor or outdoor track for this test. Record the time in minutes required to jog 1 mile and have your clients measure their postexercise HRs using the palpation technique (radial or carotid sites). Estimate the clients' $\dot{V}O_2$max using the prediction equation for the 1.0 mile steady-state jog test (see table 4.7).

Walking Test

The Rockport Walking Institute (1986) has developed a walking test to assess cardiorespiratory fitness for men and women, ages 20 to 69 years. Because this test requires only fast walking, it is useful for testing older or sedentary individuals (Fenstermaker, Plowman, and Looney 1992). The test was developed and validated for a large, heterogeneous sample of 86 women and 83 men (Kline et al. 1987). The cross-validation analysis resulted in a high validity coefficient and small standard error of estimate (SEE), indicating that the 1.0-mile walking test yields a valid submaximal assessment of estimated $\dot{V}O_2$max. Other researchers have substantiated the predictive accuracy of this equation for women 65 years of age and older (Fenstermaker, Plowman, and Looney 1992).

To administer this test, instruct your clients to walk 1.0 mile as quickly as possible and to take their heart rate immediately at the end of the test by counting the pulse for 15 seconds. It is important that clients know how to take their pulse accurately. The walking course should be a measured mile that is flat and uninterrupted, preferably a 400-meter track. Clients should stretch 5 to 10 minutes before the test and wear good walking shoes and loose fitting clothes.

To estimate your client's $\dot{V}O_2$max, use the generalized equation for the 1.0-mile walking test (see table 4.7). Alternatively, you can use the Rockport relative fitness charts (appendix B.2) to classify your client's cardiorespiratory fitness level. Locate the walking time and corresponding postexercise heart rate (bpm) on the appropriate chart for the individual's age and gender. These charts are based on body weights of 125 pounds (56.8 kg) for women and 170 pounds (77.3 kg) for men. If the client weighs substantially more than this, the cardiorespiratory fitness level will be overestimated.

Step Tests

The major advantage of using step tests to assess cardiorespiratory fitness is that they can be administered to large groups in a field situation without expensive equipment or highly trained personnel. Most of the step tests use postexercise and recovery heart rates to evaluate aerobic fitness, but they do provide an estimate of the individual's $\dot{V}O_2$max. Step test protocols and scoring procedures are described in appendix B.3.

The validity of step tests is highly dependent on the accurate measurement of pulse rate. Step tests that use recovery heart rate tend to possess lower validity than those using the time required for the heart rate to reach a specified level while performing a standardized work load (Baumgartner and

Jackson 1975). The correlation coefficients between step test performance and $\dot{V}O_2$max range between r = 0.32 to 0.77 (Cureton and Sterling 1964; deVries and Klafs 1965; Gallagher and Brouha 1943; McArdle et al. 1972).

Additional Field Tests

In addition to running, walking, and step tests, cycling and swimming tests have been devised for use in field situations (Cooper 1977). The 12-minute cycling test, using a bike with no more than three speeds, is conducted on a hard, flat surface when the wind velocity is less than 10 mph (268 m · min^{-1}). These conditions limit the effect of outside influences on the rider's performance. Five- and ten-speed bikes are not used unless use of the lower gears can be restricted. Use an odometer to measure the distance traveled in 12 minutes. In the 12-minute swimming test, the client may use any stroke and rest as needed. Norms for the 12-minute cycling test and 12-minute swimming test are available (Cooper 1977).

Of these two tests, the swimming test is least preferred because the outcome is highly dependent on skill. For example, a skilled swimmer with an average cardiorespiratory fitness level will probably be able to swim farther in 12 minutes than a poorly skilled swimmer with above average fitness. In fact, Conley and colleagues reported that the 12-minute swim has low validity (r = 0.34 to 0.42) as a cardiorespiratory field test for male and female recreational swimmers (Conley et al. 1991; Conley et al. 1992). Whenever possible, select an alternative field test and avoid using the 12-minute swim test.

EXERCISE TESTING OF CHILDREN AND OLDER ADULTS

You may need to modify the generic guidelines for exercise testing (see page 49) of apparently healthy adults when you are assessing cardiorespiratory fitness of children and older adults (ACSM 1995). You must take into account growth, maturation, and aging when selecting exercise testing modes and protocols for these groups.

Assessing Cardiorespiratory Fitness of Children

In the laboratory setting, you can assess the cardiorespiratory fitness of children using either the treadmill or bicycle ergometer. Treadmill testing is usually preferable, especially for younger children, because their shortened attention span may not allow them to maintain a constant pedaling rate during a cycle ergometer test. Also, children younger than eight years may not be tall enough to use a standard bicycle ergometer.

For treadmill testing, you should use the modified Balke protocol (see table 4.8) because the speed is constant and intensity is increased by changing the grade. For cycle ergometer testing, the ACSM (1995) recommends the McMaster protocol (see table 4.8). For this protocol the pedaling frequency is 50 rpm, and increments in work rate are based on the child's height.

Cardiorespiratory field tests, such as the 0.5- and 1.0-mile (800- and 1600-meter) run/walk, are widely used to assess the cardiorespiratory fitness of children from 5 to 17 years of age. These tests are part of the Physical Best Program (AAPHERD 1988) and Fitnessgram (Institute for Aerobics Research 1987), as well as national physical fitness surveys of children and youth (Ross and Pate 1987). To estimate $\dot{V}O_2$ peak of 8- to 17-year olds for the 1.0 mile run/walk test, you can use a generalized prediction equation (see table 4.7) (Cureton et al. 1995). For younger children (5 to 7 years of age), the 0.5-mile

run/walk test is recommended (Rikli, Petray, and Baumgartner 1992). Norms for the 0.5- and 1.0-mile tests are available elsewhere (AAHPERD 1988; Institute for Aerobics Research 1987).

Assessing Cardiorespiratory Fitness of Older Adults

To assess the cardiorespiratory fitness of elderly clients, you can use modified treadmill and bicycle ergometer protocols. The following modifications for standard GXT protocols are recommended:

- Extend the warm-up to more than 3 minutes.
- Set an initial exercise intensity of 2 to 3 METs.
- Extend the duration of each work stage (at least 3 minutes), allowing enough time for the client to attain steady state.
- Select a protocol likely to produce a total test time of 8 to 12 minutes.

Select treadmill protocols that increase grade, instead of speed, especially for older clients with poor ambulation (ACSM 1995). You can modify the standard Balke protocol (see figure 4.2) by having the

Table 4.8   GXT Protocols for Children

Modified Balke treadmill protocol

Activity classification	Speed (mph)	Initial grade (%)	Increment (%)	Duration (min)
Poorly fit	3.0	6	2	2
Sedentary	3.25	6	2	2
Active	5.0	0	2.5	2
Athletes	5.25	0	2.5	2

McMaster bicycle ergometer protocol

Height (cm)	Initial work rate kgm · min^{-1} (watts)	Increments kgm · min^{-1} (watts)	Duration (min)
<120	75 (12.5)	75 (12.5)	2
120-139.9	75 (12.5)	150 (25)	2
140-159.9	150 (25)	150 (25)	2
≥160	150 (25)	300 (50) for boys 150 (25) for girls	2

Reprinted, by permission, from American College of Sports Medicine, 1995, *ACSM's Guidelines for Exercise Testing and Prescription* (Baltimore: Williams & Wilkins), 223.

client walk at 0% grade and 3.0 mph initially and increasing the duration of each stage to at least 3 minutes. If elderly clients are more comfortable holding on to the handrails during a treadmill test, you can use the standard Bruce protocol and the McConnell and Clark (1987) prediction equation to estimate their $\dot{V}O_2max$. Alternatively, you could use bicycle ergometer GXTs for older individuals with poor balance.

Key Points

- The preferred way to assess aerobic capacity (cardiorespiratory fitness) is through a graded exercise test in which the functional $\dot{V}O_2max$ is measured.

- Unless you observe contraindications to exercise, you generally should perform a maximal exercise test for apparently healthy men (>40 yr) and women (>50 yr) before beginning a vigorous exercise program.

- Before, during, and after a maximal or submaximal exercise test, closely monitor the heart rate, BP, and RPE.

- Treadmill, bicycle ergometer, and bench stepping are the most commonly used modes for exercise testing.

- The choice of exercise mode and exercise test protocol depends on the age, gender, purpose of the test, and the health and fitness status of the individual.

- Submaximal exercise tests are used to estimate the functional aerobic capacity by predicting the $\dot{V}O_2max$ of the individual. Failure to meet the assumptions underlying submaximal exercise tests produces a ± 10% to 20% error in the prediction of $\dot{V}O_2max$ from submaximal heart rate data.

- Field tests are the least desirable way to assess aerobic capacity and should not be used for diagnostic purposes. However, field tests are useful for assessing the cardiorespiratory fitness of large groups.

- Commonly used field tests include distance runs, walking tests, and step tests.

- Distance runs should last at least 9 minutes to assess aerobic function. Distance runs usually range from 1 to 3 miles (1600-4800 meters) , or 9 to 12 minutes.

- The validity of step tests for assessing cardiorespiratory fitness is highly dependent on the accurate measurement of heart rate and is usually somewhat lower than the validity of distance run tests.

SOURCES FOR EQUIPMENT

Products	Manufacturer's Address
Bicycle ergometer (electrically braked)	Warren E. Collins, Inc. 220 Wood Rd. Braintree, MA 02184 (800) 225-5157
Bicycle ergometer (Monark)	Monark 948 Greenbay Rd. Winetka, IL 60097 (800) 359-4610
Bicycle ergometer (Bodyguard)	Thera-tronics 623 Mamaroneck New York, NY 10543 (914) 698-9802
Nordic ski machine	Nordic Track 11 Peavey Rd. Chaska, MN 55138 (800) 468-4429
Rowing ergometer	Concept II, Inc. R.R. 1, Box 1100 Morrisville, VT 05661 (800) 245-5676
Stairclimbing machines	StairMaster Sports/ Medical Products, Inc. 12421 Willows Rd. N.E., Ste. 100 Kirkland, WA 98034 (800) 635-2936
Treadmill (Quinton)	Quinton Instrument Co. 3303 Monte Villa Pkwy. Bothell, WA 98021 (800) 426-0337

REFERENCES

AAHPERD 1988. *The AAHPERD physical best program.* Reston, VA: American Alliance for Health, Physical Education, Recreation and Dance.

American College of Sports Medicine. 1991. *Guidelines for exercise testing and prescription,* 4th ed. Philadelphia: Lea & Febiger.

American College of Sports Medicine. 1995. *ACSM's guidelines for exercise testing and prescription,* 5th ed.. Baltimore: Williams & Wilkins.

American College of Sports Medicine. 1996. *ACSM health/fitness instructor certification study packet.* Baltimore: Williams & Wilkins.

Andersen, R., and Wadden, T. 1995. Validation of a cycle ergometry equation for predicting steady-rate $\dot{V}O_2$ in obese women. *Medicine and Science in Sports and Exercise* 27: 1457-1460.

Åstrand, I. 1960. Aerobic capacity in men and women with special reference to age. *Acta Physiologica Scandinavica* 49 (Suppl. 169): 1-92.

Åstrand, P.O. 1956. Human physical fitness with special reference to age and sex. *Physiological Reviews* 36: 307-335.

Åstrand, P.O. 1965. *Work tests with the bicycle ergometer.* Varberg, Sweden: AB Cykelfabriken Monark.

Åstrand, P.O., and Rodahl, K. 1977. *Textbook of work physiology.* New York: McGraw-Hill.

Åstrand, P.O., and Ryhming, I. 1954. A nomogram for calculation of aerobic capacity (physical fitness) from pulse rate during submaximal work. *Journal of Applied Physiology* 7: 218-221.

Balke, B. 1963. A simple field test for the assessment of physical fitness. *Civil Aeromedical Research Institute Report, 63-18.* Oklahoma City, OK: Federal Aviation Agency.

Balke, B. and Ware, R. 1959. An experimental study of physical fitness of Air Force personnel. *US Armed Forces Medical Journal* 10: 675-688.

Baumgartner, T.A., and Jackson, A.S. 1975. *Measurement for evaluation in physical education.* Boston: Houghton Mifflin.

Borg, G. 1982. Psychophysical bases of perceived exertion. *Medicine and Science in Sports and Exercise* 14: 377-381.

Bruce, R.A., Kusumi, F., and Hosmer, D. 1973. Maximal oxygen intake and nomographic assessment of functional aerobic impairment in cardiovascular disease. *American Heart Journal* 85: 546-562.

Burke, E.J. 1976. Validity of selected laboratory and field tests of physical working capacity. *Research Quarterly,* 47: 95-104.

Conley, D., Cureton, K., Dengel, D., and Weyand, P. 1991. Validation of the 12-min swim as a field test of peak aerobic power in young men. *Medicine and Science in Sports and Exercise* 23: 766-773.

Conley, D., Cureton, K., Hinson, B., Higbie, E., and Weyand, P. 1992. Validation of the 12-minute swim as a field test of peak aerobic power in young women. *Research Quarterly for Exercise and Sport* 63: 153-161.

Cooper, K.H. 1968. A means of assessing maximal oxygen intake. *Journal of the American Medical Association* 203: 201-204.

Cooper, K.H. 1977. *The aerobics way.* New York: Evans.

Costill, D.L., and Fox, E.L. 1969. Energetics of marathon running. *Medicine and Science in Sports* 1: 81-86.

Costill, D.L., Thomason, H., and Roberts, E. 1973. Fractional utilization of the aerobic capacity during distance running. *Medicine and Science in Sports* 5: 248-252.

Cureton, K., Sloniger, M., O'Bannon, J., Black, D., and McCormack, W. 1995. A generalized equation for prediction of $\dot{V}O_{2peak}$ from 1-mile run/walk performance. *Medicine and Science in Sports and Exercise* 27: 445-451.

Cureton, K.J., Sparling, P.B., Evans, B.W., Johnson, S.M., Kong, U.D., and Purvis, J.W. 1978. Effect of experimental alterations in excess weight on aerobic capacity and distance running performance. *Medicine and Science in Sports* 10: 194-199.

Cureton, T.K. and Sterling, L.F. 1964. Interpretation of the cardiovascular component resulting from the factor analysis of 104 test variables measured in 100 normal young men. *Journal of Sports Medicine and Physical Fitness* 4: 1-24.

deVries, H.A., and Klafs, C.E. 1965. Prediction of maximal oxygen intake from submaximal tests. *Journal of Sports Medicine and Physical Fitness* 5: 207-214.

Disch, J., Frankiewicz, R., and Jackson, A. 1975. Construct validation of distance run tests. *Research Quarterly,* 46: 169-176.

Doolittle, T.L., and Bigbee, R. 1968. The twelve minute walk-run: Test of cardiorespiratory fitness of adolescent boys. *Research Quarterly* 39: 491-495.

Ebbeling, C., Ward, A., Puleo, E., Widrick, J., and Rippe, J. 1991. Development of a single-stage submaximal treadmill walking test. *Medicine and Science in Sports and Exercise* 23: 966-973.

Falls, H.B., Ismail, A.H., and MacLeod, D.F. 1966. Estimation of maximum oxygen intake in adults from AAHPER youth fitness test items. *Research Quarterly* 37: 192-201.

Fenstermaker, K., Plowman, S., and Looney, M. 1992. Validation of the Rockport walking test in females 65 years and older. *Research Quarterly for Exercise and Sport* 63: 322-327.

Foster, C., Jackson, A.S., Pollock, M.L., Taylor, M.M., Hare, J., Sennett, S.M., Rod, J.L., Sarwar, M., and Schmidt, D.H. 1984. Generalized equations for predicting functional capacity from treadmill performance. *American Heart Journal* 107: 1229-1234.

Foster, C., Pollock, M.L., Rod, J.L., Dymond, D.S., Wible, G., and Schmidt, D.H. 1983. Evaluation of functional capacity during exercise radionuclide angiography. *Cardiology* 70: 85-93.

Fox, E.L. 1973. A simple, accurate technique for predicting maximal aerobic power. *Journal of Applied Physiology* 35: 914-916.

Gallagher, J.R., and Brouha, L. 1943. The evaluation of athletic programs by means of fitness tests. *Yale Journal of Biology and Medicine* 15: 671-677.

George, J., Vehrs, P., Allsen, P., Fellingham, G., and Fisher, G. 1993. $\dot{V}O_2$max estimation from a submaximal 1-mile track jog for fit college-age individuals. *Medicine and Science in Sports and Exercise* 25: 401-406.

Gledhill, N., and Jamnik, R. 1995. Determining power outputs for cycle ergometers with different sized flywheels. *Medicine and Science in Sports and Exercise* 27: 134-135.

Golding, L., Myers, C., and Sinning, W. (Eds.) 1989. *The Y's way to physical fitness.* Champaign, IL: Human Kinetics.

Greiwe, J., Kaminsky, L., Whaley, M., and Dwyer, G. 1995. Evaluation of the ACSM submaximal ergometer test for estimating $\dot{V}O_2$max. *Medicine and Science in Sports and Exercise* 27: 1315-1320.

Hagerman, F. 1993. *Concept II rowing ergometer nomogram for prediction of maximal oxygen consumption* [abstract]. Morrisville, VT: Concept II, Inc.

Hanson, P. 1988. Clinical exercise testing. In S. Blair, P. Painter, R. Pate, L. Smith, and C. Taylor, eds., *Resource manual for guidelines for exercise testing and prescription,* 248-255. Philadelphia: Lea & Febiger.

Hermansen, L., and Saltin, B. 1969. Oxygen uptake during maximal treadmill and bicycle exercise. *Journal of Applied Physiology* 26: 31-37.

Howley, E., Colacino, D., and Swensen, T. 1992. Factors affecting the oxygen cost of stepping on an electronic stepping ergometer. *Medicine and Science in Sports and Exercise* 24: 1055-1058.

Institute of Aerobics Research. 1987. *Fitnessgram User's Manual.* Dallas, TX: author.

Jackson, A.S., and Coleman, A.E. 1976. Validation of distance run tests for elementary school children. *Research Quarterly* 47: 86-94.

Katch, F.I., McArdle, W.D., Czula, R., and Pechar, G.S. 1973. Maximal oxygen intake, endurance running performance, and body composition in college women. *Research Quarterly* 44: 301-312.

Kattus, A.A., Hanafee, W.N., Longmire, W.P., MacAlpin, R.N. and Rivin, A.U. 1968. Diagnosis, medical and surgical management of coronary insufficiency. *Annals of Internal Medicine* 69: 115-136.

Kline, G.M., Porcari, J.P., Hintermeister, R., Freedson, P.S., Ward, A., McCarron, R.F., Ross, J. and Rippe, J.M. 1987. Estimation of $\dot{V}O_2$max from a one-mile track walk, gender, age, and body weight. *Medicine and Science in Sports and Exercise* 19: 253-259.

Lakomy, H., and Lakomy, J. 1993. Estimation of maximum oxygen uptake from submaximal exercise on a Concept II rowing ergometer. *Journal of Sports Sciences* 11: 227-232.

Lang, P., Latin, R., Berg, K., and Mellion, M. 1992. The accuracy of the ACSM cycle ergometry equation. *Medicine and Science in Sports and Exercise* 24: 272-276.

Latin, R., and Berg, K. 1994. The accuracy of the ACSM and a new cycle ergometry equation for young women. *Medicine and Science in Sports and Exercise* 26: 642-646.

Latin, R., Berg, K., Smith, P., Tolle, R., and Woodby-Brown, S. 1993. Validation of a cycle ergometry equation for predicting steady-rate $\dot{V}O_2$. *Medicine and Science in Sports and Exercise* 25: 970-974.

Latin, R., and Elias, B. 1993. Predictions of maximum oxygen uptake from treadmill walking and running. *Journal of Sports Medicine and Physical Fitness* 33: 34-39.

Lermen, J., Bruce, R.A., Sivarajan, E., Pettet, G., and Trimble, S. (1976). Low-level dynamic exercises for earlier cardiac rehabilitation: Aerobic and hemodynamic responses. *Archives of Physical Medicine and Rehabilitation* 57: 355-360.

Londeree, B., and Moeschberger, M. 1984. Influence of age and other factors on maximal heart rate. *Journal of Cardiac Rehabilitation* 4: 44-49.

Mahar, M.T., Jackson, A.S., Ross, R.M., Pivarnik, J.M., and Pollock, M.L. 1985. Predictive accuracy of single and double stage submax treadmill work for estimating aerobic capacity. *Medicine and Science in Sports and Exercise* 17: 206-207.

Maksud, M.G., and Coutts, K.D. 1971. Comparison of a continuous and discontinuous graded treadmill test for maximal oxygen uptake. *Medicine and Science in Sports* 3: 63-65.

Marley, W., and Linnerud, A. 1976. A three-year study of the Åstrand-Ryhming step test. *Research Quarterly* 47: 211-217.

McArdle, W.D., Katch, F.I., and Katch, V.L. 1996. *Exercise physiology: Energy, nutrition and human performance,* 4th ed. Baltimore: Williams & Wilkins.

McArdle, W.D., Katch, F.I., and Pechar, G.S. 1973. Comparison of continuous and discontinuous treadmill and bicycle tests for $\dot{V}O_2$max. *Medicine and Science in Sports* 5: 156-160.

McArdle, W.D., Katch, F.I., Pechar, G.S., Jacobson, L., and Ruck, S. 1972. Reliability and interrelationships between maximal oxygen intake, physical working capacity and step-test scores in college women. *Medicine and Science in Sports* 4: 182-186.

McConnell, T., and Clark, B. 1987. Prediction of maximal oxygen consumption during handrail-supported treadmill exercise. *Journal of Cardiopulmonary Rehabilitation* 7: 324-331.

McInnis, K., and Balady, G. 1994. Comparison of submaximal exercise responses using the Bruce vs modified Bruce protocols. *Medicine and Science in Sports and Exercise* 26: 103-107.

Metz, K.F., and Alexander, J.F. 1970. An investigation of the relationship between maximum aerobic capacity and physical fitness in twelve to fifteen year old boys. *Research Quarterly* 41: 75-82.

Morehouse, L.E. 1972. *Laboratory manual for physiology of exercise*. St. Louis: Mosby.

Nagle, F.S., Balke, B., and Naughton, J.P. 1965. Gradational step tests for assessing work capacity. *Journal of Applied Physiology* 20: 745-748.

Naughton, J., Balke, B., and Nagle, F. 1964. Refinement in methods of evaluation and physical conditioning before and after myocardial infarction. *American Journal of Cardiology* 14: 837.

Ng, N. 1995. *Metcalc*. Champaign, IL: Human Kinetics.

Pollock, M.L., Bohannon, R.L., Cooper, K.H., Ayres, J.J., Ward, A., White, S.R., and Linnerud, A.C. 1976. A comparative analysis of four protocols for maximal treadmill stress testing. *American Heart Journal* 92: 39-46.

Pollock, M.L., Broida, J., and Kendrick, Z. 1972. Validity of the palpation technique of heart rate determination and its estimation of training heart rate. *Research Quarterly* 43: 77-81.

Pollock, M.L., Foster, C., Schmidt, D., Hellman, C., Linnerud, A.C., and Ward, A. 1982. Comparative analysis of physiologic responses to three different maximal graded exercise test protocols in healthy women. *American Heart Journal* 103: 363-373.

Pollock, M.L., Wilmore, J.H., and Fox, S.M. III. 1978. *Health and fitness through physical activity*. New York: Wiley.

Ribisl, P.M., and Kachadorian, W.A. 1969. Maximal oxygen intake prediction in young and middle aged males. *Journal of Sports Medicine and Physical Fitness* 9: 17-22.

Rikli, R., Petray, C., and Baumgartner, T. 1992. The reliability of distance run tests for children in grades K-4. *Research Quarterly for Exercise and Sport* 63: 270-276.

Rochmis, P., and Blackburn, H. 1971. Exercise tests. A survey of procedures, safety and litigation experience in approximately 170,000 tests. *Journal of the American Medical Association* 217: 1061-1066.

Rockport Walking Institute. 1986. *Rockport fitness walking test*. Marlboro, MA: Rockport Walking Institute.

Ross, J., and Pate, R. 1987. The national children and youth fitness study II: A summary of findings. *Journal of Physical Education, Recreation, and Dance* 58: 51-56.

Shephard, R.J. 1972. *Alive man: The physiology of physical activity*. Springfield, IL: Charles C. Thomas.

Shephard, R.J. 1977. Do risks of exercise justify costly caution? *The Physician and Sportsmedicine* 5: 58-65.

Sinning, W. 1975. *Experiments and demonstrations in exercise physiology*. Philadelphia: Saunders.

Terry, J.W., Tolson, H., Johnson, D.J., and Jessup, G.T. 1977. A work load selection procedure for the Åstrand-Ryhming test. *Journal of Sports Medicine and Physical Fitness* 17: 361-366.

Vodak, P.A., and Wilmore, J.H. 1975. Validity of the 6 minute jog-walk and the 600 yard run-walk in estimating endurance capacity in boys 9-12 years of age. *Research Quarterly* 46: 230-234.

Whaley, M., Kaminsky, L., Dwyer, G., Getchell, L., and Norton, J. 1992. Predictors of over- and underachievement of age-predicted maximal heart rate. *Medicine and Science in Sports and Exercise* 24: 1173-1179.

Wilson, P.K., Winga, E.R., Edgett, J.W., and Gushiken, T.J. 1978. *Policies and procedures of a cardiac rehabilitation program—Immediate to long term care*. Philadelphia: Lea & Febiger.

Witten, C. 1973. Construction of a submaximal cardiovascular step test for college females. *Research Quarterly* 44: 46-50.

Zwiren, L., Freedson, P., Ward, A., Wilke, S., and Rippe, J. 1991. Estimation of VO$_2$ max: A comparative analysis of five exercise tests. *Research Quarterly for Exercise and Sport* 62: 73-78.

CHAPTER 5

Designing Cardiorespiratory Exercise Programs

Key Questions

- What are the basic components of an aerobic exercise prescription?
- How is the aerobic exercise prescription individualized to meet each client's goals and interests?
- What methods are used to prescribe and monitor exercise intensity?
- Which exercise modes are best suited for an aerobic exercise prescription?
- How often does a client need to exercise to improve and maintain aerobic fitness?
- How long does a client need to exercise to improve aerobic fitness?
- Is discontinuous aerobic training as effective as continuous training?
- How effective are multimodal cross-training programs?
- What are the physiological benefits of aerobic exercise training?

Once you have assessed an individual's cardiorespiratory, you are responsible for planning an aerobic exercise program to develop and maintain the cardiorespiratory endurance of that program participant—a program designed to meet the individual's needs and interests, taking into account age, gender, physical fitness level, and exercise habits. Appendix A.7 provides a lifestyle evaluation to help you determine exercise patterns and preferences.

In designing the exercise prescription, keep in mind that some people engage in aerobic exercise to improve their health status or reduce their disease risk, while others are primarily interested in enhancing their physical fitness ($\dot{V}O_2$max) levels. Given that the quantity of exercise needed to promote health is less than that needed to develop and maintain higher levels of physical fitness, you must adjust your exercise prescription according to your client's primary goal.

This chapter provides guidelines for writing individualized exercise prescriptions that promote health status as well as develop and maintain cardiorespiratory fitness. The chapter compares training methods and aerobic exercise modes, and presents examples of individualized exercise prescriptions.

THE EXERCISE PRESCRIPTION

It is important to consider your client's goals and purposes for engaging in an exercise program. The primary goal for exercising may affect the mode, intensity, frequency, duration, and progression of the exercise prescription. For example, the quantity of physical activity needed to achieve health benefits or to reduce one's risk of illness and death is less than the amount of activity typically prescribed when the client's goal is to make substantial improvements in cardiorespiratory fitness. When the primary goal for the exercise prescription is improved *health*, the following guidelines are recommended (U.S. Dept. of Health and Human Services 1996):

GUIDELINES FOR EXERCISE PRESCRIPTION FOR IMPROVED HEALTH

1. Mode: Select endurance-type physical activities, including formal aerobic exercise training, house and yard work, and physically active, recreational pursuits.

2. Intensity: Prescribe at least moderate intensity physical activities ($\geq$45% $\dot{V}O_2$max).

3. Frequency: Schedule physical activity for most, preferably all, days of the week.

4. Duration: Accumulate at least 30 minutes of activity each day. Duration varies depending on type of activity (see "Examples of Moderate Amounts of Physical Activity," chapter 1, page 3).

On the other hand, when the primary goal for the exercise prescription is to improve *cardiorespiratory fitness*, the American College of Sports Medicine (1995) suggests the following guidelines for cardiorespiratory exercise programs for healthy adults:

ACSM GUIDELINES FOR EXERCISE PRESCRIPTION FOR CARDIORESPIRATORY FITNESS

1. Mode: Select rhythmical aerobic activities that can be maintained continuously and involve large muscle groups (see "Classification of Aerobic Exercise Modalities," on the next page).

2. Intensity: Prescribe intensities between 60 to 90% of maximum heart rate or 50 to 85% of $\dot{V}O_2$max. For individuals with very low initial cardiorespiratory fitness, use intensities of 40 to 50% $\dot{V}O_2$max.

3. Frequency: Schedule exercise three to five days a week.

4. Duration: Schedule 20 to 60 minutes of continuous aerobic activity, depending on the exercise intensity.

---

5. Rate of progression: Adjust the exercise prescription for each client in accordance with the conditioning effect, participant characteristics, new exercise test results, or performance during the exercise sessions. The rate of progression depends on the individual's age, functional capacity, health status, and goals. For apparently healthy adults, the aerobic exercise prescription consists of three stages: initial, improvement, and maintenance.

Modes of Exercise

If the primary goal of the exercise program is to develop and maintain cardiorespiratory fitness, prescribe aerobic activities using large muscle groups in a continuous, rhythmical fashion. In the initial and improvement stages of the exercise program, it is important to closely monitor the exercise intensity. Therefore, you should select modes of exercise that allow the individual to maintain a constant exercise intensity and are not highly dependent on the participant's skill. Group I activities, such as walking, cycling, and simulated stairclimbing, are best suited for this purpose.

For group II activities such as aerobic dance, step aerobics, and swimming, the rate of energy expenditure is highly related to the participant's skill level. You should prescribe Group II exercise modes only in the initial and improvement stages for skilled individuals who are able to maintain constant exercise intensity while performing the activity. However, you should consider using Group II activities to add variety in the later stages (maintenance stage) of your client's exercise program.

Group III activities such as racquetball, basketball, and volleyball are highly variable in terms of exercise intensity and skill. Incorporate these activities only on a limited basis in the maintenance stage to add variety and fun to the exercise program. It is best that you not emphasize the competitive aspects of these activities, especially for high-risk and symptomatic participants.

In addition to walking, jogging, and cycling, there are other exercise modalities that provide sufficient cardiorespiratory demand for improving aerobic fitness. In recent years the emergence of new aerobic exercise modalities such as bench step aerobics, machine-based stairclimbing, rowing, and aerobic riding offer your exercise program participants a variety of options for their exercise prescription. Many individuals prefer to cross-train to add variety

Classification of Aerobic Exercise Modalities[a]

Group I activities	Group II activities	Group III activities
Cycling (indoors)	Aerobic dancing	Basketball
Jogging	Bench step aerobics	Country and western dancing
Running	Nordic skiing (outdoors)	Handball
Walking	Hiking	Racquet sports
Rowing[b]	In-line skating	Volleyball
Stairclimbing[b]	Rope skipping	Super circuit resistance training
Simulated climbing[b]	Swimming	
Nordic skiing[b]	Water aerobics	
Aerobic riding[bc]		

[a]Group I activities provide constant intensity and are not dependent on skill; Group II activities may provide constant or variable intensity, depending on skill; Group III activities provide variable intensity and are highly dependent on skill.

[b]Machine-based activities

[c]May not provide adequate training intensity for above-average fitness levels

and enjoyment to their aerobic workouts. But are these exercise modes as equally effective as traditional Group I activities (walking, jogging, and cycling)? The answer to this question is not simple and depends on the method (% $\dot{V}O_2$max or perceived exertion) used to equate different exercise modalities.

When exercising at a prescribed percentage of $\dot{V}O_2$max, Thomas et al. (1995) noted that six different aerobic exercise modes (treadmill jogging, Nordic skiing, shuffle skiing, stepping, cycling, and rowing) produced relatively similar cardiovascular responses, but cycling resulted in a significantly higher perceived exertion (RPE) compared to the other modes (see figure 5.1). Other researchers have reported that, compared to treadmill jogging, the relationship between heart rate and $\dot{V}O_2$ at constant, submaximal intensities was similar for in-line skating (Wallick et al. 1995) and aerobic dancing with arms used extensively above the head or kept below the shoulders (Berry et al. 1992). In contrast, Parker et al. (1989) reported that the average steady-state HR during 20 minutes of aerobic dancing was significantly higher than treadmill jogging when the subjects exercised at the same relative intensity (60% $\dot{V}O_2$max). Howley, Colacino, and Swensen (1992) noted that HR response during electronic stepping ergometer exercise was systematically higher than treadmill exercise at the same submaximal $\dot{V}O_2$. Also, supporting the body weight during step ergometer exercise significantly reduced the HR and oxygen consumption compared to lightly holding the handrails for balance.

When exercise modes are equated using subjective ratings of perceived exertion (RPE), research suggests that treadmill jogging may be superior to other aerobic exercise modes in terms of total oxygen consumption and rate of energy expenditure (Kravitz, Robergs, and Heyward 1996; Zeni, Hoffman, and Clifford 1996)). Subjects exercising on seven different modalities at a somewhat hard intensity (RPE = 13 to 14) for 15 to 20 minutes experienced a greater total oxygen consumption for treadmill jogging compared to stepping, rowing, Nordic skiing, cycling, shuffle skiing, and aerobic riding (Kravitz et al. 1996; Thomas et al. 1995). Also, the rate of energy expenditure for treadmill exercise was 20 to 40% greater than for stationary cycling (Kravitz et al. 1996; Zeni et al. 1996) and 57% greater than for aerobic riding (Kravitz et al. 1996). In addition, steady-state exercise HRs were higher (see figure 5.2) for treadmill jogging compared to cycling and aerobic riding (Kravitz et al. 1996; Zeni et al. 1996).

When selecting aerobic exercise modes for your client's exercise prescription, you should consider how easily the exercise intensity can be graded and adjusted in order to overload the cardiorespiratory system throughout the improvement stage. For aerobic dance and bench step aerobic exercise, work rates can be progressively increased using quicker cadences, different bench heights (Olson, Williford, Blessing, and Greathouse 1991), and upper-body exercise using light (1- to 4-pound or ~0.5-2 kg) handheld weights (Kravitz, Heyward, Stolarczyk, and

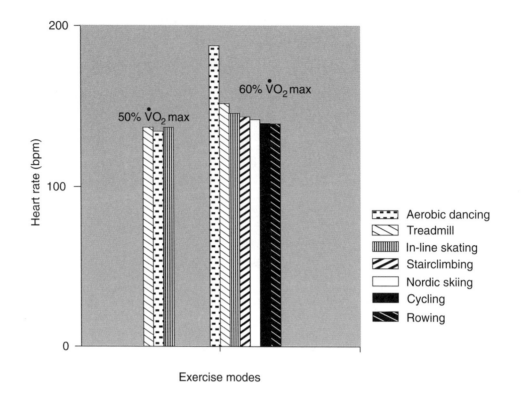

Figure 5.1   Comparison of steady-state HR response at submaximal exercise intensities for various aerobic exercise modes.

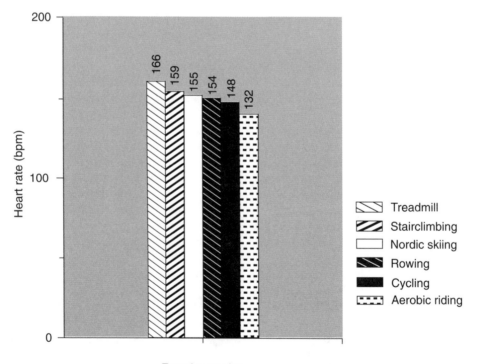

Figure 5.2   Comparison of steady-state HR response at somewhat hard intensity (RPE = 13 to 14) for various aerobic exercise modes.

Wilmerding, 1997). Intensity of in-line skating can be effectively graded by increasing the skating velocity (Wallick et al. 1995). The intensity of rowing, stairclimbing, and simulated whole-body climbing exercise can be incremented progressively using a variety of exercise machines (Brahler and Blank 1995; Howley et al. 1992).

Prescribe rope skipping activities with caution; the exercise intensity for skipping 60 to 80 skips · min^{-1} is approximately 9 METs. This value exceeds the maximum MET capacity of most sedentary individuals. Also, the exercise intensity is not easily graded because doubling the rate of skipping increases the energy requirement by only 2 to 3 METs. Town, Sol, and Sinning (1980) reported an average energy expenditure of 11.7 to 12.5 METs for skipping at rates of 125, 135, and 145 skips · min^{-1}. They concluded that rope skipping is a strenuous exercise that may not be well suited as a form of graded, aerobic exercise.

Intensity of Exercise

Exercise intensity is usually expressed as a percentage of either the individual's maximal aerobic capacity ($\dot{V}O_2max$) or functional aerobic capacity ($\dot{V}O_2peak$). Intensity and duration of exercise are inversely related. In other words, the higher the exercise intensity, the shorter the duration of exercise and vice versa.

Before prescribing the exercise intensity for aerobic exercise, carefully evaluate the individual's initial cardiorespiratory fitness classification, goals for the program, exercise preferences, and injury risks. Your client can improve cardiorespiratory fitness either with lower intensity, longer duration exercise or with higher intensity, shorter duration exercise. For most individuals, low to moderate intensities of longer duration are recommended; higher intensity exercise increases the risk of orthopedic injury and discourages continued participation in the exercise program.

Part of the art of exercise prescription is being able to select an exercise intensity that is adequate to stress the cardiovascular system without overtaxing it. According to ACSM (1995), the initial exercise intensity for apparently healthy adults is 50 to 85% $\dot{V}O_2max$. Lower intensity exercise (40 to 50% $\dot{V}O_2max$), however, may be sufficient to provide important health benefits for sedentary clients with low initial cardiorespiratory fitness levels. As a general rule, the more fit the individual, the higher the exercise intensity needs to be to produce further improvement in cardiorespiratory fitness. Exercise intensity can be prescribed using the MET, heart rate, or RPE methods.

MET Method

First, assess the client's functional aerobic capacity using a graded exercise test (see chapter 4). Use this value to determine the minimum, average, and maximum conditioning intensities. For example, if the $\dot{V}O_2max$ is 35 ml · kg^{-1} · min^{-1}, the functional capacity is 10 METs (1 MET = 3.5 ml · kg^{-1} · min^{-1}). The minimum training intensity is 50% of this value or 5 METs; the average intensity is 60 to 70% or 6 to 7 METs; the maximum exercise intensity is 85% or 8.5 METs. Thus, the exercise prescription for an apparently healthy, active individual should include activities that produce an average intensity of 6 to 7 METs.

The exercise intensities (METs) for walking, jogging, running, cycling, and bench stepping are directly related to the speed of movement, resistance, or mass lifted. Use the ACSM equations (table 4.3) to calculate the speed or work rates corresponding to a specific MET intensity. For example, to estimate how fast a woman should jog on a level course to be exercising at an intensity of 8 METs, follow these steps:

1. Convert the METs to ml · kg^{-1} · min^{-1}.

   $\dot{V}O_2$ = 8 METs × 3.5 ml · kg^{-1} · min^{-1}

   $\dot{V}O_2$ = 28 ml · kg^{-1} · min^{-1}

2. Substitute known values into the ACSM running equation and solve for speed.

   ml · kg^{-1} · min^{-1} = [speed (m · min^{-1}) × 0.2] + 3.5 ml · kg^{-1} · min^{-1}

   28.0 ml · kg^{-1} · min^{-1} − 3.5 = speed (m · min^{-1}) × 0.2

   122.5 m · min^{-1} = speed

3. Convert speed to mph.

   1 mph = 26.8 m · min^{-1}

   122.5 m · min^{-1}/26.8 m · min^{-1} = 4.57 mph

4. Convert mph to minute per mile pace.

   Pace = 60 min · hr^{-1}/mph

   = 60 min · hr^{-1}/4.57 mph

   Pace = 13.1 min · mi^{-1} (or 8.1 min · km^{-1})

When prescribing exercise intensity, be sure to consider factors such as altitude, humidity, temperature, terrain, running surface, and additional equipment. Because these factors may alter the actual exercise intensity, you may want to use the heart rate or the RPE method with the MET method to ensure that the exercise intensity does not exceed safe limits.

Heart Rate (HR) Method

There are three ways to prescribe exercise intensity for your clients using HR data. Each of these approaches is based on the assumption that HR is a linear function of exercise intensity (i.e., the higher the exercise intensity, the higher the HR).

HR vs. MET Graphing Method

When a submaximal or maximal GXT is administered, the client's steady-state HR response to each stage of the exercise test can be plotted (see figure 5.3). The HR max is the HR observed at the highest exercise intensity during a maximal GXT. For submaximal GXTs, you can estimate your client's HR max using 220 – age. From this graph, you can

obtain HRs corresponding to given percentages of the estimated functional capacity or $\dot{V}O_2$max. In our example, the functional capacity of the individual is 7.4 METs and the HR max is 195 bpm. The heart rates corresponding to exercise intensities of 4.4 and 6.3 METs (60 to 85% $\dot{V}O_2$max) are 135 and 173 bpm, respectively. During exercise workouts, the individual should measure the heart rate using heart rate monitors or palpation to verify that the appropriate exercise intensity is reached.

It is important to note that the HR response to graded exercise is somewhat dependent on the mode of exercise testing. For example, compared to treadmill testing, exercising on an electronic step ergometer elicits higher HRs, and stationary cycling typically results in somewhat lower HRs at the same relative exercise intensities. When using this method to obtain HRs for an exercise prescription, be sure to match the exercise testing and training modes by selecting a testing mode that elicits HR responses that are similar to those obtained for the training mode (see figure 5.1). For example, if your client

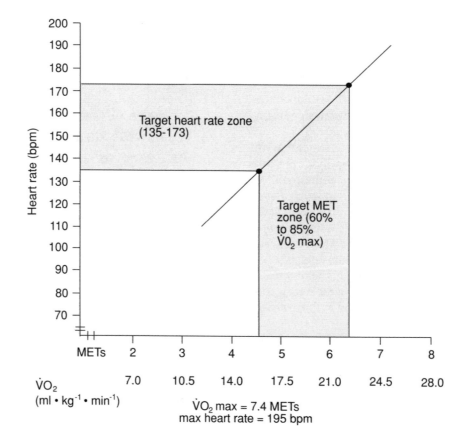

Figure 5.3   Plotting target heart rate zone using GXT data (HR vs MET).

chooses in-line skating as a training mode, you should administer a treadmill GXT given that the relationship between HR and $\dot{V}O_2$ at submaximal exercise intensities is similar for these two exercise modes (Berry et al. 1992).

Karvonen (% HRR) Method

When HR data from a GXT are not available, you can use the Karvonen, or percentage of heart rate range (% HRR), method to determine target HRs for your client's exercise prescription. This method takes into account the resting heart rate and the heart rate range (HRR), which is the difference between the maximum heart rate and resting heart rate. A percentage of HRR is added to the client's resting HR to determine the target exercise HR:

Target HR = (% HRR)(HR max – HR rest) + HR rest

The ACSM (1995) recommends using 50 to 85% HRR. For example, if

Maximum heart rate = 178 bpm

Resting heart rate = 68 bpm

Exercise intensity = 60% HRR, then

Target exercise heart rate = 0.60(178 – 68) + 68
134 bpm

Table 5.1 presents alternative guidelines for determining minimal, average, and maximal training heart rates using this method based on your client's initial fitness level (deVries 1980).

Percentage of Maximal Heart Rate (% HR max) Method

You also can use a straight percentage of maximal heart rate (% HR max) to estimate exercise intensity and determine target exercise HR. This method is based on the fact that the % HR max is related to % $\dot{V}O_2$max. In table 5.2 we can see that 69 and 89%

HR max correspond to exercise intensities of 50 and 80% $\dot{V}O_2$max. The ACSM (1995) recommends prescribing target HRs between 60 and 90% HR max depending on the fitness level of your client.

To use this technique, the actual maximal HR must be known or it must be predicted either from the HR response to submaximal work loads or from the formula, 220 – age in years. For example, if the age-predicted maximal heart rate is 180 bpm and the exercise intensity is set at 70% HR max, the target exercise heart rate is equal to 126 bpm.

% HR max × HR max = target HR

0.70 × 180 bpm = 126 bpm

Compared to the Karvonen (% HRR) method, the % HR max method tends to give a lower value when the same relative intensity is used. If in our example the client's resting HR is 80 bpm, the target HR using the Karvonen method is 150 bpm [0.70 × (180 – 80) + 80 bpm] compared to 126 bpm for the % HR max method. Therefore, the ACSM (1995) recommends correcting for this systematic underestimation by multiplying the heart rate obtained using the % HR max method by 1.15 (e.g., 126 × 1.15 = 145 bpm) to obtain a more accurate target HR.

Limitations of HR Methods

Using HR exclusively to develop intensity recommendations for your clients' exercise prescriptions may lead to large errors in estimating relative exercise intensities (% $\dot{V}O_2$max) for some individuals. This is especially true when HR max is predicted from age (220 – age) instead of being directly measured. In about 30% of the population, an age-predicted prescription of 60% HRR may be as low as 70% and as high as 80% of the actual HR max (Dishman 1994). Also, medications, emotional states, and environmental factors such as temperature, humidity, and air pollution can affect your clients' exercise training heart rates. Thus, you should

Table 5.1 Prescription of Exercise Intensity Using % HRR* Method for Various Fitness Levels			
	Low (%)	**Average (%)**	**High (%)**
Minimum HR	40	60	70
Average HR	50-60	70-75	80-85
Maximum HR	75	85	90

*Target HR = % HRR (HR$_{max}$ – HR$_{rest}$) + HR$_{rest}$

Table 5.2   Comparison of Methods for Prescribing Exercise Intensity for Healthy Adults

| Classification | Relative intensity | | | Absolute intensity | |
	% $\dot{V}O_2$max or % HRR	% HR_{max}[a]	RPE (6-20 scale)	METs[b] 20-39 yr	40-64 yr
Light	40	63	10	4.2	4.0
Moderate	50	69	11	5.5	5.0
Moderate	60	76	12	7.2	6.0
Hard	70	82	14	8.4	7.0
Hard	80	89	15	9.5	8.0
Very hard	85	92	16	10.2	8.5
Very hard	90	95	18	10.8	9.0
Maximal	100	100	20	12.0	10.0

[a]Based on data from Swain, et al. (1994)
[b]Absolute intensity (METs) values are approximate average values for men. Absolute values for women are 1-2 METs lower than those for men.

consider alternative methods for monitoring exercise intensity.

Ratings of Perceived Exertion (RPE) Method

In light of the limitations associated with using HR for setting exercise intensity, consider using a combination of HR and RPE. You can use RPEs to prescribe and monitor exercise intensity (Birk and Birk 1987). The RPE scales (see table 4.2) are valid and reliable tools for assessing the level of physical exertion during continuous, aerobic exercise (Birk and Birk 1987; Borg and Linderholm 1967; Dunbar et al. 1992).

During the graded exercise test, the client rates the intensity of each stage of the test using the RPE scale. You can use the intensities (METs) corresponding to ratings of 12 (somewhat hard) and 16 (hard) to set the minimum and maximum training intensities for the exercise prescription. Compared to the % HRR method, RPEs between 11 and 16 closely approximate 50 and 85% HRR, respectively (Dunbar et al. 1992). With practice an individual can learn to associate RPE with a specific target exercise heart rate, especially at higher exercise intensities (Smutok, Skrinar, and Pandolf 1980). Thus, the RPE can be used instead of HR, or in combination with HR, to monitor training intensity and to adjust the exercise prescription for conditioning effects.

One advantage of RPE as a method of monitoring exercise intensity is that your clients do not need to stop exercising in order to check their heart rates.

For an extensive review of research pertaining to the use of perceived exertion for prescribing exercise intensity, see Dishman (1994).

Duration of Exercise

As an exercise specialist, you must prescribe an appropriate combination of exercise intensity and duration so that the individual adequately stresses the cardiorespiratory system without overexertion. As mentioned earlier, intensity and duration of exercise are inversely related (the lower the exercise intensity, the longer the duration of the exercise). The ACSM (1995) recommends 20 to 30 minutes of continuous aerobic activity. Apparently healthy individuals usually can sustain exercise intensities of 60 to 85% $\dot{V}O_2$max for 20 to 30 minutes. During the improvement stage, duration can be increased every 2 to 3 weeks until participants can exercise continuously for 30 minutes (ACSM 1995). Poorly conditioned individuals may be able to exercise at low intensity (40% $\dot{V}O_2$max) for only 10 minutes. They may need to perform multiple sessions in a given day to accumulate 20 to 30 minutes of aerobic exercise.

An alternative way of estimating the duration of exercise is to use the caloric cost of the exercise. To achieve *health* benefits, ACSM (1995) recommends minimal caloric thresholds of 150 to 300 kilocalories (kcal) per exercise session or 800 to 900 kcal per week.

During the initial stage of the exercise program, however, weekly exercise caloric expenditure may be considerably lower (200 to 600 kcal per week). Throughout the improvement stage, the goal is to increase your client's caloric expenditure from 800 to 2000 kcal per week by gradually increasing the frequency, intensity, and duration of the exercise. For example, in order for a 60-kg (132 lb.) woman, who is exercising at an intensity of 7 METs, 5 times per week, to reach a weekly caloric threshold of 1500 kcal per week, she needs to expend 300 kcal per exercise session (1500 kcal/5 = 300 kcal). You can estimate the caloric cost of her exercise (kcal · min^{-1}) knowing her exercise intensity (7 METs) and knowing that 1 MET is equal to 1 kcal · kg^{-1}· hr^{-1}. She will expend 420 kcal · hr^{-1} (7 METs 3 60 kg of body weight) or 7 kcal · min^{-1}. Therefore, she needs to exercise approximately 43 minutes (300 kcal/7 kcal · min^{-1}), 5 times per week, in order to achieve her weekly caloric expenditure goal.

Frequency of Exercise

The frequency of the exercise sessions depends in part on the health and fitness level of the individual. Normal, sedentary individuals (functional capacity equals 5 to 8 METs) should exercise a minimum of 3 times per week to produce significant changes in cardiorespiratory endurance (ACSM 1995). As the fitness level increases, however, the frequency should be increased to 5 times per week for continued improvement (Pollock 1973). For individuals with functional capacities less than 5 METs, several daily exercise sessions are advisable. Once the desired level of cardiorespiratory fitness is reached, it may be maintained by exercising 2 to 4 days per week, providing the intensity and duration of the workouts are similar to that used to achieve the current fitness level (Brynteson and Sinning 1973; Hickson and Rosenkoetter 1981).

In terms of improving $\dot{V}O_2$max, the sequence of exercise sessions seems to be less important than the total work performed during the training. Similar improvements were noted for individuals who trained every other day (M-W-F) and 3 consecutive days (M-T-W) (Moffatt, Stamford, and Neill 1977). The ACSM (1995) recommends exercising on alternate days during the initial stages of training to lessen the chance of bone or joint injury.

Rate of Progression

Physiological changes associated with aerobic endurance training enable the individual to increase the total work performed. The greatest condition-

ing effects occur during the first 6 to 8 weeks of the exercise program. Aerobic endurance may improve as much as 3% per week during the first month, 2% per week for the second month, and 1% per week or less thereafter (Sharkey 1979). In order to make continued improvements, the cardiorespiratory system must be overloaded by adjusting the intensity and duration of the exercise to the new level of fitness. The degree of improvement is dependent on the age, health status, and initial fitness level of the participant. For the average person, aerobic training programs generally produce a 5 to 20% increase in $\dot{V}O_2$max (Pollock 1973). Sedentary, inactive persons may improve as much as 40% in aerobic fitness while elite athletes may improve only 5% because they begin at a level much closer to their genetic limits. The rate of improvement is also age-related. We do not expect older individuals entering the exercise program to improve as quickly as younger individuals even when the initial fitness levels are the same.

Physiological Changes Induced by Cardiorespiratory Endurance Training

Increases	Decreases
Cardiorespiratory System	
Heart size and volume	Resting heart rate
Blood volume and total hemoglobin	Submaximal exercise heart rate
Stroke volume—rest and exercise	Blood pressure (if high)
Cardiac Output—maximum	
$\dot{V}O_2$max	
Oxygen extraction from blood	
Lung volumes	
Musculoskeletal System	
Mitochondria—number and size	
Myoglobin stores	
Triglyceride stores	
Oxidative phosphorylation	
Other Systems	
Strength of connective tissues	Body weight (if overweight)
Heat acclimatization	Body fat
High-density lipoprotein cholesterol	Total cholesterol Low-density lipoprotein cholesterol

Stages of Progression

As discussed in chapter 3, the three stages of progression for cardiorespiratory exercise programs are the *initial conditioning, improvement, and maintenance* stages (ACSM 1995).

Initial Conditioning

The initial conditioning stage typically lasts four to six weeks and consists of stretching exercises, light calisthenics, and low-level aerobic activity. The ACSM (1995) suggests that the initial exercise intensity be set at 40 to 60% $\dot{V}O_2$max. The duration of the aerobic exercise during this stage should be at least 12 to 15 minutes, increasing to 20 minutes in 4 to 6 weeks. Active individuals with good to excellent initial cardiorespiratory fitness levels may skip the initial conditioning stage of the program.

Improvement

The improvement stage usually lasts 16 to 20 weeks. During this stage, the rate of progression is more rapid. Increase the exercise intensity gradually, and increase the duration of exercise every 2 to 3 weeks. Increase the frequency of exercise from 3 to 5 times per week. *Intensity, duration, and frequency of exercise should always be increased independently*. Rate of progression during this stage depends on a number of factors. Cardiac patients, elderly, and less fit individuals may need more time for the body to adapt to a higher conditioning intensity. In such cases, the exercise duration should be at least 20 to 30 minutes before increasing the exercise intensity (ACSM 1995).

Maintenance

After achieving the desired level of cardiorespiratory fitness, an individual enters the maintenance stage of the exercise program. This stage usually begins 6 months after the start of training and continues on a regular, long-term basis if the individual has made a lifetime commitment to exercise.

During this stage, a variety of enjoyable activities from Group II and III (see page 85) can be included in the exercise program to counteract boredom and to maintain the interest level of the participant. For example, an individual who was running 5 days per week at the end of the improvement stage may choose to run only 3 days per week and substitute in-line skating and racquetball on the other 2 days.

ESSENTIALS OF A CARDIORESPIRATORY EXERCISE WORKOUT

Each exercise session should include

- warm-up,
- aerobic conditioning, and
- cool-down phases.

The purpose of the warm-up is to increase blood flow to the working cardiac and skeletal muscles, increase body temperature, decrease the chance of muscle and joint injury, and lessen the chance of abnormal cardiac rhythms. During the warm-up, the tempo of the exercise is gradually increased to prepare the body for a higher intensity of exercise performed during the conditioning phase. The warm-up period usually lasts 5 to 10 minutes and includes stretching exercises and light calisthenics for the legs, lower back, abdomen, hips, groin, and shoulders (for specific exercises, see appendix F.1).

During the conditioning phase of the workout, the aerobic exercise is performed according to the exercise prescription. This phase usually lasts 20 to 60 minutes and is followed immediately by the cool-down phase.

During cool-down, the individual continues exercising (e.g., walking, jogging, or cycling) at a low intensity for about 5 minutes. This light activity prevents the pooling of blood in the extremities and reduces the possibility of dizziness and fainting. The continued pumping action of the muscles increases the venous return and speeds up the recovery process. Stretching exercises may be repeated during the cool-down phase to reduce the chance of muscle cramps or muscle soreness.

AEROBIC TRAINING METHODS AND MODES

Either continuous or discontinuous training methods can improve cardiorespiratory endurance. Continuous training involves one continuous, aerobic exercise bout performed at low to moderate intensities without rest intervals. Discontinuous training consists of several intermittent, low to high intensity, aerobic exercise bouts interspersed with rest periods. Research indicates that continuous training and discontinuous training are equally effective in improving cardiorespiratory fitness. However, Pollock et al. (1977) reported that the dropout rate of adults in a high-intensity interval (discontinuous) training program was twice that of those in a continuous jogging program.

Continuous Training

All of the exercise modes listed as Group I and II activities (see page 85) are suitable for continuous training. One advantage of continuous training is that a prescribed exercise intensity (e.g., 75% HR max) is maintained fairly consistently throughout the duration of the steady-paced exercise. Generally, continuous exercise at low to moderate intensities is safer, more comfortable, and better suited for individuals initiating an aerobic exercise program.

Walking, Jogging, and Cycling

The most popular modes of continuous training are walking, jogging or running, and cycling. Exercise programs using walking, jogging, and cycling provide similar cardiovascular benefits (Magel et al. 1974; Pollock, Cureton, and Greninger 1969; Pollock et al. 1971; Pollock et al. 1975; Wilmore et al 1980). Improvements in $\dot{V}O_2$max are comparable for most commonly used exercise modes. Pollock et al. (1975) compared running, walking, and cycling exercise programs of middle-aged men who trained at 85 to 90% HR max. All three groups showed significant improvements in $\dot{V}O_2$max, indicating that this improvement is independent of the mode of training when frequency, intensity, and duration of exercise are held constant and are prescribed in accordance with sound, scientific principles.

Aerobic Dance

Aerobic dance is a popular mode of exercise for improving and maintaining cardiorespiratory fitness. A number of excellent books provide detailed information about aerobic dance methods and techniques (Kuntzelman 1979; Wilmoth 1986). A typical aerobic dance workout consists of 8 to 10 minutes of stretching, calisthenics, and low-intensity exercise. This is followed by 15 to 45 minutes of either high- or low-impact aerobic dancing at the target training intensity. Hand-held weights (1 to 4 pounds or ~0.5-2 kg) can be used to increase exercise intensity. Heart rates should be monitored at least six

times during the exercise to insure that the heart rate stays within the target zone (Russell 1983). The 10 minute cool-down period usually includes more stretching and calisthenic-type exercises.

Several studies conducted to assess the cardiorespiratory effect of aerobic dance training have documented average increases in $\dot{V}O_2$max of 10% or greater (Blessing et al. 1987; Milburn and Butts 1983; Parker et al. 1989; Williford et al 1988). Milburn and Butts (1983) reported that aerobic dance was as effective as jogging for improving cardiorespiratory endurance when performed at similar intensity, frequency, and duration. The subjects trained 30 minutes, 4 days a week for 7 weeks at 83 to 84% HR max.

Bench Step Aerobics

Health and fitness clubs throughout the United States are promoting bench step training as an effective high-intensity, low-impact aerobic exercise mode. Step training uses whole-body movements on steps or benches, ranging in height from 4 to 12 inches (10.2 to 30.5 cm). Choreographed movement routines are performed to music. A typical bench step aerobic workout begins with 5 to 10 minutes of warm-up and 20 to 30 minutes of step training. This is followed by a short (3 to 5 minute) cool-down. Exercise training intensity can be graded by varying stepping cadence or bench height, and by using 1- to 4-pound handweights (Kravitz et al. 1997).

Recent studies confirm that continuous step training at bench heights ranging from 6 to 12 inches (15.2 to 30.5 cm) provides an adequate training stimulus that meets ACSM (1995) guidelines for intensity and duration (Olson et al. 1991; Petersen et al. 1993; Woodby-Brown, Berg, and Latin 1993). Following 8 to 12 weeks of step aerobic training, $\dot{V}O_2$max improves as much as 8 to 16% (Kravitz et al. 1993; Kravitz et al. 1997; Velasquez and Wilmore 1992). In a study comparing bench step exercise with and without handweights, use of 2- to 4-pound (~1-2 kg) handweights did not result in a greater improvement in $\dot{V}O_2$max compared to step training without handweights (Kravitz et al. 1997).

Step Ergometry

Step ergometry (machine-based stairclimbing) is a popular exercise mode in health and fitness clubs. Research shows a linear HR response to graded, submaximal exercise performed on stairclimbing ergometers. However, the MET levels displayed on the Stairmaster 4000 PT overestimate the actual

MET intensity of the exercise (Howley, Colacino, and Swensen 1992). When prescribing exercise intensity using this type of stairclimber, adjust the machine's estimates for each MET level using the following equation:

Actual METs = 0.556 + 0.745 (Stairmaster MET setting)

Although machine-based stairclimbing provides a sufficient training stimulus that meets guidelines for exercise intensity, presently there is no current research comparing the effectiveness of stairclimbing training with other aerobic training modes.

Aerobic Riding

Aerobic riding involves both upper- and lower-body muscle groups. Because of this, some manufacturers claim that this mode of exercise will automatically burn more calories than lower-body-only exercise modes such as jogging, cycling, and stairclimbing. A recent study, however, noted that the energy expenditure during 10 minutes of steady-state exercise at a somewhat hard intensity (RPE = 13) on an aerobic rider was significantly lower than the caloric expenditure for treadmill jogging, stationary cycling, and Nordic skiing (Kravitz, Robergs, and Heyward 1996). Subjects reported that they felt a similar workout intensity, in terms of RPE, during aerobic riding. Aerobic riding appears to challenge the muscular system (subjects complained of muscular discomfort) more than the cardiovascular system. In fact, the relative, submaximal $\dot{V}O_2$ (47% $\dot{V}O_2$max) for aerobic riding was significantly less than that for treadmill jogging (74% $\dot{V}O_2$max), Nordic skiing (68% $\dot{V}O_2$max), and stationary cycling (64% $\dot{V}O_2$max). Thus, aerobic riding may not be suitable for aerobic exercise prescriptions, particularly for individuals with above-average cardiorespiratory fitness.

Discontinuous Training

Discontinuous training involves a series of low to high intensity exercise bouts interspersed with rest or relief periods. All of the exercise modes listed as Group I and II activities (see page 85) are suitable for discontinuous training. Due to the intermittent nature of this form of training, the exercise intensity and total amount work performed can be greater than that of continuous training, making discontinuous training a versatile method that is widely used by athletes as well as by individuals with poor cardiorespiratory fitness. In fact, the ACSM (1995)

recommends the use of discontinuous (intermittent) training for symptomatic individuals who are able to tolerate only low-intensity exercise for short periods of time (3 to 5 minutes). Interval training and circuit resistance training are two types of intermittent or discontinuous training.

Interval Training

Interval training involves a repeated series of exercise work bouts interspersed with rest or relief periods. This method is popular among athletes because it allows them to exercise at higher relative intensities during the work interval than are possible with continuous training. Interval training programs also can be designed to improve speed and anaerobic endurance, as well as aerobic endurance, simply by modifying the exercise intensity and length of the work and relief intervals.

Here is an example of an interval training exercise prescription for the development of aerobic endurance:

Sets: 1

Repetitions: 3

Distance: 1100 yd

Time: 3-4 minutes

Rest-relief interval: 1.5 to 2 minutes

Each work interval consists of running at a pace so that a distance of 1100 yd is covered in 3 to 4 minutes. The work interval is followed by a rest-relief interval of 1.5 to 2 minutes. This sequence is repeated 3 times. During the rest-relief interval, the individual usually walks or jogs while recovering from the work bout. For aerobic interval training, the ratio of work to rest-relief is usually 1:1 or 1:0.5. Each work interval is 3 to 5 minutes and is repeated 3 to 7 times. The exercise intensity usually ranges between 70 and 85% $\dot{V}O_2$max. Apply the overload principle by increasing the exercise intensity or length of the work interval, decreasing the length of the rest-relief interval, or increasing the number of work intervals per exercise session. For a discussion of interval training and sample programs, including programs for developing speed and anaerobic endurance, refer to Fox and Mathews (1974).

Circuit Resistance Training

Use of circuit resistance training for development of aerobic fitness, as well as muscular strength and tone, has received much attention. An example of a circuit resistance training program is presented in chapter 7, page 128 (see figure 7.1). Circuit resistance training usually consists of several circuits of resistance training exercises with a minimal amount of rest between the exercise stations (15 to 20 seconds). Alternatively, instead of resting, you can have your clients perform 1 minute of aerobic exercise between each station. The aerobic stations may include activities such as stationary cycling, jogging in place, rope skipping, stairclimbing, bench stepping, and rowing. This modification of the circuit is known as *super circuit resistance training*.

Gettman and Pollock (1981) reviewed the research dealing with the physiological benefits of circuit resistance training. Because it produces only a 5% increase in aerobic capacity as compared with a 15 to 25% increase with other forms of aerobic training, the authors concluded that circuit resistance training should not be used to develop aerobic fitness. Rather, it may be used during the maintenance stage of an aerobic exercise program.

PERSONALIZED EXERCISE PROGRAMS

The aerobic exercise prescription should be individualized to meet each client's training goals and

Essential Elements of a Case Study

Demographic Factors

Age

Gender

Ethnicity

Occupation

Height

Body weight

Family history of CHD

Medical History

Present symptoms

Dyspnea or shortness of breath

Angina or chest pain

Leg cramps or claudication

Musculoskeletal problems or limitations

Medications

Past history

Diseases

Injruies

Surgeries

Lab tests

Lifestyle Assessment

Alcohol and caffeine intake

Smoking

Nutritional intake/eating patterns

Physical activity patterns and interests

Sleeping habits

Occupational stress level

Mental status/family lifestyle

Physical Examination

Blood pressure

Heart/lung sounds

Orthopedic problems/limitations

Laboratory Tests (Ideal or Typical Values)

Triglycerides (<200 mg $\cdot$ dl^{-1})

Total cholesterol (<200 mg $\cdot$ dl^{-1})

LDL-cholesterol (<130 mg $\cdot$ dl^{-1})

HDL-cholesterol (>35 mg $\cdot$ dl^{-1})

TC/HDL-cholesterol (<3.5)

Blood glucose (60-114 mg $\cdot$ dl^{-1})

Hemoglobin: 13.5-17.5 mg $\cdot$ dl^{-1} men
    11.5-15.5 g $\cdot$ dl^{-1} women

Hematocrit: 40-52% men
    36-48% women

Potassium (3.5-5.5 meq $\cdot$ dl^{-1})

Blood urea nitrogen (4-24 mg $\cdot$ dl^{-1})

Creatinine (0.3-1.4 mg $\cdot$ dl^{-1})

Iron: 40-190 μg $\cdot$ dl^{-1} men
    35-180 μg $\cdot$ dl^{-1} women

Calcium (8.5-10.5 mg $\cdot$ dl^{-1})

Physical Fitness Evaluation

Cardiorespiratory fitness (HR, BP, $\dot{V}O_2$max)

Body composition (% BF)

Musculoskeletal fitness (muscle and bone strength)

Flexibility

Neuromuscular tension/stress

interests. To do so, you need to consider your client's age, gender, physical fitness level, and exercise preferences. This section presents a sample case study and examples of individualized exercise prescriptions to illustrate how the exercise prescription may be personalized for each client.

Case Study

Like any preventive or therapeutic intervention, exercise should be prescribed carefully. You must assess each client's medical history, physical condition, lifestyle characteristics, and interests prior to designing the exercise program. Summarize this information in a written narrative that includes all the elements of a case study. This case study provides the information that you will need to develop an accurate and safe individualized exercise prescription (Porter 1988). Because age, gender, ethnicity, high job stress, obesity, and family history of CHD are all related to a client's risk of developing CHD, use the *demographic data* to establish a risk factor profile. The CHD risk classification (apparently healthy, at increased risk, or having known disease) dictates how closely the client's exercise program needs to be monitored.

The *medical history* and *physical examination* may reveal signs or symptoms of CHD, particularly if shortness of breath, chest pains, or leg cramps are reported or high blood pressure is detected. It is important to note the types of medication being used by the client. Drugs such as digitalis, beta-blockers, diuretics, vasodilators, bronchodilators, and insulin may alter the body's physiological responses during exercise. Musculoskeletal disorders such as arthritis, low back pain, osteoporosis, and chondromalacia also need to be considered.

The *lifestyle assessment* provides useful information regarding the individual's risk factor profile. Factors such as smoking, lack of physical activity, and diets high in saturated fats or cholesterol increase the risk of CHD, atherosclerosis, and hypertension. You often can target these factors for modification; they also can help you assess the likelihood of the client's adherence to the exercise program.

Analyze the *blood lipid profile* when you are assessing CHD risk. Individuals are at higher risk if

- triglycerides ≥ 200 mg $\cdot$ dl^{-1},
- total cholesterol ≥ 240 mg $\cdot$ dl^{-1},
- LDL-cholesterol ≥ 160 mg $\cdot$ dl^{-1},
- HDL-cholesterol < 35 mg $\cdot$ dl^{-1},

- total cholesterol / HDL ratio > 5.0, or
- blood glucose > 115 mg $\cdot$ dl^{-1}.

Use the blood pressure, heart rate, and RPE responses to the *graded exercise test* to assess the client's functional aerobic capacity and cardiorespiratory fitness level. You need to be acutely aware of the normal and abnormal physiological responses to graded exercise. After assessing your client's CHD risk and cardiorespiratory fitness level, you can design an aerobic exercise program using a personalized exercise prescription of intensity, frequency, duration, mode, and progression. To write the exercise prescription, use the results from the graded exercise test (heart rate, RPE, functional MET capacity).

Use the sample case study to test your ability to evaluate risk factors and graded exercise test results and to prescribe an accurate and safe aerobic exercise program for this individual. The results of the analysis for this case study are presented in appendix A.9.

Sample Case Study

A 28-year-old female police officer (5'5" or 165.1 cm, 140 lb or 63.6 kg, and 28% BF) has enrolled in the adult fitness program. Her job demands a fairly high level of physical fitness—a level she was able to achieve 6 years ago when she passed the physical fitness test battery used by the police department. Prior to becoming a police officer, she jogged 20 minutes usually 3 times a week. Since starting her job, she has had little or no time for exercise and has gained 15 pounds (6.8 kg). She works 8 hours a day, is divorced, and takes care of two children, ages seven and nine. At least 3 times a week, she and the children dine out, usually at fast-food restaurants like Burger King and Taco Bell. She reports that her job, along with the sole responsibility for raising her two children, is quite stressful. Occasionally, she experiences headaches and a tightness in the back of her neck. Usually, in the evening, she has one glass of wine to relax.

Her medical history reveals she smoked one pack of cigarettes per day for 4 years while she was in college. She quit smoking 3 years ago. The past 2 years she has tried some quick weight-loss diets, with little success. She was hospitalized on two occasions to give birth to her children. She reports that her father died of heart disease when he was 52 and her older brother has high blood pressure. Recently she had her blood chemistry analyzed because she was feeling light-headed and dizzy after eating. She eats only one large meal a day at dinner time in an attempt to lose weight. Results of the blood analysis were: total cholesterol = 220 mg · dl⁻¹; triglycerides = 98 mg · dl⁻¹; glucose = 82 mg · dl⁻¹; HDL-cholesterol = 37 mg · dl⁻¹; and total cholesterol/HDL ratio = 5.9.

The exercise evaluation yielded the following data:

Mode/Protocol: Treadmill/Modified Bruce

Resting data: HR = 75 bpm
                 BP = 140/82 mmHg

Stage	METs	Duration (min)	HR (bpm)	BP (mmHg)	RPE
1	2.3	3	126	145/78	8
2	3.5	3	142	160/78	11
3	4.6	3	165	172/80	14
4	7.0	3	190	189/82	18

Endpoint: Stage 4 (2.5 mph, 12% grade). Test terminated because of fatigue.

Analysis

- Evaluate the client's CHD risk profile. Be certain to address each of the positive and negative risk factors.

- Describe any special problems or limitations that need to be considered in designing an exercise program for this client.

- Were the HR, BP, and RPE responses to the graded exercise test normal? Explain.

- What is the client's functional aerobic capacity in METs? Categorize her cardiorespiratory fitness level (see table 4.1).

- Plot the HR vs METs on graph paper.

- From the graph, determine the client's target heart rate zone for the aerobic exercise program. What HRs and RPEs correspond to 60, 70, 80, and 85% of the client's V̇O₂max?

- The client expressed an interest in walking outside on a level track to develop aerobic fitness. Calculate her walking speed for each of the following training intensities: 60, 70, and 80% V̇O₂max. Use the ACSM equations presented in table 4.3.

- In addition to starting an aerobic exercise program, what suggestions do you have for this client for modifying her lifestyle?

Sample Cycling Program

The sample cycling program on page 98 shows a personalized cycling program for a 27-year-old female who was given a maximal graded exercise test on a stationary bicycle ergometer. The exercise intensity is based on a percentage of the measured V̇O₂max, and the target exercise heart rates corresponding to 50 and 80% V̇O₂max are 118 bpm and 162 bpm, respectively (see figure 5.3). Thus, the training exercise heart rate should fall within this heart rate range. During the initial stage of the exercise program, the woman will cycle at a work rates corresponding to 50% V̇O₂max (3.7 METs) for 3 weeks. The work rates corresponding to each exercise intensity are calculated using the ACSM formulas for leg ergometry (see table 4.3). During week 4, exercise intensity will be increased by 10%. In the initial stages of the program, the weekly energy expenditure is between 240 and 450 kcal. In the improvement stage, the exercise intensity, duration, and frequency are progressively increased, and the weekly caloric expenditure ranges between 425 and 1280 kcal. In the maintenance phase, tennis and aerobic dancing are added to give variety and to supplement the cycling program. The ACSM (1995) guidelines were followed to calculate each component of this exercise prescription.

Sample Jogging Program

The sample jogging program is a jogging exercise program for a 29-year-old male who has a good cardiorespiratory fitness level. Since a graded exercise test could not be administered, the V̇O₂max was predicted from performance on the 12-minute distance run test. The maximal heart rate was predicted using the formula, 220 – age. Because this client is accustomed to jogging and his cardiorespiratory fitness level is classified as excellent, he is exempted from the initial stage and enters the improvement stage of the program immediately. During this time (20 weeks), the exercise intensity is increased from 70 to 85% of the estimated V̇O₂max. The speed corresponding to each MET intensity is calculated using the ACSM formulas for running on a level course (see table 4.3). The intensity, duration, and frequency of the exercise sessions provide a weekly caloric expenditure between 700 and 2000 kcal (9.0 METs = 9.0 kcal · kg⁻¹ · hr⁻¹). Because he weighs 70 kg (154 lb), the initial energy expenditure is estimated to be

9.0 kcal 3 70 kg = 630 kcal · hr⁻¹ or 10.5 kcal · min⁻¹

During the first 4 weeks, he will expend approximately 700 kcal, jogging 22 minutes at an 11.5 minute per mile pace 3 times per week (22 min × 10.5 kcal · min⁻¹ × 3). The distance covered is figured by dividing the exercise duration by the running pace (22 min / 11.5 min · mile^{-1} = 2 miles or 3.2 km). During the improvement stage, the frequency of exercise sessions gradually progresses from 3 to 5 days a week. During the maintenance stage, the running is reduced to 3 days per week, and handball and basketball are added to the aerobic exercise program. The ACSM (1995) guidelines were followed to calculate each component of this exercise prescription

Sample Cycling Program

Client data

Age	27 yr
Gender	Female
Body weight	65 kg (143 lbs.)
Resting heart rate	67 bpm
Maximal heart rate	195 bpm (measured)
$\dot{V}O_2$max	26 ml · kg^{-1} · min^{-1} (measured) 7.4 METs
Graded exercise test	Bicycle Ergometer
Initial cardiorespiratory fitness level	Poor

Exercise prescription

Mode	Stationary cycling
Intensity	50-80% $\dot{V}O_2$max 13.0-20.6 ml · kg^{-1} · min^{-1} 3.7-5.9 METs
Exercise heart rates (from figure 5.3)	118 bpm minimum 162 bpm maximum
RPE	10-16
Duration	20-40 minutes
Frequency	3-5 times / week

Cycling program

Phase (weeks)	Intensity (% $\dot{V}O_2$)	METs	HR (bpm)	RPE	Work rate (kgm · min^{-1})	Resistance (kg)	Pedal rate (rpm)	Kcal/min	Time (min)	Freq	Weekly expenditure (kcal)
Initial											
1	50	3.7	118	10	300	1.0	50	4.0	20	3	240
2	50	3.7	118	10	300	1.0	50	4.0	25	3	300
3	50	3.7	118	10	300	1.0	50	4.0	30	3	360
4	60	4.4	135	11	385	1.3	50	4.7	30	3	425
Improvement											
5-8	60-70	4.4-5.2	135-146	11-12	385-480	1.3-1.6	50	4.7-5.6	30	3-4	425-675
9-12	60-70	4.4-5.2	135-146	11-12	385-480	1.3-1.6	50	4.7-5.6	35	3-4	495-785
13-16	70-75	5.2-5.6	146-158	12-14	480-523	1.6-1.7	50	5.6-6.1	35	3-4	585-850
17-20	70-75	5.2-5.6	146-158	12-14	480-523	1.6-1.7	50	5.6-6.1	40	4-5	900-1220
21-24	75-80	5.6-5.9	158-162	14-16	523-557	1.7-1.9	50	6.1-6.4	40	4-5	975-1280
25-28	75-80	5.6-5.9	158-162	14-16	523-557	1.7-1.9	50	6.1-6.4	40	4-5	975-1280
Maintenance											
29+											
Cycling	75-80	5.6-5.9	158-162	14-16	523-557	1.7-1.9	50	6.1-6.4	40	1	730-770
Aerobic Dance	65% HRR	5.0	150	13-14				5.4	30	1	200
Tennis		5.0		12-13				5.4	60	1	325

Sample Jogging Program

Client data

Age	29 yr
Gender	Male
Body weight	70 kg (154 lbs.)
Resting heart rate	50 bpm
Maximal heart rate	191 bpm (age-predicted)
$\dot{V}O_2max$	45 ml · kg^{-1}· min^{-1} (predicted)
Graded exercise test	None
Initial cardiorespiratory fitness level	Excellent

Exercise prescription

Mode	Jogging and running
Intensity	70-85% $\dot{V}O_2max$ 31.5-38.1 ml · kg^{-1}· min^{-1} 9.0-10.9 METs
Exercise heart rates	147 bpm minimum (70% HRR) 170 bpm maximum (85% HRR)
RPE	12-16
Duration	22-32 minutes
Frequency	3-5 times / week

Jogging program

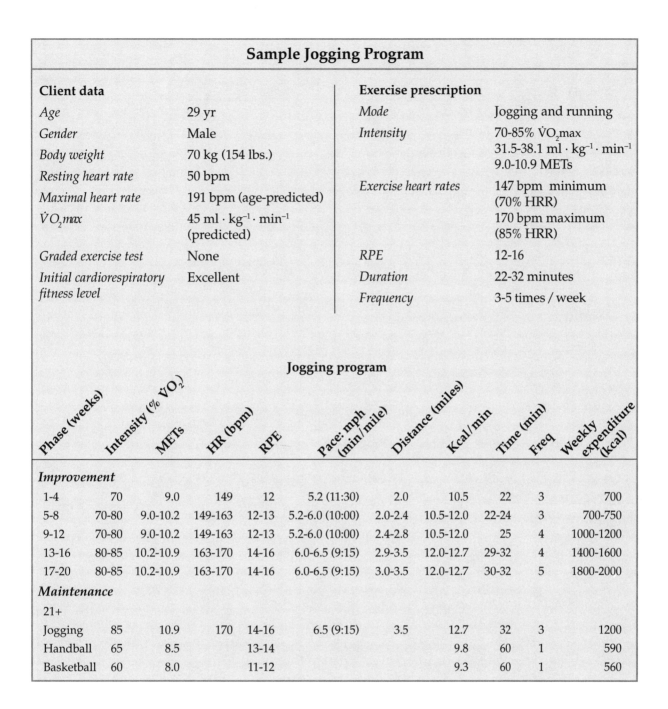

Phase (weeks)	Intensity (% $\dot{V}O_2$)	METs	HR (bpm)	RPE	Pace: mph (min/mile)	Distance (miles)	Kcal/min	Time (min)	Freq	Weekly expenditure (kcal)
Improvement										
1-4	70	9.0	149	12	5.2 (11:30)	2.0	10.5	22	3	700
5-8	70-80	9.0-10.2	149-163	12-13	5.2-6.0 (10:00)	2.0-2.4	10.5-12.0	22-24	3	700-750
9-12	70-80	9.0-10.2	149-163	12-13	5.2-6.0 (10:00)	2.4-2.8	10.5-12.0	25	4	1000-1200
13-16	80-85	10.2-10.9	163-170	14-16	6.0-6.5 (9:15)	2.9-3.5	12.0-12.7	29-32	4	1400-1600
17-20	80-85	10.2-10.9	163-170	14-16	6.0-6.5 (9:15)	3.0-3.5	12.0-12.7	30-32	5	1800-2000
Maintenance										
21+										
Jogging	85	10.9	170	14-16	6.5 (9:15)	3.5	12.7	32	3	1200
Handball	65	8.5		13-14			9.8	60	1	590
Basketball	60	8.0		11-12			9.3	60	1	560

Sample Multimodal Exercise Program

Some clients may prefer to engage in a variety of exercise modes (cross training) to develop their cardiorespiratory fitness (see "Multimodal Exercise Program" on pages 100-101). For these cases, it is difficult to systematically prescribe increments in exercise intensity using METs or target heart rates.

Although MET equivalents for various activities are available (ACSM 1995), typically a range of values is given, making it difficult for you to accurately prescribe work rates corresponding to specific intensity recommendations in an exercise prescription. Also, the HR response to a given MET level is highly dependent on the exercise mode.

Sample Multimodal Exercise Program

Client data

Age	44 yr
Gender	Female
Body weight	68 kg (150 lbs.)
Resting heart rate	70 bpm
Maximal heart rate	170 bpm measured
$\dot{V}O_2max$ *(measured)*	30 ml · kg⁻¹ · min⁻¹ 8.6 METs
Graded exercise test	Treadmill maximal GXT (Bruce protocol)
Initial cardiorespiratory fitness level	Fair

Exercise prescription

Modes and estimates of caloric expenditure (kcal · min⁻¹)	Stationary cycling: 6.8 Step aerobics: 8.2 Walking: 5.4 In-line skating: 6.5 Stairclimbing: 5.9 Hiking: 5.6 Resistance training 7.8
Intensity	RPE: 10 to 16
Duration	20 to 60 minutes
Frequency	3 to 5 days / week
Weekly caloric expenditure	400 to 1400 kcal per week

Multimodal exercise program

Phase (weeks)	Intensity (RPE)	Minimal duration (min)	Minimal frequency	Average kcal/workout	Weekly caloric goal
Initial					
1-2	10	20	3	133	400
3-4	10	25	3	166	500
Improvement					
5-8	12	25	3	200	600
9-12	12	30	3	230	700
13-16	12-13	30	4	230	900
17-20	14-15	30	4	250	1000
20-24	15-16	30	5	280	1400
Maintenance					
25+	15-16	30	5	280	1400

(cont.)

Examples

Week 1	Activity	Kcal · min⁻¹ estimates	Time (min)	Freq	Kcal per workout	Activity groupᵃ
Monday	Indoor cycling	6.8	20	1	136	I
Wednesday	Step aerobics	8.2	20	1	164	II
Friday	Walking	5.4	30	1	162	I
	*Totals:		70	3	462	3
	Goals:		60	3	400	3

Week 17	Activity	Kcal · min⁻¹ estimates	Time (min)	Freq	Kcal per workout	Activity groupᵃ
Monday	In-line skating	6.5	35	1	227	II
Tuesday	Walking	5.4	40	1	216	I
Wednesday	Stairclimbing	5.9	30	1	177	I
Friday	Resistance training	7.8	20	1	156	III
Sunday	Hiking	5.6	40	1	224	II
	*Totals:		165	5	1000	4
	Goals:		150	4	1000	4

ᵃ Check all Group I and II activities
* Compare weekly totals to weekly goals.

The degree of muscle mass involved in the activity, as well as whether the body weight is supported during exercise, can affect the HR response to a prescribed exercise intensity. For example, whole-body exercise modes, such as Nordic skiing and aerobic dancing, involve both upper- and lower-body musculature. These produce higher submaximal HRs compared to lower-body exercise modes (e.g., cycling and jogging). Also, at any given exercise intensity, the HR response during weight-bearing exercise, like jogging, is greater than that of non-weight-bearing exercise (e.g., cycling).

Therefore, you should use ratings of perceived exertion (RPE) to progressively increase exercise intensity throughout the improvement stage of a multimodal aerobic exercise program (see table 4.2). To use the RPE safely and effectively, you will need to teach your clients to focus on and learn to monitor important exertional cues such as breathing effort (rate and depth of breathing) and muscular sensations (e.g., pain, warmth, and fatigue).

Guidelines for developing multimodal exercise prescriptions are presented on page 102. For multimodal exercise programs (see the Sample Multimodal Program) you should set exercise frequency and weekly caloric expenditure goals for each client. Provide your clients with estimates of energy expenditure (kcal · min⁻¹) for each of the aerobic activities they select for their exercise prescriptions. The exercise duration to achieve a specified weekly caloric expenditure goal will vary depending on the activity mode chosen for each exercise session. Any combination of Group I and II activities can be used, providing the client is able to maintain the prescribed RPE intensity for at least 20 minutes.

Guidelines for Multimodal Exercise Prescriptions

Modes: Select at least 3 per week from Group I and II activities.

Frequency: 3 to 7 sessions a week. Engage in either Group I or II activities at least 3 times per week.

Intensity: RPE between 10 and 16.

Duration: At least 15 minutes, preferably 20 to 30 minutes. Duration depends on energy cost (kcal · min^{-1}) of exercise mode.

Caloric expenditure: 700 to 800 kcal · wk^{-1}, preferably 1000 to 2000 kcal · wk^{-1}. Group III activities can be used to reach weekly caloric expenditure goal but cannot be counted as one of the required aerobic workouts.

Flexibility is the key to successful multimodal exercise prescriptions. Clients should be free not only to select exercise modes of interest but to decide on various combinations of frequency and duration as long as they meet the caloric thresholds specified in their exercise prescriptions for each week.

The primary benefits of multimodal exercise programs for your clients are

- greater likelihood of engaging in a safe and effective exercise program,
- overall greater enjoyment of physical activity and exercise,
- better understanding of how their bodies respond to exercise,
- more direct involvement and sense of control in developing and monitoring their exercise programs, and
- increased likelihood of incorporating physical activity and exercise into their lifestyles.

Key Points

- Always personalize cardiorespiratory exercise programs to meet the needs, interests, and abilities of each participant.
- The exercise prescription includes mode, frequency, intensity, duration, and progression of exercise.
- Aerobic endurance activities involving large muscle groups are well suited for developing cardiorespiratory fitness. Group I activities such as walking, jogging, and cycling allow the individual to maintain steady-state exercise intensities and are not highly dependent on skill.
- You can prescribe exercise intensity using the heart rate, MET, or RPE methods, or a combination of these methods.
- For the average person, the cardiorespiratory exercise program should be at an intensity of 60 to 85% functional aerobic capacity, a duration of 20 to 60 minutes, and a frequency of 3 to 5 days per week.
- The cardiorespiratory exercise program includes three stages of progression: initial conditioning, improvement, and maintenance.
- Each exercise session includes warm-up, aerobic conditioning exercise, and cool-down.
- Continuous and discontinuous training methods are equally effective for improving cardiorespiratory fitness.
- Multimodal exercise prescriptions use a variety of Group I and II aerobic activities to improve cardiorespiratory endurance.

REFERENCES

American College of Sports Medicine. 1995. *ACSM's guidelines for exercise testing and prescription*. Baltimore: Williams & Wilkins.

Berry, M.J., Cline, C.C., Berry, C.B., and Davis, M. 1992. A comparison between two forms of aerobic dance and treadmill running. *Medicine and Science in Sports and Exercise* 24: 946-951.

Birk, T.J., and Birk, C.A. 1987. Use of ratings of perceived exertion for exercise prescription. *Sports Medicine* 4: 1-8.

Blessing, D.L., Wilson, D.G., Puckett, J.R., and Ford, H.T. 1987. The physiological effects of 8 weeks of aerobic dance with and without hand-held weights. *American Journal of Sports Medicine* 15: 508-510.

Borg, G.V., and Linderholm, H. 1967. Perceived exertion and pulse rate during graded exercise in various age groups. *Acta Medica Scandinavica* 472(Suppl.): 194-206.

Brahler, C.J., and Blank, S.E. 1995. VersaClimbing elicits higher $\dot{V}O_2$max than does treadmill running or rowing ergometry. *Medicine and Science in Sports and Exercise* 27: 249-254.

Brynteson, P., and Sinning, W.E. 1973. The effects of training frequencies on the retention of cardiovascular fitness. *Medicine and Science in Sports* 5: 29-33.

deVries, H.A. 1980. *Physiology of exercise for physical education and athletics*. Dubuque, IA: William C. Brown.

Dishman, R.K. 1994. Prescribing exercise intensity for healthy adults using perceived exertion. *Medicine and Science in Sports and Exercise* 26: 1087-1094.

Dunbar, C.C., Robertson, R.J., Baun, R., Blandin, M.F., Metz, K., Burdett, R., and Goss, F.L. 1992. The validity of regulating exercise intensity by ratings of perceived exertion. *Medicine and Science in Sports and Exercise* 24:, 94-99.

Fox, E.L., and Mathews, D.K. 1974. *Interval training: Conditioning for sports and general fitness*. Philadelphia: W.B. Saunders.

Gettman, L.R., and Pollock, M.L. 1981. Circuit weight training: A critical review of its physiological benefits. *The Physician and Sportsmedicine* 9: 44-60.

Hickson, R.C., and Rosenkoetter, M.A. 1981. Reduced training frequencies and maintenance of increased aerobic power. *Medicine and Science in Sports and Exercise* 13: 13-16.

Howley, E.T., Colacino, D.L., and Swensen, T.C. 1992. Factors affecting the oxygen cost of stepping on an electronic stepping ergometer. *Medicine and Science in Sports and Exercise* 24: 1055-1058.

Kravitz, L., Cizar, C., Christensen, C., and Setterlund, S. 1993. The physiological effects of step training with and without handweights. *Journal of Sports Medicine and Physical Fitness* 33: 348-358.

Kravitz, L., Heyward, V., Stolarczyk, L., and Wilmerding, V. 1997. Effects of step training with and without handweights on physiological profiles of women. *Journal of Strength and Conditioning Research* 11:194-199.

Kravitz, L., Robergs, R., and Heyward, V. 1996. Are all aerobic exercise modes equal? *Idea Today* 14: 51-58.

Kuntzelman, B.A. 1979. *The complete guide to aerobic dancing*. Skokie, IL: Publications International.

Magel, J.R., Foglia, G.F., McArdle, W.D., Gutin, B., Pechard, G.S., and Katch, F.I. 1974. Specificity of swim training on maximum oxygen uptake. *Journal of Applied Physiology* 38: 151-155.

Milburn, S., and Butts, N.K. 1983. A comparison of the training responses to aerobic dance and jogging in college females. *Medicine and Science in Sports and Exercise* 15: 510-513.

Moffatt, R.J., Stamford, B.A., and Neill, R.D. 1977. Placement of tri-weekly training sessions: Importance regarding enhancement of aerobic capacity. *Research Quarterly* 48: 583-591.

Olson, M.S., Williford, H.N., Blessing, D.L., and Greathouse, R. 1991. The cardiovascular and metabolic effects of bench stepping exercise in females. *Medicine and Science in Sports and Exercise* 23: 1311-1318.

Parker, S.B., Hurley, B.F., Hanlon, D.P., and Vaccaro, P. 1989. Failure of target heart rate to accurately monitor intensity during aerobic dance. *Medicine and Science in Sports and Exercise* 21: 230-234.

Petersen, T., Verstraete, D., Schultz, W., and Stray-Gundersen, J. 1993. Metabolic demands of step aerobics. *Medicine and Science in Sports and Exercise* 25: S79 [abstract].

Pollock, M.L. 1973. The quantification of endurance training programs. In J.H. Wilmore, ed., *Exercise and sport sciences reviews* 1: 155-188. New York: Academic Press.

Pollock, M., Cureton, T.K., and Greninger, L 1969. Effects of frequency of training on working capacity, cardiovascular function, and body composition of adult men. *Medicine and Science in Sports* 1: 70-74.

Pollock, M., Dimmick, J., Miller, H., Kendrick, Z., and Linnerud, A.C. 1975. Effects of mode of training on cardiovascular function and body composition of adult men. *Medicine and Science in Sports* 7: 139-145.

Pollock, M., Gettman, L., Milesis, C., Bah, M., Durstine, L., and Johnson, R. 1977. Effects of frequency and duration of training on attrition and incidence of injury. *Medicine and Science in Sports* 9: 31-36.

Pollock, M.L., Miller, H.S., Janeway, R., Linnerud, A.C., Robertson, B., and Valentino, R. 1971. Effects of walking on body composition and cardiovascular function of middle-aged men. *Journal of Applied Physiology* 30: 126-130.

Porter, G.H. 1988. Case study evaluation for exercise prescription. In S.N. Blair, P. Painter, R.R. Pate, L.K. Smith, and C.B. Taylor, eds., *Resource manual for guidelines for exercise testing and prescription*, 248-255. Philadelphia: Lea & Febiger.

Russell, P.J. 1983. Aerobic dance programs: Maintaining quality and effectiveness. *Physical Educator* 40: 114-120.

Sharkey, B.J. 1979. *Physiology of fitness*. Champaign, IL: Human Kinetics.

Smutok, M.A., Skrinar, G.S., and Pandolf, K.B. 1980. Exercise intensity: Subjective regulation by perceived exertion. *Archives of Physical Medicine and Rehabilitation* 61: 569-574.

Swain, D.P., Abernathy, K.S., Smith, C.S., Lee, S.J., and Bunn, S.A. 1994. Target heart rates for the development of cardiorespiratory fitness. *Medicine and Science in Sports and Exercise* 26: 112-116.

Thomas, T.R., Ziogas, G., Smith, T., Zhang, Q., and Londeree, B.R. 1995. Physiological and perceived exertion responses to six modes of submaximal exercise. *Research Quarterly for Exercise and Sport* 66: 239-246.

Town, G.P., Sol, N., and Sinning, W. 1980. The effect of rope skipping rate on energy expenditure of males and females. *Medicine and Science in Sports and Exercise* 12: 295-298.

U.S. Department of Health and Human Services. 1996. *Physical activity and health: A report of the Surgeon General*. Atlanta, GA: U.S. Department of Health and Human Services, Centers for Disease Control and Prevention, National Center for Chronic Disease Prevention and Health Promotion.

Velasquez, K.S., and Wilmore, J.H. 1992. Changes in cardiorespiratory fitness and body composition after a 12-week bench step training program. *Medicine and Science in Sports and Exercise* 24: S78 [abstract].

Wallick, M.E., Porcari, J.P., Wallick, S.B., Berg, K.M., Brice, G.A., and Arimond, G.R. 1995. Physiological responses to in-line skating compared to treadmill running. *Medicine and Science in Sports and Exercise* 27: 242-248.

Williford, H.N., Blessing, D.L., Barksdale, J.M., and Smith, F.H. 1988. The effects of aerobic dance training on serum lipids, lipoproteins, and cardiopulmonary function. *Journal of Sports Medicine and Physical Fitness* 28: 151-157.

Wilmore, J.H., Davis, J.A., O'Brien, R.S., Vodak, P.A., Walder, G.R., and Amsterdam, E.A. 1980. Physiological alterations consequent to 20-week conditioning programs of bicycling, tennis and jogging. *Medicine and Science in Sports and Exercise* 12: 1-9.

Wilmoth, S.K. 1986. *Leading aerobic dance-exercise*. Champaign, IL: Human Kinetics.

Woodby-Brown, S., Berg, K., and Latin, R.W. 1993. Oxygen cost of aerobic bench stepping at three heights. *Journal of Strength and Conditioning Research* 7: 163-167.

Zeni, A.I., Hoffman, M.D., and Clifford, P.S. 1996. Energy expenditure with indoor exercise machines. *Journal of the American Medical Association* 275: 1424-1427.

CHAPTER 6

Assessing Strength and Muscular Endurance

Key Questions

- How are strength and muscular endurance assessed?
- How does the type of muscle contraction (concentric, eccentric, and isokinetic) affect force production?
- What test protocols can be used to assess a client's muscular fitness?
- What are the advantages and limitations of using free weights and exercise machines to assess muscular strength?
- What are sources of measurement error for muscular fitness tests, and how are they controlled?
- What are the recommended procedures for administering strength tests?
- Is it safe to give strength tests to children and older adults?

Muscular strength and endurance are two important components of physical fitness. Minimal levels of muscular fitness are needed to perform activities of daily living, to maintain functional independence as one ages, and to partake in active leisure-time pursuits without undue stress or fatigue. Adequate levels of muscular fitness lessen the chance of developing low back problems, osteoporotic fractures, and musculoskeletal injuries.

This chapter describes a variety of laboratory and field tests for assessing all forms of muscular strength and endurance. In addition, the chapter compares types of exercise machines, addresses factors affecting muscular fitness tests, and discusses sources of measurement error.

DEFINITION OF TERMS

Strength is defined as the ability of a muscle group to develop maximal contractile force against a resistance in a single contraction. The force generated by a muscle or muscle group, however, is highly dependent on the velocity of movement. Maximal force is produced when the limb is not rotating (i.e., zero velocity). As the speed of joint rotation increases, the muscular force decreases. Thus, *strength for dynamic movements* is defined as the maximal force generated in a single contraction at a specified velocity (Knuttgen and Kraemer 1987). *Muscular endurance* is the ability of a muscle group to exert submaximal force for extended periods.

Both strength and muscular endurance can be assessed for static and dynamic muscular contractions. If the resistance is immovable, the muscle contraction is *static* or *isometric* (*iso*, same; *metric*, length), and there is no visible movement of the joint. *Dynamic contractions*, in which there is visible joint movement, are either concentric, eccentric, or isokinetic (see figure 6.1, *a* and *b*).

If the resistance is less than the force produced by the muscle group, the contraction is *concentric,*

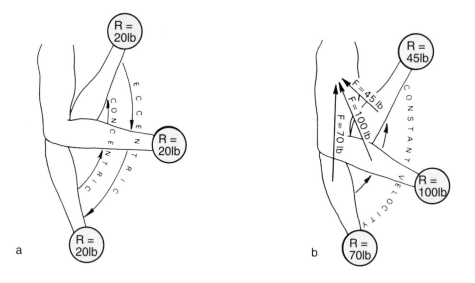

Figure 6.1 Types of muscle contraction: (**a**) dynamic and (**b**) isokinetic.

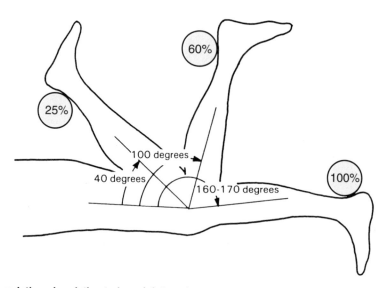

Figure 6.2 Strength variations in relation to knee joint angle.

allowing the muscle to shorten as it exerts tension to move the bony lever. The muscle also is capable of exerting tension while lengthening. This is known as *eccentric contraction* and typically occurs when the muscles produce a braking force to decelerate rapidly moving body segments or to resist gravity (e.g., slowly lowering a barbell). Both concentric and eccentric contractions are sometimes called *isotonic (iso*, same; *tonic*, tension*)*. The term isotonic contraction is a misnomer, because the tension produced by the muscle group fluctuates greatly even though the resistance is constant throughout the

range of motion (ROM). This fluctuation in muscular force is due to the change in muscle length and angle of pull as the bony lever is moved, creating a strength curve that is unique for each muscle group (Kreighbaum and Barthels 1981). For example, the strength of the knee flexors is maximal at 160° to 170° (see figure 6.2).

In regular (concentric and eccentric), dynamic exercise, the muscle group is not contracting maximally throughout the ROM due to the change in mechanical and physiological advantage as the limb is moved. Thus, the greatest resistance that can be used during regular, dynamic exercise is equal to the maximum weight that can be moved at the *weakest* point in the range of motion.

Isokinetic contraction (see figure 6.1*b*) is a maximal contraction of a muscle group at a constant velocity throughout the entire range of joint motion (*iso*, same; *kinetic*, motion). The velocity of contraction is controlled mechanically so that the limb rotates at a set velocity (e.g., $120° \cdot sec^{-1}$). Electromechanical devices vary the resistance to match the muscular force produced at each point in the ROM. Thus, isokinetic exercise machines allow the muscle group to encounter variable but maximal resistances during the movement.

STRENGTH AND MUSCULAR ENDURANCE ASSESSMENT

Static strength and muscular endurance are measured using dynamometers, cable tensiometers, and load cells. Free weights (barbells and dumbbells), as well as constant-resistance, variable-resistance and isokinetic exercise machines, are used to assess dynamic strength and endurance (see table 6.1). The testing procedures vary depending on the type of test (i.e., strength or endurance) and equipment.

Isometric Muscle Testing Using Dynamometers

You can use isometric dynamometers to measure static strength and endurance of the grip squeezing muscles and leg and back muscles (see figure 6.3). The handgrip dynamometer has an adjustable handle to fit the size of the hand and measures forces between 0 and 100 kilograms, in 1-kg increments. The back and leg dynamometer consists of a scale that

measures forces ranging from 0 to 2500 pounds in 10-lb increments. Both dynamometers are spring devices. As force is applied to the dynamometer, the spring is compressed and moves the indicator needle a corresponding amount.

Grip-Strength Testing Procedures

Before using the handgrip dynamometer, adjust the handgrip size to a position that is comfortable for the individual. Alternatively, you can measure the hand width with a caliper, and use this value to set the optimum grip size (Montoye and Faulkner 1964). The individual stands erect, with the arms at the sides. The client should hold the dynamometer parallel to the side, with the dial facing away from the body, then squeeze the dynamometer as hard as possible without moving the arm. Administer three trials for each hand, allowing a 1-minute rest between trials, and use the best score as the client's static strength.

Grip Endurance Testing Procedures

Once the grip size is adjusted, instruct the client to squeeze the handle as hard as possible and to continue squeezing for one minute. Record the initial force and the final force exerted at the end of one minute. The greater the endurance, the less the rate and degree of decline in force. The relative endurance score is the final force divided by the initial force times 100.

Alternatively, you can assess static grip endurance by having your client exert a submaximal force, which is a given percentage of the individual's maximum voluntary contractile (MVC) strength (e.g., 50% MVC). The relative endurance score is the amount of time that this force level is maintained. To monitor the appropriate force level, the subject must watch the dial of the dynamometer during the test.

Table 6.1 Strength Testing Modes		
Testing mode	**Equipment**	**Measure***
Static	Isometric dynamometers, cable tensiometers, and load cells	MVC (kg)
Dynamic Constant-resistance	Free weights (barbells and dumbbells) and exercise machines	1-RM (lb or kg)
Variable-resistance	Exercise machines	NA
Isokinetic and omnikinetic	Isokinetic and omnikinetic dynamometers	Peak torque (Nm or ft-lb)

*MVC = maximal voluntary contraction; NA = not applicable; Nm = newton-meter; ft-lb = foot-pound.

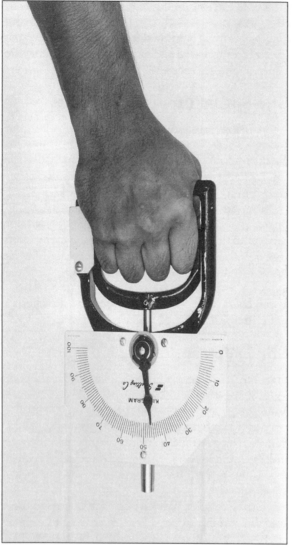

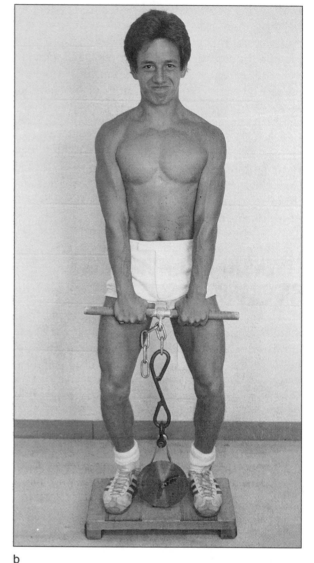

a   b

Figure 6.3   Dynamometers for measuring static strength and endurance: (*a*) Stoelting hand grip dynamometer and (*b*) back and leg dynamometer. Photos courtesy of Swede Scholer.

Leg Strength Testing Procedures

Using the back and leg dynamometer, the individual stands on the platform with trunk erect and the knees flexed to an angle of 130° to 140°. The client holds the handbar using a pronated grip and positions it across the thighs by adjusting the length of the chain (see figure 6.3*b*). If a belt is available, attach it to each end of the handbar after positioning the belt around the client's hips. The belt helps to stabilize the bar and to reduce the stress placed on the hands during the leg lift. Without using the back, the client slowly but vigorously extends the knees. The maximum indicator needle remains at the peak force achieved. Administer two or three trials with

a 1-minute rest interval. Divide the maximum score (in pounds) by 2.2 to convert it to kilograms.

Back Strength Testing Procedures

Using the back and leg dynamometer, the individual stands on the platform with the knees fully extended and the head and trunk erect. The client grasps the handbar using a pronated (right hand) and supinated (left hand) grip. Position the handbar across the client's thighs. Without leaning backward, the client pulls the handbar straight upward using the back muscles and is instructed to roll the shoulders backward during the pull. Clients should be reminded prior to lifting to flex the trunk minimally and to keep the head and trunk erect during the test. Administer two trials with a 1-minute rest between the trials. Divide the maximum score (in pounds) by 2.2 to convert it to kilograms.

Static Strength Norms

You can use the norms, developed for men and women, to assess your client's static strength for each dynamometric test item (see table 6.2). Calculate your client's total strength score by adding the right grip, left grip, leg strength, and back strength scores. Before doing this, convert the leg and back strength scores (measured in lb) to kilograms. To calculate the relative strength score, divide the total strength score by body weight (expressed in kilograms).

Isometric Muscle Testing Using Cable Tensiometers

You can use cable tensiometry to assess the static strength of 38 different muscle groups throughout the body. Standardized testing procedures have been described elsewhere in detail and should be followed closely to ensure the validity and reliability of the test results (Clarke 1966). The instrumentation includes a tensiometer, steel cables, testing table, wall hooks, straps, and goniometer. Attach one end of the cable to the wall or table hooks and the other end to the body part to be tested using a strap. Always position the cable at a right angle to the pulling bony lever. Use a goniometer to measure the appropriate joint angle. Place the tensiometer on a taut cable. As the individual exerts force on the cable, the riser of the tensiometer is depressed and a maximum indicator needle registers the static strength score. Tensiometers measure forces ranging between 0 and 400 pounds (0-181.8 kg). However, the larger tensiometers are less accurate in the lower range; therefore you should use a small tensiometer, which measures forces between 0 and 100 pounds (0-45.4 kg), to obtain greater accuracy in the lower range.

Cable tensiometry tests can be used to assess strength impairment at specific joint angles and to monitor progress during rehabilitation. As with all forms of static strength testing, you should be aware that strength is specific to the joint angle and muscle group being tested. Therefore, test at least three to four muscle groups to provide an adequate estimation of static strength.

Test batteries and norms have been developed for males and females, nine years old through college age (Clarke 1975; Clarke and Monroe 1970). The test battery for males of all ages includes the same three strength tests: shoulder extension, knee extension, and ankle plantar flexion. For elementary and junior high school girls, the test battery includes shoulder extension, hip extension, and trunk flexion. The three test items in the battery developed for senior high school and college women are shoulder flexion, hip flexion, and ankle plantar flexion.

Table 6.2 Static Strength Norms

Classification	Left grip (kg)	Right grip (kg)	Back strength (kg)	Leg strength (kg)	Total strength (kg)	Relative strength*
Men						
Excellent	>68	>70	>209	>241	>587	>7.50
Good	56-67	62-69	177-208	214-240	508-586	7.10-7.49
Average	43-55	48-61	126-176	160-213	375-507	5.21-7.09
Poor	39-42	41-47	91-125	137-159	307-374	4.81-5.20
Very poor	<39	<41	<91	<137	<307	<4.81
Women						
Excellent	>37	>41	>111	>136	>324	>5.50
Good	34-36	38-40	98-110	114-135	282-323	4.80-5.49
Average	22-33	25-37	52-97	66-113	164-281	2.90-4.79
Poor	18-21	22-24	39-51	49-65	117-163	2.10-2.89
Very poor	<18	<22	<39	<49	<117	<2.10

*Relative strength is determined by dividing total strength by body weight (in kilograms).

Data from Corbin et al. (1978). For persons over age 50, reduce scores by 10% to adjust for muscle tissue loss due to aging.

Dynamic Muscle Testing Using Constant-Resistance and Variable-Resistance Modes

Although either a *constant-resistance* or a *variable-resistance exercise* mode can be used to assess dynamic (concentric and eccentric) muscle strength and endurance, you will be better served if you use either free weights or constant-resistance exercise machines. A major disadvantage of free weights, dumbbells, and constant-resistance exercise machines, however, is that they measure dynamic strength only at the weakest point in the range of motion. This is because the resistance cannot be varied to account for fluctuations in muscular force caused by the changing mechanical (angle of pull of muscle) and physiological (length of muscle) advantage of the musculoskeletal system during the movement.

In an attempt to overcome the above-mentioned deficiency, researchers have designed variable-resistance machines that vary the resistance during the range of motion. Variable-resistance machines have a moving connection (i.e., lever, cam, or pulley) between the resistance and the point of force application. As the weight is lifted, the mechanical advantage of the machine decreases. Therefore, more force must be applied to continue moving the resistance. The variable-resistance mode of exercise attempts to match the force capability of the musculoskeletal system throughout the range of motion. However, many variable-resistance exercise machines fail to match the strength curves of different muscle groups. Also, with variable-resistance machines, it is difficult to assess the client's maximal force or strength because the resistance is modified by the levers, pulleys, and cams, causing the movement velocity to vary. Variable-resistance exercise machines therefore have limited usefulness for maximal testing. Still, these types of machines are well suited for resistance training.

Although free weights and constant-resistance exercise machines are generally recommended for muscular fitness testing, there are advantages and limitations for each of these modalities. Compared to exercise machines, free weights require more neuromuscular coordination in order to stabilize body parts and maintain balance while lifting the barbell or dumbbell. While exercise machines reduce the need for spotting during the test, these machines limit the individual's range of joint motion and plane of movement. Also, some exercise machines have relatively large weight plate increments, so that you must attach smaller weights to the weight stack in order to measure your client's strength accurately. Although most exercise machines have adjustable seats and lever arms, some cannot accommodate individuals with short limbs. Machines designed specifically for children and smaller adults must be used to standardize such clients' starting positions for testing. Body size and weight increments are less of a problem with free weights. The following dynamic strength and muscular endurance test protocols were specifically developed for constant-resistance exercise machines.

Dynamic Strength Tests

Dynamic strength is usually measured as the *maximum weight that can be lifted for one complete repetition of the movement (1-RM)*. The *1-RM* strength value is obtained through trial and error.

STEPS FOR 1-RM TESTING

The following basic steps are recommended for 1-RM testing (Kraemer and Fry, 1995):

1. Have your client warm up by completing 5 to 10 repetitions of the exercise at 40 to 60% of the estimated 1-RM.

2. During a 1-minute rest, have the client stretch the muscle group. This is followed by 3 to 5 repetitions of the exercise at 60 to 80% of the estimated 1-RM.

3. Then increase the weight conservatively, and have the client attempt the 1-RM lift. If the lift is successful, the client should rest 3 to 5 minutes before attempting the next weight increment. Follow this procedure until the client fails to complete the lift. The 1-RM typically is achieved within 3 to 5 trials.

4. Record the 1-RM value as the maximum weight lifted for the last successful trial.

The ACSM (1995) recommends the bench press and leg press (upper plate of constant-resistance exercise machine) for assessing strength of the upper and lower body, respectively. To determine relative strength, divide the 1-RM values by the client's body weight. Norms for men and women are provided in tables 6.3 and 6.4.

Another test of dynamic strength includes six test items: bench press, arm curl, latissimus pull, leg press, leg extension, and leg curl. For each exercise, express and evaluate the 1-RM as a percentage of body weight. For example, if a 120-pound (54.5 kg)

Table 6.3   Age-Gender Norms for 1-RM Bench Press

Rating	<20 yr	20-29 yr	30-39 yr	40-49 yr	50-59 yr	60+ yr
Men						
Superior	≥1.34	≥1.32	≥1.12	≥1.00	≥0.90	≥0.82
Excellent	1.20-1.33	1.15-1.31	0.99-1.11	0.89-0.99	0.80-0.89	0.72-0.81
Good	1.07-1.19	1.00-1.14	0.89-0.98	0.81-0.88	0.72-0.79	0.67-0.71
Fair	0.90-1.06	0.89-0.99	0.79-0.88	0.730-.80	0.64-0.71	0.58-0.66
Poor	≤0.89	≤0.88	≤0.78	≤0.72	≤0.63	≤0.57
Women						
Superior	≥0.78	≥0.81	≥0.71	≥0.63	≥0.56	≥0.55
Excellent	0.66-0.77	0.71-0.80	0.61-0.70	0.55-0.62	0.49-0.55	0.48-0.54
Good	0.59-0.65	0.60-0.70	0.54-0.60	0.51-0.54	0.44-0.48	0.43-0.47
Fair	0.54-0.58	0.52-0.59	0.48-0.53	0.44-0.50	0.40-0.43	0.39-0.42
Poor	≤0.53	≤0.51	≤0.47	≤0.43	≤0.39	≤0.38

The Physical Fitness Specialist Certification Manual, The Cooper Institute for Aerobics Research, Dallas, TX, revised 1997.

Table 6.4   Age-Gender Norms for 1-RM Leg Press

Rating	<20 yr	20-29 yr	30-39 yr	40-49 yr	50-59 yr	60+ yr
Men						
Superior	≥2.28	≥2.13	≥1.93	≥1.82	≥1.71	≥1.62
Excellent	2.05-2.27	1.98-2.12	1.78-1.92	1.69-1.81	1.59-1.70	1.50-1.61
Good	1.91-2.04	1.84-1.97	1.66-1.77	1.58-1.68	1.47-1.58	1.39-1.49
Fair	1.71-1.90	1.64-1.83	1.53-1.65	1.45-1.57	1.33-1.46	1.26-1.38
Poor	≤1.70	≤1.63	≤1.52	≤1.44	≤1.32	≤1.25
Women						
Superior	≥1.71	≥1.68	≥1.47	≥1.37	≥1.25	≥1.18
Excellent	1.60-1.70	1.51-1.67	1.34-1.46	1.24-1.36	1.11-1.24	1.05-1.17
Good	1.39-1.59	1.38-1.50	1.22-1.33	1.14-1.23	1.00-1.10	0.94-1.04
Fair	1.23-1.38	1.23-1.37	1.10-1.21	1.03-1.13	0.89-0.99	0.86-0.93
Poor	≤1.22	≤1.22	≤1.09	≤1.02	≤0.88	≤0.85

The Physical Fitness Specialist Certification Manual, The Cooper Institute for Aerobics Research, Dallas, TX, revised 1997.

woman bench presses 60 pounds, (27.2 kg) her strength-to-body weight ratio is 0.50 (60 divided by 120), and she scores 3 points for that exercise. Follow this procedure for each exercise, then add the total points to determine the overall strength and fitness category of the individual. Strength-to-body weight ratios with corresponding point values for college-age men and women are presented in table 6.5.

Although you can safely administer 1-RM strength tests to individuals of all ages, you should take precautions to decrease the risk of injury when clients attempt to lift maximal loads. Be certain that your client warms up prior to attempting the lift and starts with a weight that is below the individual's expected 1-RM. When you administer these tests, you should spot your clients and closely monitor their lifting technique and breathing.

Dynamic Muscle Endurance Tests

You can assess your client's dynamic muscle endurance by having the individual perform as many repetitions as possible using a weight that is a set percentage of the body weight or maximum strength (1-RM). Pollock, Wilmore, and Fox (1978) recommend using a weight that is 70% of the 1-RM value for each exercise. Although norms for this test have not been established, these authors suggest, based on their testing and research findings, that the average individual should be able to complete 12 to 15 repetitions.

Table 6.5   Strength-to-Body Weight Ratios for Selected 1-RM Tests[a]

Bench press	Arm curl	Lat pull-down	Leg press	Leg extension	Leg curl	Points
Men						
1.50	0.70	1.20	3.00	0.80	0.70	10
1.40	0.65	1.15	2.80	0.75	0.65	9
1.30	0.60	1.10	2.60	0.70	0.60	8
1.20	0.55	1.05	2.40	0.65	0.55	7
1.10	0.50	1.00	2.20	0.60	0.50	6
1.00	0.45	0.95	2.00	0.55	0.45	5
0.90	0.40	0.90	1.80	0.50	0.40	4
0.80	0.35	0.85	1.60	0.45	0.35	3
0.70	0.30	0.80	1.40	0.40	0.30	2
0.60	0.25	0.75	1.20	0.35	0.25	1
Women						
0.90	0.50	0.85	2.70	0.70	0.60	10
0.85	0.45	0.80	2.50	0.65	0.55	9
0.80	0.42	0.75	2.30	0.60	0.52	8
0.70	0.38	0.73	2.10	0.55	0.50	7
0.65	0.35	0.70	2.00	0.52	0.45	6
0.60	0.32	0.65	1.80	0.50	0.40	5
0.55	0.28	0.63	1.60	0.45	0.35	4
0.50	0.25	0.60	1.40	0.40	0.30	3
0.45	0.21	0.55	1.20	0.35	0.25	2
0.35	0.18	0.50	1.00	0.30	0.20	1

Total points	Strength fitness category[b]
48-60	Excellent
37-47	Good
25-36	Average
13-24	Fair
0-12	Poor

[a]Refer to appendix C.3 for descriptions of exercises.

[b]Based on data compiled by author for 250 college-age men and women

The YMCA (Golding, Meyers, and Sinning 1989) recommends using a bench press test to assess dynamic muscular endurance of the upper body. For this absolute endurance test, use a flat bench and barbell. The client performs as many repetitions as possible at a set cadence of 30 repetitions per minute. Use a metronome to establish the exercise cadence. Male clients lift an 80-pound (36.4 kg) barbell, whereas female clients use a 35-pound (15.9 kg) barbell. Terminate the test when the client is unable to maintain the exercise cadence. Table 6.6 presents norms for this test.

Alternatively, you can use a test battery of seven items to assess dynamic muscular endurance. Set the weight as a set percentage of the individual's body weight, to be lifted up to a maximum of 15 repetitions. Table 6.7 provides percentages for each test item, as well as the scoring system and norms for college-age men and women.

Dynamic Muscle Testing Using Isokinetic and Omnikinetic Exercise Modes

Isokinetic dynamometers provide an accurate and reliable assessment of strength, endurance, and power of muscle groups (see figure 6.4). The speed of limb movement is kept at a constant preselected

Table 6.6   YMCA Bench Press Test Norms*

Percentile	18-25	26-35	36-45	46-55	56-65	>65
Men						
95	42	40	34	28	24	20
75	30	26	24	20	14	10
50	22	20	17	12	8	6
25	13	12	10	6	4	2
5	2	2	2	1	0	0
Women						
95	42	40	32	30	30	22
75	28	25	21	20	16	12
50	20	17	13	11	9	6
25	12	9	8	5	3	2
5	2	1	1	0	0	0

Column headers span **Age group (yr)**.

*Score is number of repetitions completed using 80-lb barbell for men and 35-lb barbell for women.

Data from Golding, Meyers, and Sinning (1989). *The Y's way to physical fitness* (3rd ed.) Champaign, IL: Human Kinetics. Reprinted from *The Y's way to physical fitness* with permission of the YMCA of the USA, 101 N. Wacker Drive, Chicago, IL 60606.

Table 6.7   Dynamic Muscular Endurance Test Battery

Exercise[a]	Men	Women	Repetitions (max = 15)
Arm curl	0.33	0.25	_____
Bench press	0.66	0.50	_____
Lat pull-down	0.66	0.50	_____
Triceps extension	0.33	0.33	_____
Leg extension	0.50	0.50	_____
Leg curl	0.33	0.33	_____
Bent-knee sit-up	—	—	_____

Men/Women columns are under **% body weight to be lifted**.

Total repetitions (max = 105) _____

Total repetitions	Fitness category[b]
91-105	Excellent
77-90	Very good
63-76	Good
49-62	Fair
35-48	Poor
<35	Very poor

[a]Refer to appendix C.3 for descriptions of exercises.
[b]Based on data compiled by author for 250 college-age men and women

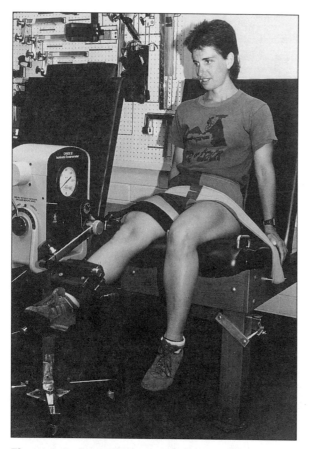

Figure 6.4   Cybex II™ isokinetic dynamometer.

velocity. Any increase in muscular force produces an increased resistance rather than increased acceleration of the limb. Thus, fluctuations in muscular force throughout the ROM are matched by an equal counterforce or *accommodating resistance*.

Isokinetic dynamometers measure muscular torque production at speeds of 0° to 300° · sec^{-1}. From the recorded output, you can evaluate peak torque, total work, and power. Some less expensive isokinetic dynamometers lack this recording capability but are suitable for training and rehabilitation exercise.

Omnikinetic exercise dynamometers (see figure 6.5) provide maximum overload at every joint angle throughout the ROM at whatever speed the individual is capable of generating. This testing system provides an accommodating resistance that adjusts to both the force and velocity output of the individual and is not limited to a preset velocity of limb movement. Thus, at any one setting, the individual maximally overloads both the force and velocity production capabilities of the contractile elements. The stronger the individual, the faster the speed of limb movement at any given setting. Also, increasing limb velocity results in increased resistance. Even as the muscle fatigues, the individual receives optimal overload with each repetition because the limb speed and resistance decrease. Theoretically, movement at slower speeds will allow recruitment of motor units that were not contributing to the total

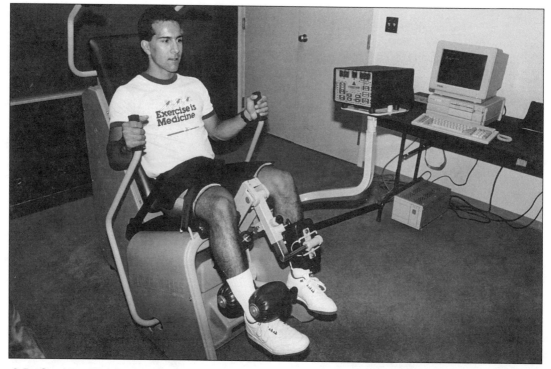

Figure 6.5   Omni-tron™ dynamometer.

force production in earlier repetitions performed at faster speeds. Self-accommodating, variable resistance–variable velocity exercise devices therefore assess the isokinetic strength and endurance of both fast-twitch and slow-twitch motor units in the muscle group.

Table 6.8 summarizes isokinetic and omnikinetic test protocols for assessing strength, endurance, and power. For detailed descriptions of isokinetic test protocols and test norms, see Perrin (1993). Appendix C.1 provides omnikinetic performance norms for young and middle-aged men and women, as well as male and female weight trainers.

CALISTHENIC-TYPE STRENGTH AND MUSCULAR ENDURANCE TESTS

In certain field situations, you may not have access to dynamometers, free weights, or exercise machines to assess muscular fitness. As an alternative, you may use calisthenic-type strength and endurance tests to assess your client's strength and muscular endurance.

Dynamic Strength Tests

You can measure dynamic strength using calisthenic-type exercises by determining the maximum weight, in excess of body weight, that an individual can lift for one repetition of the movement. Because strength is related to the size and body weight of the individual, Johnson and Nelson (1986) recommend using relative strength scores. For each test, attach weight plates (2-1/2, 5, 10, and 25 pounds or 1, 2.3, 4.5, and 11.4 kg) to the individual. The relative strength score is the amount of additional weight divided by the body weight. For example, if a 150-pound (68.2 kg) man successfully performs one pull-up with a 30-pound (13.6 kg) weight attached to the waist belt, his relative strength score is 0.20 (30 lb/150 lb). Test protocols and performance norms for the pull-up, dip strength, sit-up, and bench squat are described elsewhere (Johnson and Nelson 1986).

Dynamic Endurance Tests

You can assess dynamic muscular endurance by measuring the maximum number of repetitions for each calisthenic-type exercise. Test protocols and

Table 6.8   Isokinetic and Omnikinetic Test Protocols

Isokinetic tests	Speed setting	Protocol	Measure[*]
Strength	30° to 60° · sec⁻¹	2 submax practice trials, followed by 3 maximal trials	Peak torque (ft-lb or Nm)
Endurance	120° to 180° · sec⁻¹	1 maximal trial	Number of repetitions until torque reaches 50% of initial value
Power	120° to 300° · sec⁻¹	2 submax practice trials, followed by 3 maximal trials	Peak torque (ft-lb or Nm)

Omnikinetic tests	Resistance setting	Protocol	Measure[*]
Strength	10	2 submax trials at resistance setting 2, followed by 5 maximal trials	Peak torque (ft-lb)
Endurance	3	3 practice trials at resistance setting 2, followed by 20 maximal repetitions	Total work output (ft-lb)
Power	6	3 submax trials, followed by 1 maximal trial	Peak torque or total work (ft-lb)

[*]ft-lb = foot-pound; Nm = newton-meter; 1 ft-lb = 0.138 Nm.

norms for some commonly-used muscular endurance tests (e.g., pull-ups, sit-ups, and dips) are presented elsewhere (Johnson and Nelson 1986).

Because many women and children are unable to perform even one pull-up, the timed flexed arm hang is commonly used for these groups. However, the flexed arm hang measures isometric endurance. To assess dynamic endurance of the arm and shoulder girdle musculature, Baumgartner (1978) developed a modified pull-up test that uses an inclined board (30° angle to floor) with a pull-up bar at the top. A scooter board was modified to slide along garage door tracks attached to the inclined board (Baumgartner et al. 1984). While lying prone on the scooter board and grasping the pull-up bar, the individual pulls up until the chin is over the pull-up bar. Detailed testing procedures, equipment design, and performance norms for children, adolescents and college-age men and women are available (Baumgartner 1978; Baumgartner et al. 1984).

The ACSM (1995) recommends using a push-up test to assess endurance of the upper body musculature. When you are testing men, have the client assume a standard push-up position, with back straight, head up, and hands placed shoulder width apart. Place your fist on the floor beneath the client's chest, and count the repetition only if his chest contacts your fist during each repetition. For women, modify the standard push-up position by having the client assume a kneeling position with the knees flexed to 90° and the ankles crossed. There is no set criterion for determining how far the body must be lowered during each repetition. Score the push-up test for men and women as the maximum number

of consecutive repetitions performed without rest. Table 6.9 provides norms for the push-up test.

MUSCULAR FITNESS TESTING: SOURCES OF MEASUREMENT ERROR

The validity and reliability of strength and muscular endurance measures are affected by client factors, equipment, technician skill, and environmental factors. You must control each of these factors to ensure the accuracy and precision of muscular fitness scores.

Client Factors

Prior to measuring your clients' strength or muscular endurance, familiarize them with the equipment and testing procedures. Clients with limited or no prior weightlifting experience need time to practice each lift to control for the effects of learning on performance. Even experienced weight lifters should be given time to practice so you can correct any improper lifting techniques prior to testing.

Muscular fitness tests require each client to give a maximal effort. Therefore, adequate sleep is needed, and you should restrict client's use of drugs and medications that may adversely affect their performance. It is also important that you motivate your clients during testing by encouraging them to do their best and by giving them positive feedback

Table 6.9 Age-Gender Norms for Push-Up Test					
Classification	**20-29 yr**	**30-39 yr**	**40-49 yr**	**50-59 yr**	**60+ yr**
Men					
Superior	≥48	≥40	≥31	≥26	≥24
Excellent	38-47	31-39	25-30	20-25	19-23
Good	30-37	25-30	19-24	14-19	11-18
Fair	23-29	18-24	12-18	10-13	7-10
Poor	≤22	≤17	≤11	≤9	≤6
Women*					
Superior	≥37	≥32	≥25	≥21	≥15
Excellent	31-36	25-31	19-24	18-20	13-14
Good	24-30	20-24	14-18	13-17	6-12
Fair	18-23	12-19	7-13	7-12	3-5
Poor	≤17	≤11	≤6	≤6	≤2

*Norms for modified push-ups

The Physical Fitness Specialist Certification Manual, The Cooper Institute for Aerobics Research, Dallas, TX, revised 1997.

after each trial. Adequate rest between trials is necessary in order to obtain a score that truly represents your client's maximal effort.

Equipment

The design of testing equipment may also affect your client's test scores. Most of the dynamic strength and muscular endurance protocols and norms in this chapter were developed using constant-resistance exercise machines. Therefore, you should not use free weights and variable-resistance machines when administering the tests. It is also important to calibrate the equipment and make sure that it is in proper working condition prior to testing. Inspection and maintenance of equipment will increase accuracy and decrease the risk of accidents. When selecting exercise machines, make sure that the equipment can be properly adjusted to accommodate varying limb lengths and body sizes. Use equipment specifically designed for smaller individuals when testing children and smaller adults.

Technician Skill

All strength testing should be done by qualified, trained technicians who are knowledgeable about proper lifting and spotting techniques and familiar with standardized testing procedures. After explaining and demonstrating the proper lifting technique, give your client ample time to practice the lift, correcting any performance errors you see as the client practices. During the test, clients may inadvertently "cheat" by moving extraneous body parts to help lift the weight. Carefully observe the client during the test, focusing on the grip used and starting position. The type of grip (pronated vs supinated) has a substantial effect on performance. For example, using a narrow grip instead of a wide grip during a lat-pulldown exercise increases the amount of weight that can be lifted. Likewise, the client will be able to produce more force during an arm curl using a supinated grip compared to a pronated grip. The client's starting position may also affect strength scores. During the bench press, for example, eccentric movement (i.e., lowering the weight) prior to the concentric phase of the lift will increase maximal muscular force due to the stretch reflex and the tendency for the client to "bounce" the weight off the chest. To obtain accurate assessments of your client's strength, it is important to standardize starting positions and to follow all testing procedures carefully.

Environmental Factors

Factors such as room temperature and humidity may affect test scores. The room temperature should be 70° to 74° F (21° to 23° C) to maximize client comfort during testing. Ideally, you want a quiet, clean environment with limited distractions (e.g., avoid an overcrowded weight room). When assessing improvements due to training, remember to pretest and posttest your client at the same time of day to control for diurnal variations in strength.

ADDITIONAL CONSIDERATIONS FOR MUSCULAR FITNESS TESTING

A number of additional factors and questions need to be addressed when assessing static and dynamic muscle strength and endurance of your clients.

Can Strength or Muscular Endurance Be Assessed by a Single Test?

Strength and endurance are specific to the muscle group, the type of muscular contraction (static or dynamic), the speed of muscular contraction (slow or fast), and the joint angle being tested (static contraction). There is no single test to evaluate total body muscle strength or endurance. Minimally, the strength test battery should include a measure of abdominal, lower-extremity, and upper-extremity strength. In addition, if the individual trains dynamically, select a dynamic, not static, test to assess strength or endurance levels before and after training.

You should also use caution in selecting test items to measure muscle strength. The maximum number of sit-ups, pull-ups, or push-ups that an individual can perform measures muscular endurance; yet, maximum repetition tests have been included in some strength test batteries. This may lead to misinterpretation of the test results.

Is It Safe to Give 1-RM Tests to Children and Older Adults?

It is safe to administer 1-RM tests to clients of all ages if appropriate procedures are used (Kraemer and Fleck 1993; Shaw, McCully, and Posner 1995). The risk of injury in older adults (55 to 80 years) is low, with only 2.4% of older adults experiencing an injury during 1-RM assessments (Shaw et al. 1995). However, some experts recommend using 6-RM tests to assess the strength of children (Kraemer and Fry 1995).

Alternatively, you can estimate the 1-RM of older clients, children, and adolescents from submaximal muscle endurance tests. Research demonstrates a strong relationship between muscle endurance (measured as the number of repetitions to fatigue) and the percentage of 1-RM lifted (Brzycki 1993). Muscular strength (1-RM) therefore can be predicted from muscular endurance tests with a fair degree of accuracy (Ball and Rose 1991; Braith et al. 1993; Invergo, Ball, and Looney 1991; Kuramato and Payne 1995; Mayhew et al. 1992). For this purpose, use the Brzycki (1993) equation to estimate 1-RM of men. This equation can be used for any combination of submaximal weights and repetitions to fatigue providing that the repetitions to fatigue do not exceed 10.

1-RM = weight lifted (lb)/[1.0278 − (reps to fatigue × 0.0278)]

For example, if your client completes 7 repetitions to fatigue during a bench press exercise using a 100-pound barbell, the estimated 1-RM is calculated as follows:

1-RM = 100 pounds/[1.0278 − (7 reps × 0.0278)]

1-RM = 120 pounds (54.5 kg)

For middle-aged and older women, Kuramoto and Payne (1995) developed prediction equations to estimate 1-RM from a submaximal muscular endurance test. For this endurance protocol, the client completes as many repetitions as possible using a weight equivalent to 45% of her body weight. To estimate 1-RM, use the following equations:

Middle-Aged Women (40 to 50 years)

1-RM = (1.06 × weight lifted in kg) + (0.58 × repetitions) − (0.20 × age) − 3.41

R^2_{mc} = .95, SEE = 1.85 kg

Older Women (60 to 70 years)

1-RM = (0.92 × weight lifted in kg) + (0.79 × repetitions) − 3.73

R^2_{mc} = .91, SEE = 2.04 kg

How Is Muscle Balance Assessed?

Muscle strength is important for joint stability; however, a strength imbalance between opposing muscle groups (e.g., quadriceps femoris and hamstrings) may compromise joint stability and increase the risk of musculoskeletal injury. For this reason, experts recommend maintaining a balance in strength between agonist and antagonistic muscle groups.

Muscle balance ratios differ among muscle groups and are affected by the force-velocity of muscle groups at specific joints. To control limb velocity during muscle balance testing, you will do best to use isokinetic dynamometers. In field settings, however, you can obtain a crude index of muscle balance by comparing 1-RM values of muscle groups. Based on isokinetic tests of peak torque production at slow speeds (30° to 60° · sec⁻¹), the following muscle balance ratios are recommended for agonist and antagonistic muscle groups:

Muscle groups	Muscle balance ratio
Hip extensors and flexors	1:1
Elbow extensors and flexors	1:1
Trunk extensors and flexors	1:1
Ankle invertors and evertors	1:1
Shoulder flexors and extensors	2:3
Knee extensors and flexors	3:2
Shoulder internal and external rotators	3:2
Ankle plantar flexors and dorsiflexors	3:1

Muscle balance between other pairs of muscle groups is also important. The difference in strength between contralateral (right vs left sides) muscle groups should be no more than 10 to 15%, and the relative strength of the upper-body (bench press 1-RM/BW) should be at least 40 to 60% of the lower-body relative strength (leg press 1-RM/BW). If you detect imbalances, prescribe additional exercises for the weaker muscle groups.

Additional Questions

1. Should absolute or relative measures be used to classify a client's muscle strength?

Because strength is directly related to the body weight and lean body weight of the individual, you should express the test results in relative terms. This is especially true for making group comparisons and for assessing individual improvement due to training.

2. How can the influence of strength on muscular endurance be controlled?

Performance on some endurance tests (e.g., pull-ups and push-ups) is highly dependent on the strength of the individual. It is recommended that you use relative endurance tests that are proportional to the body weight or maximum strength of the individual to assess muscle endurance. You cannot use a pull-up test to assess muscular endurance if the individual is not strong enough to lift the body weight for one repetition of that exercise. Therefore, select a modified or submaximal (percentage of body weight) endurance test.

3. Are there comprehensive norms that can be used to classify muscular fitness levels of diverse population subgroups?

There are no up-to-date endurance norms for men and women, especially for older adults. New norms need to be established for this population in particular.

Key Points

- Strength is the ability of a muscle group to exert maximal contractile force against a resistance in a single contraction.
- Muscular endurance is the ability of a muscle group to exert submaximal force for an extended duration.
- Both strength and muscular endurance are specific to the muscle group and to the type of muscle contraction—static, concentric, eccentric, or isokinetic.
- The greatest resistance that can be used during dynamic, concentric muscular contraction with a constant-resistance exercise mode is equal to the maximum weight that can be moved at the weakest point in the range of motion.
- Dynamometers, cable tensiometers, and load cells are used to measure static strength and endurance.
- Constant-resistance modes of exercise (free weights and exercise machines) are used to assess dynamic (i.e., concentric and eccentric) strength and endurance.
- The accommodating resistance mode of exercise is used to assess isokinetic and omnikinetic strength, endurance, and power.

- Calisthenic-type exercise tests provide a crude index of strength and endurance but can be used when other equipment is not available.
- Strength should be expressed relative to the body weight or lean body weight of the individual.
- Muscular endurance tests should take into account the body weight or maximal strength of the individual.
- Test batteries should include a minimum of three to four items that measure upper-body, lower-body, and abdominal strength or endurance.
- It is important to follow standardized testing procedures and to control for extraneous variables (e.g., motivation level, time of testing, isolation of body parts, and joint angles) when assessing strength and muscular endurance.
- It is safe to give 1-RM strength tests to children and older adults if appropriate testing procedures are followed.
- Although strength can be predicted from submaximal endurance tests, 1-RM assessments are preferable.

SOURCES FOR EQUIPMENT

Product	Manufacturer's Address
Body masters (constant and variable resistance)	Body Masters Sports Industry 700 E. Texas Ave. Rayne, LA 70578 (800) 325-8964
Cable tensiometer (static)	Pacific Scientific Co., Inc. 110 Fordham Rd. Wilmington, MA 01887 (888) 772-6284
CAM II (variable resistance)	Keiser Sports Health Equipment 411 S. West Ave. Fresno, CA 93706 (800) 888-7009
CYBEX II, Orthotron (isokinetic)	Cybex 2100 Smithtown Ave. Ronkonkoma, NY 11779 (800) 645-5392

Free weights (constant resistance)	York Barbell Co. 3300 Boar Rd. York, PA 17402 (800) 358-YORK
Handgrip dyna-mometer (static)	Creative Health Products 5148 Saddle Ridge Rd. Plymouth, MI 48170 (800) 742-4478
Leg / back dyna-mometer (static)	Best Priced Products P.O. Box 1174 White Plains, NY 10602 (800) 824-2939
Nautilus (variable resistance)	Nautilus International P.O. Box 708 Independence, VA 24348 (800) 628-8458
Omni-tron Total Power (omnikinetic)	Hydra-fitness 120 Industrial Blvd. Sugarland, TX 77478 (800) 433-3111
Total Gym machines (variable resistance)	Total Gym/EFI 7766 Arjons Dr., Ste B San Diego, CA 92126 (800) 541-4900
Universal Gym Machines (constant and variable resistance)	Universal Gym Equipment, Inc. 515 N. Flaggler, 4th Floor Pavilion W. Palm Beach, FL 33406 (800) 843-3906

REFERENCES

American College of Sports Medicine. 1995. *ACSM's guidelines for exercise testing and prescription*. Baltimore: Williams & Wilkins.

Ball, T.E., and Rose, K.S. 1991. A field test for predicting maximum bench press lift of college women. *Journal of Applied Sport Science Research* 5: 169-170.

Baumgartner, T.A. 1978. Modified pull-up test. *Research Quarterly* 49: 80-84.

Baumgartner, T.A., East, W.B., Frye, P.A., Hensley, L.D., Knox, D.F., and Norton, C.J. 1984. Equipment improvements and additional norms for the modified pull-up test. *Research Quarterly for Exercise and Sport* 55: 64-68.

Braith, R.W., Graves, J.E., Leggett, S.H., and Pollock, M.L. 1993. Effect of training on the relationship between maximal and submaximal strength. *Medicine and Science in Sports and Exercise* 25: 132-138.

Brzycki, M. 1993. Strength testing—Predicting a one-rep max from reps-to-fatigue. *Journal of Physical Education, Recreation, and Dance* 64 (1): 88-90.

Clarke, D.H. 1975. *Exercise physiology*. Englewood Cliffs, NJ: Prentice-Hall.

Clarke, H.H. 1966. *Muscular strength and endurance in man*. Englewood Cliffs, NJ: Prentice-Hall.

Clarke, H.H., and Monroe, R.A. 1970. *Test manual: Oregon cable-tension strength test batteries for boys and girls from fourth grade through college*. Eugene, OR: University of Oregon.

Corbin, C.B., Dowell, L.J., Lindsey, R., and Tolson, H. 1978. *Concepts in physical education*. Dubuque, IA: Brown.

Golding, L.A., Meyers, C.R., and Sinning, W.E. 1989. *The Y's way to physical fitness*, 3rd ed. Champaign, IL: Human Kinetics.

Invergo, J.J., Ball, T.E., and Looney, M. 1991. Relationship of pushups and absolute muscular endurance to bench press strength. *Journal of Applied Sport Science Research* 5: 121-125.

Johnson, B.L., and Nelson, J.K., eds. 1986. *Practical measurements for evaluation in physical education*. Minneapolis, MN: Burgess.

Knuttgen, H.G., and Kraemer, W.J. 1987. Terminology and measurement in exercise performance. *Journal of Applied Sport Science Research* 1: 1-10.

Kraemer, W.J., and Fleck, S.J. 1993. *Strength training for young athletes*. Champaign, IL: Human Kinetics.

Kraemer, W.J., and Fry, A.C. 1995. Strength testing: Development and evaluation of methodology. In P.J. Maud and C. Foster, eds., *Physiological assessment of human fitness*, 115-138. Champaign, IL: Human Kinetics.

Kreighbaum, E., and Barthels, K.M. (1981). *Biomechanics: A qualitative approach for studying human movement*. Minneapolis, MN: Burgess.

Kuramoto, A.K., and Payne, V.G. (1995). Predicting muscular strength in women: A preliminary study. *Research Quarterly for Exercise and Sport* 66: 168-172.

Mayhew, J.L., Ball, T.E., Arnold, M.D., and Bowen, J.C. (1992). Relative muscular endurance performance as a predictor of bench press strength in college men and women. *Journal of Applied Sport Science Research* 6: 200-206.

Montoye, H.J., and Faulkner, J.A. (1964). Determination of the optimum setting of an adjustable grip dynamometer. *Research Quarterly* 35: 29-36.

Perrin, D.H. (1993). *Isokinetic exercise and assessment*. Champaign, IL: Human Kinetics.

Pollock, M.L., Wilmore, J.H., and Fox, S.M. III. (1978). *Health and fitness through physical activity*. New York: Wiley.

Shaw, C.E., McCully, K.K., and Posner, J.D. (1995). Injuries during the one repetition maximum assessment in the elderly. *Journal of Cardiopulmonary Rehabilitation* 15: 283-287.

CHAPTER 7

Designing Resistance Training Programs

Key Questions

- How do training principles specifically apply to the design of resistance training programs?
- Which type of resistance training (static, dynamic, or isokinetic) is most effective for improving strength and muscle endurance?
- How are resistance training programs modified to optimize the development of strength, muscular endurance, muscle tone, or muscle size?
- What factors need to be considered when designing individualized exercise prescriptions?
- Is resistance training recommended for children, adolescents, and older adults?
- What methods can be used to design advanced resistance training programs?
- What are the outcomes and health benefits of resistance training?
- What is the cause of delayed-onset muscle soreness, and can it be prevented?

Muscular strength and endurance are important to the overall health and physical fitness of your clients, enabling them to engage in physically active leisure-time pursuits, to perform activities of daily living more easily, and to maintain functional independence later in life. Weight resistance training is a systematic program of exercise for development of the muscular system. Although the primary outcome of weight resistance training is improved strength and muscular endurance, a number of health benefits also are derived from this form of exercise. Resistance exercise builds bone mass, thereby counteracting the loss of bone mineral (osteoporosis) and risk of falls as one ages. This form of training also lowers blood pressure in hypertensive individuals, reduces body fat levels, and may prevent the development of low back syndrome.

While resistance training is widely used by bodybuilders, powerlifters, and competitive athletes to develop strength and muscle size, participation in weightlifting by individuals of all ages and levels of athletic interest has increased dramatically over the past 15 years. The popularity and widespread appeal of weightlifting exercise for general muscle conditioning challenge exercise specialists and personal trainers to develop resistance training programs that can meet the diverse needs of their clients.

This chapter shows you how to apply basic training principles (see chapter 3) to the design of resistance training programs for novice, intermediate, and advanced weightlifters. The chapter also presents guidelines for developing programs for general muscle toning and conditioning, for strength

121

and muscular endurance, and for muscle hypertrophy. There is also a discussion of common concerns and misconceptions about weightlifting.

APPLICATION OF TRAINING PRINCIPLES TO WEIGHT RESISTANCE EXERCISE

To develop effective weight resistance training programs, you must apply the training principles presented in chapter 3. By varying the combination of intensity, duration, and frequency of exercise, you can design programs that meet the unique goals and needs of each client.

Specificity Principle

The development of muscular fitness is specific to the muscle group that is exercised, the type of contraction, and the training intensity. To increase the dynamic strength of the elbow flexors, for example, you must select exercises that involve the concentric and eccentric contractions of that particular muscle group. For strength, the exercises are performed at a high intensity with low repetitions; exercising at a low intensity with high repetitions stimulates the development of muscular endurance.

Strength and endurance gains are also specific to the speed and range of motion used during the training. With isometric training, strength gains at angles other than the training angle are typically 50% less than those at the exercised angle (Gardner 1963). Similarly, with isokinetic training, the strength gain may be limited to velocities at or below the training velocity (Lesmes et al. 1978; Moffroid and Whipple 1970).

Overload Principle

To promote strength and endurance gains, the muscle group must be exercised at work loads that are greater than normal for the client. The exercise intensity should be at least 60% of maximum to stimulate the development of strength (McArdle, Katch, and Katch 1996). More rapid strength gains may be achieved, however, by exercising the muscle at or near maximum (80 to 100%) resistance (Stone and Kroll 1978). To stimulate endurance gains, intensities as low as 30% of maximum may be used;

however, at low intensities the muscle group should be exercised to the point of fatigue.

Progression Principle

Throughout the resistance training program you must periodically increase the training volume, or total amount of work performed, to continue overloading the muscle so that further improvements in strength and muscular endurance can be made. The progression needs to be gradual, because doing too much too soon may cause musculoskeletal injuries and excessive muscle soreness. Typically, muscle groups are progressively overloaded by increasing the resistance or amount of weight lifted. As clients adapt to the training stimulus, they will be able to perform more repetitions at the prescribed resistance. Thus, the number of repetitions a client is able to perform will indicate when the resistance needs to be increased throughout the training program.

Additional Principles

Individuals with lower initial strength will show greater relative gains and a faster rate of improvement in response to resistance training compared to those starting out with higher strength levels (principles of initial values and individual variability). However, the rate of improvement slows, and eventually plateaus, as clients progress through the program and move closer to their genetic ceiling (principle of diminishing returns). Also, when the individual reduces the training volume or stops resistance training, the physiological adaptations and improvements in muscle structure and function are reversed (principle of reversibility). Using periodization techniques (for description, see variations for training volume and intensity on page 126), you can lessen the effects of detraining on athletes and maintain strength during the competitive period by manipulating the intensity and volume of the resistance training exercise (see Wathen 1994).

TYPES OF RESISTANCE TRAINING

Muscular fitness can be improved using various types of resistance training—static (isometric), dynamic (concentric and eccentric), and isokinetic. Although there are general guidelines for designing static, dynamic, and isokinetic resistance training programs, you need to individualize each exercise prescription to meet the specific needs and goals of your client.

Static (Isometric) Training

In 1953, Hettinger and Muller reported that significant gains in static strength (5% per week) are produced by holding one 6-second contraction at 2/3 of maximum intensity, 5 days a week. This type of training became popular in the late 1950s and early 1960s because the exercises could be performed anywhere and at any time with little or no equipment. A major disadvantage is that strength gains are specific to the joint angle used during training (Gardner 1963). Thus, to increase strength throughout the range of motion, the exercise needs to be performed at a number of different joint angles (e.g., 30°, 60°, 90°, 120°, and 180° of knee flexion).

Static exercise is widely used in rehabilitation programs to counteract strength loss and muscle atrophy, especially for cases in which the limb is temporarily immobilized. This type of training, however, is contraindicated for coronary-prone and hypertensive individuals because the static contraction may produce large increases in intrathoracic pressure. This reduces the venous return to the heart, increases the work of the heart, and causes a substantial rise in blood pressure.

After further research, Hettinger and Muller modified their original exercise prescription. Table 7.1 presents general guidelines for designing training programs to develop static strength and endurance. For descriptions and illustrations of static exercises for different muscle groups, see appendix C.2.

Dynamic Resistance Training

In recent years, the popularity of dynamic resistance training has risen in the United States. This type of training is suitable for developing muscular fitness of men and women of all ages, as well as children. Dynamic resistance training involves concentric and eccentric contractions of the muscle group performed against a constant or variable resistance. For this type of training, people typically use free weights (barbells and dumbbells) and constant- or variable-resistance machines.

Several important concepts used to prescribe dynamic resistance training programs are intensity, repetitions, set, training volume, and order of exercises (Fleck and Kraemer 1997). *Intensity* is expressed either as a percentage of the individual's *1-RM* or as the maximum weight that can be lifted for a given number of repetitions of an exercise (e.g., 8-RM equals the maximum weight that can be lifted for 8 repetitions). The number of repetitions corresponding to various percentages of 1-RM are as follows:

60% 1-RM = 15 to 20-RM	**85% 1-RM = 6-RM**
65% 1-RM = 14-RM	**90% 1-RM = 4-RM**
70% 1-RM = 12-RM	**95% 1-RM = 2-RM**
75% 1-RM = 10-RM	**100% 1-RM = 1-RM**
80% 1-RM = 8-RM	

Intensity is inversely related to *repetitions*. In other words, individuals are able to perform more repetitions using lighter resistances or weights and vice versa. A *set* consists of a given number of consecutive repetitions of the exercise. *Training volume* is the total amount of weight lifted during the workout and is calculated by summing the products of the weight lifted, repetitions, and sets for each exercise.

The optimal training stimulus for strength development is *high intensity-low repetitions*; whereas, *low intensity-high repetitions* optimize muscular endurance gains. Although novice weightlifters will

Table 7.1   Guidelines for Designing Static (Isometric) Training Programs

Type	Intensity	Duration	Repetitions	Frequency	Length of program
Static strength	100% MVC[*]	5 sec/contraction	5-10	5 days/week	4 weeks or more
Static endurance	60% MVC or less	Until fatigued	1/session	5 days/week	4 weeks or more

[*]Maximal voluntary contraction

experience muscular fitness gains from low training volumes (1 to 2 sets using moderate resistances and repetitions, 2 days per week), large training volumes (5 to 6 sets, 5 to 6 days per week) are prescribed for advanced resistance training programs.

Table 7.2 presents the ACSM (1995b) guidelines for apparently healthy adults, older adults, and children who are beginning a resistance training program. For clients with resistance training experience, you need to modify these guidelines based on the client's goals, initial muscular fitness level, and time available for exercising.

You can tailor dynamic resistance training programs to optimize the development of muscle strength, tone, size (hypertrophy), or endurance by varying the intensity, repetitions, sets, and frequency of training. Table 7.3 presents guidelines for designing these types of resistance training programs for novice and advanced weightlifters. For descriptions and illustrations of dynamic resistance training exercises, see appendix C.3.

Intensity

To optimize strength gains, the intensity should be set at 80 to 85% 1-RM. At this intensity, most individuals are able to perform 6 to 8 repetitions (6- to 8-RM) of the exercise. However, when your client's primary goal is to develop muscular endurance, prescribe an intensity of ≤60% 1-RM (15 to 20-RM) Although low-to-moderate intensity is best suited for muscle endurance and toning, your clients also will experience some strength gains. The degree and rate of strength gain, however, will be less compared to a program designed specifically to optimize strength development (specificity principle). For advanced strength training and hypertrophy programs, large training volumes are achieved by increasing the number of sets, performing multiple exercises for each muscle group, and increasing the frequency of training. For programs designed specifically to increase muscle size, you also can maximize the client's training volume by

Table 7.2   ACSM (1995) Guidelines for Resistance Training

Group	Intensity	Repetitions	Sets	Frequency	No. of exercises per muscle group
Apparently healthy adults	70-80% 1-RM	8-12	1	≥2	1
Older adults[a]	70-80% 1-RM	8-12	1	≥2	1
Children[a, b]	≤70% 1-RM	≥8-12	1-2	2	1

[a]Multi-joint exercises are recommended for older adults and children.
[b]Programs for children and adolescents should be closely supervised by trained personnel.

Table 7.3   Guidelines for Designing Dynamic Resistance Training Programs

Type	Intensity	Repetitions	Sets	Frequency	Length of program
Strength (novice)	80-85% 1-RM or 6-8 RM	6-8	3	3	6 weeks or more
Strength (advanced)	80-90% 1-RM or 4-8 RM	4-8	5-6	5-6	12 weeks or more
Toning	60-70% 1-RM or 12-15 RM	12-15	3	3	6 weeks or more
Endurance	≤60% 1-RM or 15-20 RM	15-20	3	3	6 weeks or more
Hypertrophy (advanced)	70-75% 1-RM or 10-12 RM	10-12	5-6	5-6	12 weeks or more

using a combination of moderate intensities and repetitions.

Sets

Although improvements in muscular fitness may result from performing only one set of a given exercise, research suggests that multiple sets (3 or more) are more beneficial for optimal gains in muscular fitness (Berger 1962a; Berger 1962b; Berger and Hardage 1967; Clarke 1973; Clarke 1974). The number of sets and individual exercises for each muscle group in the prescription depends not only on your client's goal but also on the time available for each workout. For clients who are pressed for time, one set for each of the major muscle groups (total of 8 to 10 exercises) can be effective, particularly for those with low initial muscular fitness levels. In contrast, you should prescribe 5 to 6 sets of multiple (2 to 3) exercises for each muscle group for advanced strength training and hypertrophy programs.

Frequency

Improvements in muscular fitness may result from exercising just one day per week, especially for clients with below-average muscular fitness. However, research suggests that exercising 3 times per week improves both the rate and amount of strength gain. For advanced resistance training programs, a frequency of 5 to 6 days per week will provide the high training volume necessary to stimulate further gains in muscle strength and size.

Order of Exercises

For a well-rounded resistance training program, include at least one exercise for each of the major muscle groups. In this way your client will maintain muscle balance—that is, the ratio of strength between opposing muscle groups (agonists vs antagonists), contralateral muscle groups (right vs left side), and upper- and lower-body muscle groups. Order the exercises so that your client first executes multi-joint exercises—such as the seated leg press, bench press, and lat pull-down—that involve larger muscles (e.g., gluteus maximus, pectoralis major, and latissimus dorsi) and more muscle groups. Then have your client progress to single-joint exercises for smaller muscle groups (see table 7.4). To avoid muscle fatigue in novice weightlifters, arrange the exercises so that successive exercises do not involve the same muscle group. This allows time for the muscle to recover.

Dynamic Resistance Training Methods

You can use a variety of methods to design dynamic resistance training programs. The majority of these methods are best suited for advanced programs. Each uses a different approach for prescribing sets, order of exercises, or frequency of workouts.

Variations for Sets

You can use either a *single set* or *multiple sets* of exercises. For multiple sets, have your client execute the designated number of sets (usually 3 or more) for each exercise consecutively. For circuit resistance training, however, have your client complete one set at each of 10 to 15 different exercise stations, and then repeat this circuit 1 or 2 times.

A client performing multiple sets may choose to lift the same weight for each of the sets or vary the intensity of each set by lifting progressively heavier *(light-to-heavy sets)* or lighter *(heavy-to-light sets)* weights. *Pyramiding* is a light-to-heavy system in which the client performs as many as 6 sets of each exercise. In the first set, the client lifts a relatively lighter weight for 10 to 12 repetitions (10- to 12-RM). In subsequent sets, the individual lifts progressively heavier weights (e.g., 8-RM, 6-RM, 4-RM, 2-RM, and 1-RM). Because this involves such a large volume of work, prescribe the pyramid system only for experienced weightlifters. This system is commonly used by bodybuilders to develop muscle size.

Variations for Order and Number of Exercises

Exercise scientists generally recommend exercising large muscle groups at the beginning of a workout, progressing to smaller muscle groups later in the workout. To maximize the overload of muscle groups, however, some clients may choose to *pre-exhaust* muscle groups by reversing this order. To do this, the individual first fatigues smaller muscles by using single-joint exercises prior to performing multi-joint exercises.

When you prescribe two or more exercises for a specific muscle group, instruct the average individual to *alternate muscle groups* so that the muscle can rest and recover between exercises. For example, your client should not perform leg press and leg extension exercises consecutively because the quadriceps femoris is used in both of these exercises. Instead, intersperse one or more exercises using different muscle groups between these two exercises.

In contrast, most *advanced* weightlifters prefer to do *compound sets* or *tri-sets* in order to completely

Table 7.4   Examples of Exercise Order for a Basic Resistance Training Program

Body segment	Type of exercise*	Joint actions	Exercise
1. Hips and thighs	Multi-joint	Hip extension and knee extension	Seated leg press
2. Chest	Multi-joint	Shoulder horizontal flexion and elbow extension	Flat bench press
3. Upper- and mid-back	Multi-joint	Shoulder extension/adduction and elbow flexion	Lat pull-down
4. Legs	Single-joint	Knee extension	Leg extension
5. Shoulders and upper arms	Multi-joint	Shoulder abduction and elbow flexion	Upright row
6. Lower back	Multi-joint	Trunk extension and hip extension	Back extension
7. Upper arms	Single-joint	Elbow extension	Triceps push-down
8. Leg	Single-joint	Knee flexion	Leg curl
9. Upper arms	Single-joint	Elbow flexion	Arm curl
10. Calves	Single-joint	Ankle plantar flexion	Toe raise
11. Forearms	Single-joint	Wrist flexion and extension	Wrist curl
12. Abdomen	Single-joint	Trunk flexion	Curl-up

*Multi-joint exercises involving larger muscle groups are followed by single-joint exercises for smaller muscle groups.

fatigue a targeted muscle group. To use this system, the client performs 2 (compound sets) or 3 (tri-sets) exercises consecutively for the same muscle group, with little or no rest between the exercises. Many bodybuilders also use a training system called *supersetting.* For supersets, the client exercises agonistic and antagonistic muscle groups consecutively without resting. For example, to superset the quadriceps femoris and hamstrings, follow a leg extension set immediately with a leg curl set.

Variations for Frequency

Traditionally, exercise scientists have recommended resistance training 3 times per week, on alternate days (e.g., M-W-F), to allow the muscles time to recover. One study, however, reported that exercising 3 consecutive days resulted in greater strength gains compared to alternate days (Hunter 1985). Until more definitive studies are done, encourage your clients to workout 3 times a week on the days that best fit their schedules. For advanced resistance training programs, prescribe a frequency of 5 to 6 days a week. Most exercise specialists advocate a *split routine*, in which different muscle groups are targeted on consecutive days, in order to allow at least one day of recovery for each muscle group. For example, a bodybuilder may exercise the chest and shoulders on Monday and Thursday, the hips and legs on Tuesday and Friday, and the back and arms on Wednesday and Saturday.

Variations for Training Volume and Intensity

To prevent overtraining and to optimize strength and power gains for peak performance, many athletes who train year-round divide their resistance training program into cycles. This method is known as *periodization.* Each *macrocycle* (usually one year), for example, can be divided into four, 3-month *mesocycles:* preparation, first transition, competition, and second transition phases (McArdle, Katch, and Katch 1996). The length and amount of mesocycles vary with the number of competitions. You will need to modify the training volume and intensity for each mesocycle (see table 7.5). During the *preparatory phase* (mesocycle I), prescribe high-volume, low-intensity exercise to increase muscle mass and muscular endurance. Gradually decrease the volume of training as the intensity is increased during the *transition phase* (mesocycle II), culminating in "peak" performance during the *competition phase* (mesocycle III). For the *second transition phase* (mesocycle IV), have the athlete engage in low-intensity physical activities which may not include resistance training. A detailed example illustrating the application of periodization in resistance training programs is available (see Wathen 1994).

Circuit Resistance Training

Circuit resistance training is a method of dynamic resistance training designed to increase strength,

Table 7.5   General Guidelines for Periodization

Mesocycle	Volume		Intensity	
	Sets	Repetitions	% 1-RM	Goals
I Preparation	3-5	8-20	50-80%	Muscle mass Muscular endurance
II 1st transition	3-5	5-8	80-90%	Strength
III Competition	3-5	2-4	90-95%	Power Peak performance
IV 2nd transition	Low*		Low	Physical and psychological recovery

*Athlete engages in low-intensity physical activities which may not necessarily include resistance training.

muscular endurance, and cardiorespiratory endurance (Gettman and Pollock 1981). Circuit resistance training compares favorably with traditional resistance training programs for increasing muscle strength, especially if low-repetition, high-resistance exercises are used (Gettman et al. 1978; Wilmore et al. 1978).

A circuit resistance training program usually has 10 to 15 stations per circuit (see figure 7.1). Have your client repeat the circuit 2 to 3 times so that the total time of continuous exercise is 20 to 30 minutes. At each exercise station, select a resistance that fatigues the muscle group in approximately 30 seconds (as many repetitions as possible at approximately 40 to 55% of 1-RM). Include a 15- to 20-second rest period between exercise stations. You should generally have a client perform circuit resistance training 3 days a week for at least 6 weeks. This method of training is ideal for people with a limited amount of time for exercise. As mentioned in chapter 5, you can add aerobic exercise stations to the circuit between each weightlifting station (i.e., super circuit resistance training) to obtain additional cardiorespiratory benefits.

Isokinetic Training

You can use isokinetic training to increase strength, power, and muscular endurance. Isokinetic training involves dynamic, shortening contractions of a muscle group against an accommodating resistance that matches the force produced by the muscle group throughout the entire range of motion. The speed of movement is controlled mechanically by the isokinetic exercise device. Isokinetic dynamometers are used for isokinetic training. If this equip-

ment is not available, your clients can work with partners who offer accommodating resistance to the movement. In this case, however, the speed of the movement is not precisely controlled.

Isokinetic training is done at speeds that vary between 24° and 300° · sec^{-1}, depending on the needs of the individual. The carryover effect appears to be greater when a person trains at faster speeds (180° to 300° · sec^{-1}) as compared with slower speeds (such as 30° to 60° · sec^{-1}). In some studies, strength gains have been limited to velocities at or below the training velocity (Lesmes et al. 1978; Moffroid and Whipple 1970). Other researchers have reported significant strength gains at all testing velocities (30° to 300° · sec^{-1}) for high velocity training groups (240° to 300° · sec^{-1}) (Coyle et al. 1981; Jenkins, Thackaberry, and Killian 1984). Table 7.6 presents general guidelines for designing isokinetic training programs for development of strength and endurance.

COMPARISON OF RESISTANCE TRAINING METHODS

All of the resistance training methods (static, dynamic, and isokinetic) are effective for developing strength and muscle endurance. Comparing methods is difficult because the amount of work performed during the three types of exercise cannot easily be equated. Because of the specificity of training, it also is difficult to find an unbiased testing device. For example, if you are comparing dynamic and static training programs and use a constant-resistance exercise machine as the testing device, the results most likely will favor the group that trained using that equipment.

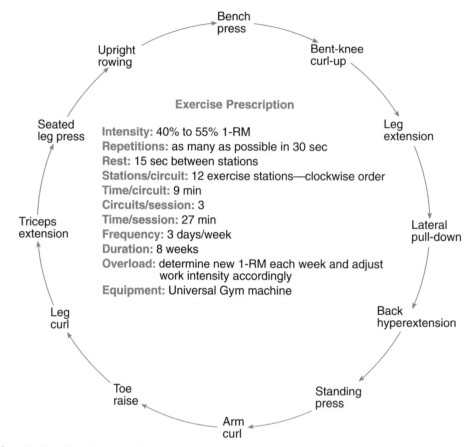

Figure 7.1   Sample circuit resistance training program.

Table 7.6   Guidelines for Designing Isokinetic Training Programs

Type	Intensity	Repetitions	Sets	Speed	Frequency	Length of program
Isokinetic strength	Maximum contraction	2-15	3	24-180°/sec	3-5 days/week	6 weeks or more
Isokinetic endurance	Maximum contraction	Until fatigued	1	≥180°/sec	3-5 days/week	6 weeks or more

Static Versus Dynamic Training

In a review of research dealing with various forms of strength and muscular endurance training, Clarke (1974) reported the following:

- Dynamic training is preferable to static (isometric) training because the former develops greater strength and muscular endurance.

- Motivation is generally superior with dynamic training, because the individual receives visual feedback concerning the amount of weight lifted, and can set explicit goals.

- Static exercise can effectively counteract strength loss and muscular atrophy when a body part is temporarily immobilized due to injury. It is also especially useful when circumstances do not allow the use of dynamic exercise (e.g., limited space and equipment).

Either method of training effectively increases strength; thus, it is difficult to state absolutely that one method is superior to the other (Clarke 1971). Your choice of method depends, in part, on factors such as time, expense, and the purpose of the training.

Dynamic Versus Isokinetic Training

Isokinetic exercise combines the advantages of dynamic (full range of motion) and static (maximum force exerted) exercise. Since the resistance is accommodating, isokinetic training overcomes the weakness of using either a constant- or variable-resistance exercise mode.

Research comparing traditional forms of training with isokinetic training is limited. Thistle, Hislop, and Moffroid (1967) reported peak force gains of 47, 29, and 13%, respectively, for isokinetic, dynamic, and static training methods. Sharkey (1990) compared dynamic, isokinetic, and fitness trail (calisthenic) training in young women. He reported that individuals in the dynamic training group improved the most on the weightlifting tests, while the fitness trail group performed best on the calisthenic tests. The isokinetic training group did not improve as much on either type of test.

A major advantage of isokinetic training over traditional forms of training is that little or no muscle soreness results because the muscles do not contract eccentrically. In addition, isokinetic training at fast speeds apparently produces strength gains not only at the training velocity but also at speeds slower than the training velocity (Lesmes et al. 1978). Isokinetic training is not the best choice, however, when the goal of training is an increase in muscle size. Eccentric contractions apparently are essential for muscle hypertrophy (Cote et al. 1988; Hather et al. 1991). Cote et al. (1988) reported no change in muscle fiber cross-sectional area even when the strength of the quadriceps femoris increased 54% during isokinetic training.

DEVELOPING THE RESISTANCE TRAINING PROGRAM

After assessing your client's muscular fitness, you can individualize the resistance training exercise prescription to meet the needs and interests of each person by using the following steps:

STEPS FOR DEVELOPING A RESISTANCE TRAINING PROGRAM

These steps were used to design the sample dynamic resistance training programs on pages 130-133.

1. In consultation with your clients, identify the primary goal of the program (i.e., strength, muscular endurance, muscle size, or muscle toning) and ask clients how much time they are willing to commit to this program.

2. Based on your client's goal, time commitment, and access to equipment, determine the type of resistance training program (i.e., dynamic, static, or isokinetic).

3. Using results from your client's muscular fitness assessment, identify specific muscle groups that need to be targeted in the exercise prescription.

4. In addition to core exercises for the major muscle groups, select additional exercises for those muscle groups targeted in step 3.

5. For novice weightlifters, order the exercises so the same muscle group is not exercised consecutively.

6. Based on your client's goals, determine appropriate starting loads, repetitions, and sets for each exercise, as well as frequency of the workouts.

7. Set guidelines for progressively overloading each muscle group.

The first example, on next page, describes a beginning resistance training program for an older man (70 years) with no previous weightlifting experience. The primary goal is to develop adequate muscular fitness so that he can retain functional independence. This program followed the ACSM

(1995b) recommendations. During the first 8 weeks of training, low-intensity (30 to 40% 1-RM), high-repetition (15 to 20 repetitions) exercises are prescribed to familiarize the client with weightlifting and reduce the chance of injury and excessive muscle soreness. He gradually increases the resistance so

Sample Resistance Training Program for Older Adult

Client data

Age	70 yr	*Frequency*	2 days/week, at least 48 hr between workouts (e.g., M-Th)
Gender	Male		
Body weight	160 lb (72.7 kg)	*Duration*	16+ weeks
Program goal	Muscular fitness and functional independence	*Overload*	Increase reps first; only increase resistance when he is able to complete >15 reps at prescribed intensity
Time commitment	20-30 min/workout		
Equipment	Exercise machines	*Rest*	2-3 minutes between exercises
Intensity	30-60% 1-RM for first 8 weeks, 70-80% 1-RM thereafter		

Training program

Exercise[a]	1-RM (lb)*	Weeks[b]	Intensity[c] (% 1-RM)	Weight (lb)*	Reps	Sets	Muscle groups
Leg press (seated)	180	1-4	30-40	55-70	15-20	1	Hip extensors, knee extensors
		5-8	50-60	90-110	15-20	1	
		9-12	70	125	8-12	1	
		13-16	80	145	8-12	1	
Bench press (flat)	90	1-4	30-40	25-35	15-20	1	Shoulder horizontal flexors, elbow extensors
		5-8	50-60	45-55	15-20	1	
		9-12	70	60	8-12	1	
		13-16	80	70	8-12	1	
Lat pull-down (shoulder-width grip)	100	1-4	30-40	30-40	15-20	1	Shoulder extensors, elbow extensors
		5-8	50-60	50-60	15-20	1	
		9-12	70	70	8-12	1	
		13-16	80	80	8-12	1	
Leg curl (seated)	45	1-4	30-40	15-20	15-20	1	Knee flexors
		5-8	50-60	20-25	15-20	1	
		9-12	70	30	8-12	1	
		13-16	80	35	8-12	1	
Shoulder press (seated, overhead)	50	1-4	30-40	15-20	15-20	1	Shoulder flexors and adductors
		5-8	50-60	20-35	15-20	1	
		9-12	70	35	8-12	1	
		13-16	80	40	8-12	1	
Heel (calf) raises (seated)	90	1-4	30-40	25-35	15-20	1	Ankle plantar flexors
		5-8	50-60	50-60	15-20	1	
		9-12	70	65	8-12	1	
		13-16	80	70	8-12	1	
Abdominal curl	—	1-4	—	Body weight	5-10	1-2	Trunk flexors
		5-8			10-15	1-2	
		9-12			15-20	1-2	
		13-16			20-25	1-2	

[a]Multi-joint exercise machines are used for most exercises. Seated and lying (instead of standing) positions are recommended to stabilize the body while lifting. Do exercises in the order listed.

[b]During first 2 weeks, closely monitor and supervise workouts. Initial training phase lasts 8 weeks.

[c]Intensity is gradually increased every 2 weeks, only after client is able to do more than the prescribed number of repetitions at each target intensity.

*1 lb = 0.45 kg

that, by the end of the initial phase, the exercise intensity is 60% 1-RM. After 8 weeks, the intensity starts at 70% 1-RM and gradually increases to 80% 1-RM. He does one to 2 sets of 8 to 12 repetitions for each exer-cise. To overload the muscles during this phase, he increases the resistance gradually, but only after he is able to complete 15 or more repetitions at the prescribed relative intensity. This program in-cludes multi-joint exercises using exercise machines only (no free weights). The client exercises twice a week, allowing at least 2 days of rest between each workout.

The second program, below, is for a 35-year-old woman whose primary goal is to improve muscle strength. Although this client has some previous weightlifting experience, she has not lifted weights for more than 2 years. Results from her 1-RM tests indicate that her upper-body strength (particularly the shoulder flexor and forearm flexor muscle groups) is below average. Therefore, 2 exercises are prescribed for each of the weaker muscle groups. The strength of all other muscle groups is aver-age or above average; therefore, only one exer-cise is prescribed for each of these muscle groups.

Sample Resistance Training Program for Novice

Client data

Age	35 yr	Intensity	80% 1-RM
Gender	Female	Frequency	3 days/week, alternate days
Body weight	155 lb (70.4 kg)	Duration	12 weeks or longer
Program goal	Muscle strength	Overload	Increase weight when able to complete 10-12 reps at the prescribed exercise intensity
Time commitment	45-50 min/workout		
Equipment	Variable resistance machines and free weights	Rest	1 minute between sets

Training program[a]

Exercise[b]	1-RM (lb)[c]	Intensity (% 1-RM)	Weight (lb)[c]	Reps	Sets	Muscle groups
Leg press	200	80	160	8	3	Hip extensors, knee extensors
Bench press*	75	80	60	8	3	Shoulder flexors and adductors, elbow extensors
Leg curl (lying)	70	80	55	8	3	Knee flexors
Lat pull-down	125	80	100	8	3	Shoulder extensors and adductors, elbow flexors
Dumbbell fly* (flat bench)	20	80	15	8	3	Shoulder flexors and adductors
Heel (calf) raises (standing)	160	80	125	8	3	Ankle plantar flexors
Abdominal curl	—	—	—	15-20	3	Trunk flexors
Arm curl (incline bench)*	45	80	35	8	3	Elbow flexors
Lateral raises (dumbbell)	20	80	15	8	3	Shoulder abductors
Triceps press-down	60	80	45	8	3	Elbow extensors
Hammer curls* (dumbbells)	40	80	30	8	3	Elbow flexors

[a]Do exercises in the order listed, using larger muscle groups first. Multi-joint exercises are done before single-joint exercises.
[b]Other exercises that work the same muscle groups may be substituted to add variety to the program (see appendix C.3).
[c]1 lb = 0.45 kg
*Two exercises prescribed for each of the weaker muscle groups (shoulder flexors and elbow flexors) identified from her strength assessment.

Given her initial strength levels and previous weightlifting experience, 3 sets of each exercise are prescribed, and the exercise intensity is set at 80% 1-RM to maximize the development of strength. The client completes about 8 repetitions at the prescribed intensity for each set and gradually increases the weight when she is able to complete 10 to 12 repetitions at that intensity. She devotes 45 to 50 minutes, 3 days a week to her workouts.

The third example, below, illustrates an advanced resistance training program developed for an ex-perienced weightlifter (28-year-old male with su-perior strength) whose long-term goal is competi-tive bodybuilding. He engages in a high-volume training program, using moderate intensity (70-75% 1-RM) and moderate repetitions (10-12 reps), in order to maximize the development of muscle size. To achieve a high training volume, he performs 3 exercises for each muscle group and 5 to 6 sets of each exercise. To effectively overload the muscles, he does the 3 exercises for each muscle group con-secutively (tri-sets) with little or no rest between the

Sample Advanced Resistance Training Program for Bodybuilder

Client data

Age	28 yr
Gender	Male
Body weight	190 lb (86.4 kg)
Program goal	Muscle size for body-building
Time commitment	90 min/workout
Equipment	Free weights and exercise machines

Training methods	High volume, tri-sets; split routine
Intensity	70-75% 1-RM
Frequency	6 days/week
Duration	24 weeks or longer
Overload	Increase weight when able to complete >12 reps
Rest	1 min between tri-sets

Training program

Exercise	1-RM (lb)[*]	Intensity (% 1-RM)	Weight (lb)[*]	Reps	Sets	Muscles
Monday and Thursday[a]						
Chest[b]						
Flat bench press (barbell)	250	70-75	175-185	10-12	5-6	Pectoralis major (mid-sternal portion), triceps brachii
Incline dumbbell fly	80	70-75	55-60	10-12	5-6	Pectoralis major (clavicular portion), anterior deltoid
Decline bench press (barbell)	180	70-75	125-135	10-12	5-6	Pectoralis major (lower sternal portion)
Shoulders[b]						
Upright row (barbell)	140	70-75	100-105	10-12	5-6	Middle deltoid
Front dumbbell raises	80	70-75	55-60	10-12	5-6	Anterior deltoid
Posterior cable pull (horizontal plane)	100	70-75	70-75	10-12	5-6	Posterior deltoid
Tuesday and Friday[a]						
Hips and Thighs[b]—1st tri-set						
Squats	300	70-75	210-225	10-12	3	Gluteus maximus, quadriceps femoris, upper hamstrings
Leg extension	150	70-75	105-110	10-12	3	Quadriceps femoris
Leg curl (standing, unilateral)	90	70-75	60-65	10-12	3	Hamstrings (mid-to-lower portions)

(continued)

Training program *(continued)*

Exercise	1-RM (lb)*	Intensity (% 1-RM)	Weight (lb)*	Reps	Sets	Muscles
Tuesday and Friday[a] (continued)						
Hips and Thighs[b]—2nd tri-set						
Leg press	400	70-75	280-300	10-12	3	Gluteus maximus, quadriceps femoris, upper hamstrings
Leg curl (lying)	130	70-75	90-100	10-12	3	Hamstrings (mid-to-lower portions)
Glute-ham raise	—	—	—	10-15	3	Gluteus maximus, hamstrings
Legs and Calves[b]						
Standing calf (heel) raise	250	70-75	175-185	10-12	5-6	Gastrocnemius, soleus
Ankle flexion exercise (seated)	90	70-75	60-65	10-12	5-6	Tibialis anterior
Seated calf raise	180	70-75	125-135	10-12	5-6	Soleus, gastrocnemius
Wednesday and Saturday[a]						
Back[b]						
Lat pull-down (wide grip)	225	70-75	155-170	10-12	5-6	Latissimus dorsi (lateral portions), biceps brachii, brachialis
Seated row (narrow grip)	240	70-75	170-180	10-12	5-6	Latissimus dorsi (mid portion), biceps brachii, brachialis
Dumbbell row	90	70-75	60-65	10-12	5-6	Latissimus dorsi (mid portion), biceps brachii, brachialis
Elbow Flexors[b]						
Standing barbell curl	130	70-75	90-100	10-12	3-4	Biceps brachii, brachialis, brachioradialis
Preacher curl (dumbbells)	100	70-75	70-75	10-12	3-4	Biceps brachii (mid portion), brachialis
Hammer curl (dumbbells)	80	70-75	55-60	10-12	3-4	Brachioradialis, brachialis
Elbow Extensors[b]						
Lying triceps extension (barbell)	120	70-75	85-90	10-12	3-4	Triceps brachii (long head)
Triceps pushdown	150	70-75	105-110	10-12	3-4	Triceps brachii (short and lateral heads)
Triceps pull-down with lateral flair (cables)	130	70-75	90-100	10-12	3-4	Triceps brachii (lateral head)

[a]Other exercises that work the same muscles may be substituted on the second day to add variety to the program (see appendix C.3).

[b]For tri-sets, the 3 exercises listed are performed consecutively without rest and then the tri-set is repeated for the prescribed number of sets for that body part.

*1 lb = 0.45 kg

sets. He lifts weights 6 days a week, splitting the routine so that he is not exercising the same muscle groups on consecutive days. Each muscle group is exercised 2 times a week. He increases the resistance when he is able to complete more than 12 repetitions in the set.

Several excellent references discuss the design of advanced resistance training programs (Baechle 1994; Fleck and Kraemer 1997; Zatsiorsky 1995) and give examples of sport-specific, resistance training programs for athletes (Chu 1996; Stone and Kroll 1978).

DESIGNING RESISTANCE TRAINING PROGRAMS FOR CHILDREN

Children can safely participate in resistance training if special precautions and recommended guidelines (see table 7.2) are carefully followed (ACSM 1995b). Because children are anatomically and physiologically immature, heavy weights may cause damage to the developing bones and joints. Exercise intensity should not exceed 70% 1-RM, which equates to 8 or more repetitions per set. Prescribe 1 to 2 sets of 8 to 10 multi-joint (no single-joint) exercises. To progressively overload the muscle groups, increase the number of repetitions gradually before increasing the resistance. Instruct the child about proper weightlifting (e.g., no fast or jerky movements) and breathing techniques (no breath-holding). A trained exercise leader should closely supervise and monitor the weightlifting activity of the child during every workout.

DESIGNING RESISTANCE TRAINING PROGRAMS FOR OLDER ADULTS

Resistance training provides many health benefits, especially for older adults. The primary goal of resistance training is to develop sufficient muscular fitness so that older people may carry out daily activities without undue stress or fatigue and retain their functional independence. The general guidelines for resistance training programs for older adults are similar to those recommended by the ACSM (1995b) for apparently healthy adults and children who are beginning a resistance training program (see table 7.2). However, some additional guidelines and precautions are recommended (ACSM 1995b):

- During the first 8 weeks of training, use minimal resistance (30 to 50% 1-RM) for all exercises.

- Instruct older adults about proper weightlifting and breathing techniques.

- Trained exercise leaders, who have experience working with older adults, should closely supervise and monitor the clients' weightlifting techniques and resistance training during the first few sessions.

- Prescribe multi-joint, rather than single joint, exercises.

- Use exercise machines to stabilize body position and control the range of joint motion. Avoid using free weights with older adults.

- Each exercise session should be approximately 20 to 30 minutes and should never exceed 60 minutes.

- Older adults should rate their perceived exertion (RPE) during exercise. RPEs should be between 12 and 13 (somewhat hard).

- Allow at least 48 hours of rest between the exercise workouts.

- Never allow arthritic clients to lift weights when they are actively experiencing joint pain or inflammation.

- When returning to resistance training following a lay-off of more than one month, start with a low resistance that is less than 50% of the weight that the individual was lifting prior to the lay-off.

EFFECTS OF RESISTANCE TRAINING PROGRAMS

Resistance training improves muscular fitness by increasing both strength and muscular endurance. This section addresses the morphological, neurological, and biochemical effects of resistance training.

Summary of Effects of Resistance Training

Morphological Factors

- Muscle hypertrophy due to increase in contractile proteins, number and size of myofibrils, connective tissues, and size of Type II muscle fibers

- No change in relative amounts of Type I and II muscle fibers

- Little or no change in the number of muscle fibers (<5%)

- Increase in size and strength of ligaments and tendons

- Increase in bone density and bone strength

- Increase in muscle capillary density

Neural Factors

- Increase in motor unit activation and recruitment

- Increase in discharge frequency of motoneurons

- Decrease in neural inhibitions

Biochemical Factors

- Minor increase in ATP and CP stores

- Minor increase in activity of creatine phosphate kinase (CPK), myosin ATPase, and myokinase

- Decrease in mitochondrial volume density

- Increase in testosterone, growth hormone, IGF, and catecholamines during resistance training exercises

Additional factors

- Little or no change in body weight
- Increase in fat-free mass
- Decrease in fat mass and relative body fat
- Improved bone health

Morphological Effects of Resistance Training on Skeletal Muscle

Resistance training leads to morphological adaptations in skeletal muscles. Structural changes in muscle fibers account for a large portion of the strength gains resulting from resistance training. The following questions address these adaptations:

What Is Exercise-Induced Muscle Hypertrophy?

One effect of strength training is an increase in the size of the muscle tissue. This adaptation is known as *exercise-induced hypertrophy* and results from an increase in the total amount of contractile proteins, the number and size of myofibrils per fiber, and amount of connective tissue surrounding the muscle fibers (Goldberg et al. 1975).

Is It Possible to Increase the Number of Muscle Fibers by Resistance Training?

Heavy resistance training has been reported to increase the number of muscle fibers (i.e., hyperplasia) in animals due to longitudinal splitting and satellite cell proliferation (Antonio and Gonyea 1993; Edgerton 1970; Gonyea, Ericson, and Bonde-Petersen 1977). Such processes, however, have not been clearly demonstrated in human skeletal muscle tissue (Taylor and Wilkinson 1986; Tesch 1988). Although there are some data suggesting that human skeletal muscle has the potential to increase muscle fiber number (Alway et al. 1989; Sjostrom et al. 1992), hyperplasia probably contributes less than 5% to overall muscle growth in response to heavy resistance training (Kraemer, Fleck, and Evans 1996). The major factor contributing to exercise-induced hypertrophy for humans apparently is an increase in the size of existing muscle fibers.

Does Resistance Training Alter Muscle Fiber Type From Slow-Twitch to Fast-Twitch?

Although strength training produces greater hypertrophy in fast-twitch (Type II) muscle fibers than in slow twitch (Type I) fibers (Tesch 1988; Thorstensson et al. 1976), there is no evidence to support the conversion of slow-twitch to fast-twitch fibers (Costill et al. 1979; Dons et al. 1979; Mikesky et al. 1991). Resistance training does not alter the percentage of Type I and II muscle fibers. However, heavy resistance training appears to increase the percentage of Type IIA (fast-twitch-glycolytic) muscle fibers, while decreasing the percentage of Type IIB (fast-twitch-oxidative) fibers in both men and women (Kraemer et al. 1995; Staron et al. 1994).

Is the Relationship Between Muscle Size and Strength the Same for Men and Women?

Muscle strength is directly related to the cross-sectional area of the muscle tissue. Ikai and Fukunaga (1968) noted that the static strength per unit of cross-sectional area of the elbow flexors was similar for young men and women. These values ranged between 4.5 and 8.9 kg/cm^2, with the average values being 6.2 and 6.7 kg/cm^2 for women and men, respectively. Cureton et al. (1988) also reported that the dynamic strength per unit of cross-sectional area (CSA) was similar for men and women. Post-training ratios of elbow flexor/extensor strength to upper arm CSA were 1.65 kg/cm^2 and 1.85 kg/cm^2, respectively, for men and women. Likewise, the post-training ratios for leg strength to thigh CSA were 1.10 kg/cm^2 for men and 0.90 kg/cm^2 for women.

How Much Do Women's Muscles Hypertrophy in Response to Resistance Training?

In the past it was believed that resistance training produces less muscle hypertrophy in women compared to men even though their relative strength gains were similar (Brown and Wilmore 1974; Mayhew and Gross 1974; Wilmore 1974). In these studies, muscle hypertrophy was assessed indirectly using anthropometric and body composition measures. Cureton et al. (1988), using computerized tomography to directly assess muscle hypertrophy in a heavy resistance training program (70-90% 1-RM, 3 days per week for 16 weeks), found significant increases in cross-sectional area of the upper arms of men (7 cm² or 15%) and women (5 cm² or 23%). Although the absolute change was slightly larger in men, the relative degree of hypertrophy was similar for men and women.

Is It Possible for Older Adults to Increase the Size of Their Muscles by Resistance Training?

Electromyographic (EMG) evidence led Moritani and deVries (1979) to conclude that increased strength in older men engaged in resistance training is highly dependent on neural changes, such as increased frequency of motoneuron discharge and recruitment of motor units. Because of studies such as this, it was long believed that strength gains from resistance training in older individuals were due primarily to neural adaptation rather than muscle hypertrophy.

However, Frontera et al. (1988) reported that resistance training produces muscle hypertrophy in men ages 60 to 72 years. The men trained in a high-intensity program for knee extensors and flexors (3 sets at 80% 1-RM) for 12 weeks, 3 days per week. Computerized tomography revealed significant increases in total thigh area (4.8%), total muscle area (11.4%), and quadriceps area (9.3%). The relative increase in total muscle area was similar to values reported for young men (Luthi et al. 1986). Research also shows significant increases in muscle size in older women, as well as in very old (87 to 96 years) men and women, due to high-intensity (80% 1-RM) resistance training (Charette et al. 1991; Fiatarone et al. 1990).

Exercise-induced hypertrophy appears to be an important mechanism underlying strength gains in older women and men. This implies that age-related loss in muscle mass can be countered effectively by participating in a vigorous resistance training program.

Biochemical Effects of Resistance Training

The morphological changes in skeletal muscles due to resistance training are caused by hormones. This section addresses questions regarding hormonal responses to resistance exercise, as well as changes in the metabolic profile of skeletal muscles.

What Causes the Increase in Muscle Size With Resistance Training?

Exercise-induced hypertrophy occurs through hormonal mechanisms. Anabolic (protein-building) hormones such as testosterone, growth hormone, and insulin-like growth hormone (IGH) increase in response to heavy resistance exercise and interact to promote protein synthesis. The magnitude of testosterone and growth hormone release, however, is related to the size of the muscle groups used, exercise intensity (% 1-RM), and the length of rest between sets, with larger increases observed for high-intensity (5- to 10-RM) and short (1 minute) rest periods involving large muscle groups (Kraemer et al. 1991). In men, high-intensity resistance training produces significant increases in testosterone and growth hormone (Fahey et al. 1976; vanHelder, Radomski, and Goode 1984; Weiss, Cureton, and Thompson 1983). Levels of catecholamines (norepinephrine, epinephrine, and dopamine), which augment the release of testosterone and IGF, also increase in men in response to heavy resistance exercise (Kraemer, Noble, Clark, and Culver 1987). In women, the growth hormone response to resistance exercise varies over stages of the menstrual cycle (Kraemer et al. 1991).

Does Resistance Training Alter the Metabolic Profile of Skeletal Muscles?

Although high-intensity resistance training results in substantial increases in muscle proteins, it appears to have little or no effect on muscle substrate stores and enzymes involved with the generation of ATP. Although stores of ATP and creatine phosphate (CP) may increase significantly in response to strength training (MacDougall et al. 1979), the changes are not large enough to have practical significance. Strength training produces only minor alterations in myosin ATPase activity (Tesch 1992) and other ATP turnover enzymes, such as CPK (Costill et al. 1979; Komi et al., 1978; Thorstensson et al. 1976). Strength training using heavy resistance and explosive exercises results in decreased activities for hexokinase, myofibrillar ATPase, and citrate synthase (Tesch 1988).

Does Resistance Training Decrease Aerobic Capacity and Endurance Performance?

The mitochondrial volume density following heavy resistance training has been reported to decrease due to a disproportionate increase of contractile protein in comparison with mitochondria. In theory, this could be detrimental to aerobic capacity and endurance performance. A review of studies of this phenomenon, however, concluded that participation in heavy resistance training does not negatively affect aerobic power (Dudley and Fleck 1987). Also, capillary density has been shown to increase, which in turn enhances the potential to remove lactate produced by the muscles during moderate-intensity, high-volume resistance exercise (Kraemer, Fleck, and Evans 1996).

Neurological Effects of Resistance Training

The nervous system also responds to resistance training. Neurological adaptations account for much of the improvement in muscle strength in the early stages of resistance training, leading to the following question: How long does it take to show substantial improvements in muscle strength and size?

The answer is somewhat complex. Increased muscle size alone cannot account for the rate of strength gain due to resistance training (Dons et al. 1979; Moritani and deVries 1979). In the early stages (2 to 8 weeks) of resistance training, neural factors are also involved. These factors include learning to disinhibit motoneurons and to increase activation levels of motor units (Kraemer, Deschenes, and Fleck 1988; Sale 1988). At about 8 to 10 weeks of resistance training, muscle hypertrophy contributes more than neural adaptations to strength gains, but eventually levels off (Sale 1988). Staron et al. (1994) noted that at least 16 resistance training workouts are needed in order to produce substantial increases in muscle contractile proteins (hypertrophy).

Additional Effects of Resistance Training

Resistance training also positively affects bone health and overall body composition. The following questions address these adaptations.

Does Resistance Training Improve Bone Health and Joint Integrity?

Resistance training has beneficial effects on bone health that may decrease the risk of osteoporosis and bone fractures, particularly in women. Bone mineral density of the lumbar spine and femur in premenopausal women significantly increased after 12 to 18 months of strength training (Lohman et al. 1995). Also, lumbar bone mineral density of early, postmenopausal women was improved following nine months of strength training (Pruitt et al. 1992). However, in a study of older women (65 to 79 years), 12 months of high-intensity (80% 1-RM) and low-intensity (40% 1-RM) resistance training did not significantly improve the bone mineral density of the lumbar spine and hip (Pruitt, Taaffe, and Marcus 1995). Still, evidence suggests that resistance training and higher-intensity, weight-bearing activities (not walking) may slow the decline of bone loss even if there is no significant increase in bone mineral density. Physical activity, however, should not be substituted for hormonal replacement therapy at the time of menopause (ACSM 1995a).

Resistance training also improves the size and strength of ligaments and tendons (Edgerton 1973; Fleck and Falkel 1986; Tipton et al. 1975). These changes may increase joint stability, thereby reducing the risk of sprains and dislocations.

Is Resistance Training Effective for Weight Control?

Resistance training positively alters body composition and preserves lean body tissues. Although total body weight undergoes little change, the lean body mass increases as the absolute and relative amounts of body fat decrease (Brown and Wilmore 1974; Mayhew and Gross 1974; Wilmore 1974). For weight-loss programs, exercise science and nutrition professionals recommend using resistance training, in combination with aerobic exercise, to maximize the loss of body fat while maintaining lean body tissues (see chapter 9).

MUSCULAR SORENESS

Muscular soreness may develop as a result of resistance training, because isolated muscle groups are being overloaded beyond normal use. *Acute soreness* occurs during or immediately following the exercise and is usually caused by ischemia and the accumulation of metabolic waste products in the muscle tissue. The pain and discomfort may persist up to 1 hour after the cessation of the exercise.

In *delayed-onset muscle soreness* (DOMS), the pain occurs 24 to 48 hours after exercise. The causes of DOMS are not known (Armstrong 1984; Smith

1991); however, it appears to be related to the type of muscle contraction. Eccentric exercise produces a greater degree of delayed muscular soreness than either concentric or isometric exercise (Byrnes, Clarkson, and Katch 1985; Schwane et al. 1983; Talag 1973). Little or no muscular soreness occurs with isokinetic exercise (Byrnes, et al., 1985). This is most likely related to the fact that isokinetic exercise devices offer no resistance to the recovery phase of the movement, and therefore the muscle does not contract eccentrically.

Theories of DOMS

Although the precise causes of DOMS remains unclear, several theories have been proposed. The more widely recognized theories suggest that exercise, particularly eccentric exercise, causes damage to skeletal muscle cells and connective tissues, producing an acute inflammation.

Connective Tissue Damage

Abraham (1977) extensively studied the factors related to delayed-onset muscular soreness. He suggested that DOMS most likely results from disruption in the connective tissue of the muscle and its tendinous attachments. Abraham noted that urinary excretion of hydroxyproline, a specific by-product of connective tissue breakdown, was higher in subjects who experienced muscular soreness than in those who did not. Because a significant rise in urinary hydroxyproline levels indicates an increase in both collagen degradation and synthesis, he concluded that more strenuous exercise damages the connective tissue, which increases the degradation of collagen and creates an imbalance in collagen metabolism. To compensate for this imbalance, the rate of collagen synthesis increases.

Skeletal Muscle Damage

Skeletal muscle damage induced through exercise has been assessed by examining micrographs of myofibrils from biopsy samples. Friden, Sjostrom, and Ekblom (1983) observed structural damage to myofibrillar Z-bands resulting from intense eccentric exercise. The damage to fast-twitch fibers was more extensive than that of slow-twitch fibers.

Researchers also have examined markers of muscle damage such as serum CPK, lactate dehydrogenase, and myoglobin. Schwane et al. (1983) noted a significant increase in plasma CPK levels produced by downhill running. They suggested that the me-

chanical stress from eccentric exercise causes cellular damage that results in an enzyme efflux. Clarks on et al. (1986) reported similar increases in serum CPK levels following concentric (37.6%), eccentric (35.8%), and isometric (34%) arm curl exercises. They concluded that muscle damage occurred with all 3 types of contraction; however, the subjects perceived greater muscle soreness with eccentric and isometric exercises. Likewise, Byrnes et al. (1985) observed that both concentric and eccentric resistance training elevated serum CPK levels, but individuals who trained concentrically did not develop DOMS.

Armstong's Model of DOMS

Based on an extensive literature review, Armstrong (1984) proposed the following model of DOMS:

- The structural proteins in muscle cells and connective tissue are disrupted by high mechanical forces produced during exercise, especially eccentric exercise.

- Structural damage to the sarcolemma alters the permeability of the cell membrane, allowing a net influx of calcium from the interstitial space. Abnormally high levels of calcium inhibit cellular respiration, thereby lessening the cell's ability to produce ATP for active removal of calcium from the cell.

- High calcium levels within the cell activate a calcium-dependent proteolytic enzyme that degrades Z-discs, troponin, and tropomyosin.

- This progressive destruction of the sarcolemma (postexercise) allows intracellular components to diffuse into the interstitial space and plasma. These substances attract monocytes and activate mast cells and histocytes in the injured area.

- Histamine, kinins, and potassium accumulate in the interstitial space due to the active phagocytosis and cellular necrosis. These substances, as well as increased tissue edema and temperature, may stimulate pain receptors resulting in the sensation of DOMS.

Acute Inflammation Theory

Smith (1991) suggested that acute inflammation, in response to muscle cell and connective damage caused by eccentric exercise, is the primary mechanism underlying DOMS. Many of the signs and symptoms of acute inflammation, such as pain, swelling, and loss of function, are also present with DOMS. Based on research about acute inflammation and DOMS, she proposed the following sequence of events:

- Connective tissue and muscle tissue disruption occurs during eccentric exercise, especially when the individual is not accustomed to eccentric exercise.
- Within a few hours, neutrophils in the blood are elevated and migrate to the site of injury for several hours post-injury.
- Monocytes also migrate to the injured tissues at 6 to 12 hours post-injury.
- Macrophages synthesize prostaglandins (Series E).
- The prostaglandins sensitize Type III and IV pain afferents, resulting in the sensation of pain in response to intramuscular pressure caused by movement or palpation.
- The combination of increased pressure and hypersensitization produces the sensation of DOMS.

Prevention of Muscular Soreness

To prevent muscular soreness, you should prescribe warm-up exercises for your clients. The warm-up exercises are done at the beginning of the resistance training workout and usually include slow, static stretching exercises for all major muscle groups. This form of stretching may be effective in preventing the onset of muscular soreness (deVries 1961). Using a gradual progression of exercise intensity when beginning a resistance training program also may help to prevent muscular soreness. McArdle, Katch, and Katch (1996) suggest using 12- to 15-RM during the beginning phases of strength training. After 2 weeks, increase the exercise intensity to 6- to 8-RM. Avoiding eccentric contractions during dynamic resistance training also may lessen the chance of muscular soreness. Have an assistant or exercise partner return the weight to the starting position.

COMMON MISCONCEPTIONS AND QUESTIONS ABOUT RESISTANCE TRAINING

Because of the overwhelming amount of misinformation about resistance training in popular maga-

zines, your clients will have many questions and concerns.

1. Will my muscles be stiff and sore after I lift weights?

It is highly likely that you will experience some muscle soreness 1 to 2 days after your workout, especially if you are a beginning weightlifter or have not been lifting weights on a regular basis. To lessen the chance of developing sore muscles, warm up before each workout by slowly and statically stretching each muscle group. If you have never lifted weights, you should begin by using light weights (≤60% of your 1-RM) during the first few weeks of training. As your muscles get stronger, progressively but gradually increase the amount of weight for each exercise. Avoid doing too much, too soon.

2. What can I do to relieve my muscle soreness?

If your muscles are sore, do not lift weights. Sometimes slow, static stretching of the sore muscles will help to relieve some of the pain. Nonprescription painkillers such as aspirin and ibuprofen often help. If the soreness persists for more than 48 hours, you should contact your physician.

3. Is it okay to lift weights every day?

During weightlifting, your muscles are exercised at greater than normal workloads, producing microscopic tears in the muscle cells and connective tissues. Your body responds by producing new muscle proteins. This causes muscle growth and increased strength. For these changes to occur, you need to rest the exercised muscles between workouts. Also, most people can show substantial improvements in strength when they lift weights every other day, just 2 to 3 times a week. If you lift weights every day, you run the risk of overtraining your muscles. This may cause muscle strains, tendinitis, bursitis, and other injuries to your muscles and joints. Experienced weightlifters who work out every day split their exercise routine, so that the same muscle groups are not exercised on consecutive days. This type of routine reduces the risk of developing excessive muscle soreness and overuse injuries if you lift weights every day.

4. Can I use calisthenic exercises, like push-ups and pull-ups, to improve my strength?

Calisthenic exercises can increase strength. Exercise professionals often prescribe push-ups and pull-ups, in addition to free weights and machine exercises, to build the strength of chest, arm, and back muscles.

When you do calisthenic exercises, your body weight provides the resistance. Therefore, if you are unable to lift your body weight, you will need to modify the calisthenic exercise. For example, doing push-ups with your body weight supported by the knees and hands is easier than doing standard push-ups where your body is fully extended and the weight is supported by the hands and feet. As your strength improves, you may increase the difficulty of the push-up by placing the hands wider than shoulder width.

If you are unable to lift your body weight, you can modify pull-ups by using a spotter. As you pull up, you can assist your movement by extending your knees as the spotter supports your lower legs or ankles. To increase the difficulty of a pull-up, place your hands wider than shoulder width and use an overhand (pronated) grip instead of an underhand (supinated) grip.

5. Are exercise devices more effective than calisthenic exercises for strengthening my abdominal muscles?

No scientific evidence currently justifies claims that doing calisthenic exercises with the aid of an abdominal exercise device is more effective than simply doing calisthenic exercises, like abdominal curls, without these devices. As your strength improves, you can modify abdominal exercises to overload the muscles by changing your body position (e.g., abdominal curls done on a decline bench are more difficult than on a flat bench), holding weight plates across your chest, or changing your arm position. Abdominal exercises get progressively more difficult as your arms are moved from along your sides to behind your head and overhead.

6. Will I get "muscle-bound" and lose joint flexibility if I lift weights?

It is a common misconception that resistance training decreases your joint flexibility. Studies of elite bodybuilders and powerlifters indicate that these athletes have excellent levels of flexibility. The key to remaining flexible is performing each exercise throughout the entire range of motion. Also, you should statically stretch muscle groups before and after each workout to ensure that flexibility is maintained.

7. Will my strength improve if I train aerobically at the same time I am resistance training?

If you do aerobic training concurrently with resistance training, your muscle growth and strength improvement may be lessened because of the increased energy demands and protein requirements for endurance training. Although this is an important consideration for competitive bodybuilders and power athletes, the decision to participate in both forms of training depends on the overall goal of your exercise program. If your goal is improved health or weight loss, experts recommend including both aerobic training and resistance training in your exercise program.

8. Are protein and amino acid supplements necessary to maximize my muscle growth and strength during resistance training?

Providing that your diet is well-balanced and nutritionally sound, you do not need supplements. Although the protein needs of resistance-trained individuals (1.2 to 1.6 g/kg/day) are slightly higher than the recommended dietary allowance for inactive individuals (0.9 g/kg/day), a well-balanced diet containing 12 to 15% protein is adequate to meet the increased protein need while weightlifting. Protein intake in excess of this level does not increase protein synthesis. Instead, excess protein is metabolized by the body. So your muscle size and strength will not be enhanced by a high protein intake. Also, there is no scientific evidence to justify the claim that amino acid supplements stimulate muscle growth or increase muscle strength and performance.

9. I have followed my exercise prescription closely; but, over the last several weeks, I haven't seen any change in my strength. What should I do?

At the beginning of your program, your strength gains were dramatic and rapid because your initial strength level was less than it is now. As you get closer to your genetic limit, the rate and degree of improvement in strength slows down, and eventually you reach a plateau. It may be helpful if you periodically change the training stimulus by using a different combination of intensity, repetitions, and sets. For example, if you are presently doing high-intensity, low-repetition exercises, you may want to try decreasing your intensity (from 80 to 70% 1-RM) and increasing your repetitions from 6-8 to 10-12 reps for several weeks. Selecting different exercises for the muscle groups may also help.

Key Points

- The specificity principle states that muscular fitness development is specific to the muscle group, type of contraction, training intensity, speed, and range of movement.

- The overload principle states that the muscle group must be exercised at greater than normal work loads to promote muscular strength and endurance development.

- Throughout the training program, the training volume must be progressively increased to overload the muscle groups for continued gains in strength and muscular endurance.

- In most programs, resistance training exercises should be ordered so that successive exercises do not involve the same muscle group. For advanced programs, however, exercises for the same muscle group should be done consecutively.

- Dynamic resistance training can be used to develop muscular strength, tone, size, or endurance by modifying the intensity, repetitions, sets, and frequency of the exercise.

- Strength and endurance gains resulting from resistance training are due to morphological, neurological, and biochemical changes in the muscle tissue.

- Eccentric exercise produces a greater degree of DOMS than either concentric, isometric, or isokinetic exercise

- Little or no muscular soreness is produced by isokinetic training.

- The precise cause of DOMS is unknown; however, connective tissue and muscle damage, as well as acute inflammation, have been proposed as possible causes.

REFERENCES

Abraham, W.M. 1977. Factors in delayed muscle soreness. *Medicine and Science in Sports* 9: 11-20.

Alway, S.E., Grumbt, W.H., Gonyea, W.J., and Stray-Gundersen, J. 1989. Contrasts in muscle and myofibers of elite male and female bodybuilders. *Journal of Applied Physiology* 67: 24-31.

American College of Sports Medicine. 1995a. ACSM Position stand on osteoporosis and exercise. *Medicine and Science in Sports and Exercise* 27 (4): i-vii.

American College of Sports Medicine. 1995b. *ACSM's guidelines for exercise testing and prescription.* Baltimore: Williams & Wilkins.

Antonio, J., and Gonyea, W.J. 1993. Skeletal muscle fiber hyperplasia. *Medicine and Science in Sports and Exercise* 25: 1333-1345.

Armstrong, R.B. 1984. Mechanisms of exercise-induced delayed onset muscular soreness: A brief review. *Medicine and Science in Sports and Exercise* 16: 529-538.

Baechle, T.R. 1994. *Essentials of strength training and conditioning.* Champaign, IL: Human Kinetics.

Berger, R.A. 1962a. Comparison of static and dynamic strength increases. *Research Quarterly* 33: 329-333.

Berger, R.A. 1962b. Optimum repetitions for the development of strength. *Research Quarterly* 33: 334-338.

Berger, R.A., and Hardage, B. 1967. Effect of maximum loads for each of ten repetitions on strength improvement. *Research Quarterly* 38: 715-718.

Brown, C.H., and Wilmore, J.H. 1974. The effects of maximal resistance training on the strength and body composition of women athletes. *Medicine and Science in Sports* 6: 174-177.

Byrnes, W.C., Clarkson, P.M., and Katch, F.I. 1985. Muscle soreness following resistive exercise with and without eccentric contraction. *Research Quarterly for Exercise and Sport* 56: 283-285.

Charette, S.L., McEvoy, L., Pyka, G., Snow-Harter, C., Guido, D., Wiswell, R.A., and Marcus, R. 1991. Muscle hypertrophy response to resistance training in older women. *Journal of Applied Physiology* 70: 1912-1916.

Chu, D.A. 1996. *Explosive power and strength.* Champaign, IL: Human Kinetics.

Clarke, D. 1973. Adaptations in strength and muscular endurance resulting from exercise. In J.H. Wilmore, ed., *Exercise and sport sciences reviews* 1:73-102. New York: Academic Press.

Clarke, H.H. 1971. Isometric versus isotonic exercises. *Physical Fitness Research Digest*, series 1, no. 1(July). Washington, DC: President's Council on Physical Fitness and Sports.

Clarke, H.H. 1974. Development of muscular strength and endurance. *Physical Fitness Research Digest*, series 4, no. 1 (January). Washington, DC: President's Council on Physical Fitness and Sports.

Clarkson, P.M., Byrnes, W.C., McCormick, K.M., Turcotte, L.P., and White, J.S. 1986. Muscle soreness and serum creatine kinase activity following isometric, eccentric and concentric exercise. *International Journal of Sports Medicine* 7: 152-155.

Costill, D.L., Coyle, E.F., Fink, W.F., Lesmes, G.R., and Witzmann, F.A. 1979. Adaptations in skeletal muscle following strength training. *Journal of Applied Physiology* 46: 96-99.

Cote, C., Simoneau, J.A., Lagasse, P., Bouley, M., Thibault, M.C., Marcotte, M., and Bouchard, C.1988. Isokinetic strength training protocols: Do they induce skeletal muscle fiber hypertrophy? *Archives of Physical Medicine and Rehabilitation* 69: 281-285.

Coyle, E.F., Feiring, D.C., Rotkis, T.C., Cote, R.W. III, Roby, F.B., Lee, W., and Wilmore, J.H. 1981. Specificity of power improvements through slow and fast isokinetic training. *Journal of Applied Physiology* 51: 1437-1442.

Cureton, K.J., Collins, M.A., Hill, D.W., McElhannon, F.M. Jr. 1988. Muscle hypertrophy in men and women. *Medicine and Science in Sports and Exercise* 20: 338-344.

deVries, H.A. 1961. Prevention of muscular distress after exercise. *Research Quarterly* 32: 177-185.

Dons, B., Bollerup, K., Bonde-Petersen, F., and Hancke, S. 1979. The effect of weight-lifting exercise related to muscle fiber composition and muscle cross-sectional area in humans. *European Journal of Applied Physiology* 40: 95-106.

Dudley, G.A. and Fleck, S.J. 1987. Strength and endurance training: Are they mutually exclusive? *Sports Medicine* 4: 79-85.

Edgerton, V.R. 1970. Morphology and histochemistry of the soleus muscle from normal and exercised rats. *American Journal of Anatomy* 127: 81-88.

Edgerton, V.R. 1973. Exercise and the growth and development of muscle tissue. In G.L. Rarick, ed., *Physical activity, human growth and development*, 1-31. New York: Academic Press.

Fahey, T.D., Rolph, R., Moungmee, P., Nagel, J., and Mortara, S. 1976. Serum testosterone, body composition, and strength of young adults. *Medicine and Science in Sports* 8: 31-34.

Fiatarone, M.A., Marks, E.C., Ryan, N.D., Meredith, C.N., Lipstiz, L.A., and Evans, W.J. 1990. High-intensity strength training in nonagenarians. Effects on skeletal muscle. *Journal of the American Medical Association* 263: 3029-3034.

Fleck, S.J., and Falkel, J.E. 1986. Value of resistance training for the reduction of sports injuries. *Sports Medicine* 3: 61-68.

Fleck, S.J., and Kraemer, W.J. 1997. *Designing resistance training programs*, 2nd ed. Champaign, IL: Human Kinetics.

Friden, J., Sjostrom, M., and Ekblom, B. 1983. Myofibrillar damage following intense eccentric exercise in man. *International Journal of Sports Medicine* 4: 170-176.

Frontera, W.R., Meredith, C.N., O'Reilly, K.P., Knuttgen, H.G., and Evans, W.J. 1988. Strength conditioning in older men: Skeletal muscle hypertrophy and improved function. *Journal of Applied Physiology* 64: 1038-1044.

Gardner, G.W. 1963. Specificity of strength changes of the exercised and non-exercised limb following isometric training. *Research Quarterly* 34: 98-101.

Gettman, L.R., Ayres, J.J., Pollock, M.L., and Jackson, A. 1978. The effect of circuit weight training on strength,

cardiorespiratory function, and body composition of adult men. *Medicine and Science in Sports* 10: 171-176.

Gettman, L.R., and Pollock, M.L. 1981. Circuit weight training: A critical review of its physiological benefits. *The Physician and Sportsmedicine* 9: 44-60.

Goldberg, A., Etlinger, J., Goldspink, D., and Jablecki, C. 1975. Mechanism of work-induced hypertrophy of skeletal muscle. *Medicine and Science in Sports* 7: 185-198.

Gonyea, W.J., Ericson, G.C., and Bonde-Petersen, F. 1977. Skeletal muscle fiber splitting induced by weight-lifting exercise in cats. *Acta Physiologica Scandinavica* 99: 105-109.

Hather, B.M., Tesch, P.A., Buchanan, P., and Dudley, G.A. 1991. Influence of eccentric actions on skeletal muscle adaptations to resistance training. *Acta Physiologica Scandinavica* 143: 177-185.

Hettinger, T., and Muller, E.A. 1953. Muskelleistung und muskeltraining. *European Journal of Applied Physiology* 15: 111-126.

Hunter, G.R. 1985. Changes in body composition, body build and performancee associated with different weight training frequencies in males and females. *National Strength and Conditioning Association Journal.* 7:26-28.

Ikai, M., and Fukunaga, T. 1968. Calculation of muscle strength per unit cross-sectional area of human muscle by means of ultrasonic measurement. *European Journal of Applied Physiology* 26: 26-32.

Jenkins, W.L., Thackaberry, M., and Killian, C. 1984. Speed-specific isokinetic training. *Journal of Orthopaedic and Sports Physical Therapy* 6: 181-183.

Komi, P.V., Viitasalo, J.T., Rauramaa, R., and Vihko, V. 1978. Effect of isometric strength training on mechanical, electrical, and metabolic aspects of muscle function. *European Journal of Applied Physiology* 40: 45-55.

Kraemer, W.J., Deschenes, M.R., and Fleck, S.J. 1988. Physiological adaptations to resistance exercise: Implications for athletic conditioning. *Sports Medicine* 6: 246-256.

Kraemer, W.J., Fleck, S.J., and Evans, W.J. 1996. Strength and power training: Physiological mechanisms of adaptation. In J.O. Holloszy, ed., *Exercise and sport sciences reviews* 24: 363-397. Baltimore: Williams & Wilkins.

Kraemer, W.J., Gordon, S.E., Fleck, S.J., Marchitelli, L.J., Mello, R., Dziados, J.E., Friedl, K., Harman, E., Maresh, C., and Fry, A.C. 1991. Endogenous anabolic hormonal and growth factor responses to heavy resistance exercise in males and females. *International Journal of Sports Medicine* 12: 228-235.

Kraemer, W.J., Noble, B.J., Clark, M.J., and Culver, B.W. 1987. Physiologic responses to heavy-resistance exercise with very short rest periods. *International Journal of Sports Medicine* 8: 247-252.

Kraemer, W.J., Patton, J., Gordon, S.E., Harman, E.A., Deschenes, M.R., Reynolds, K., Newton, R.U., Triplett, N.T., and Dziados, J.E. 1995. Compatibility of high intensity strength and endurance training on hormonal and skeletal muscle adaptations. *Journal of Applied Physiology* 78: 976-989.

Lesmes, G.R., Costill, D.L., Coyle, E.F., and Fink, W.J. 1978. Muscle strength and power changes during maximal isokinetic training. *Medicine and Science in Sports* 10: 266-269.

Lohman, T.G., Going, S., Pamenter, R., Hall, M., Boyden, T., Houtkooper, L., Ritenbaugh, C., Bare, L., Hill, A., and Aickin, M. 1995. Effects of resistance training on regional and total bone mineral density in premenopausal women: A randomized prospective study. *Journal of Bone Mineral Research* 10: 1015-1024.

Luthi, J.M., Howald, H., Claasen, H., Rosler, K., Vock, P., and Hoppeler, H. 1986. Structural changes in skeletal muscle tissue with heavy resistance exercise. *International Journal of Sports Medicine* 7: 123-127.

MacDougall, J.D., Sale, D.G., Moroz, J.R., Elder, G.C., Sutton, J.R., and Howalk, H. 1979. Mitochondrial volume density in human skeletal muscle following heavy resistance training. *Medicine and Science in Sports* 11: 164-166.

Mayhew, J.L., and Gross, P.M. 1974. Body composition changes in young women with high resistance weight training. *Research Quarterly* 45: 433-440.

McArdle, W.D., Katch, F.I., and Katch, V.L. 1996. *Exercise physiology.* Baltimore: Williams & Wilkins.

Mikesky, A.E., Giddings, C.J., Matthews, W., and Gonyea, W.J. 1991. Changes in fiber size and composition in response to heavy-resistance exercise. *Medicine and Science in Sports and Exercise* 23: 1042-1049.

Moffroid, M.T., and Whipple, R.H. 1970. Specificity of speed of exercise. *Physical Therapy* 50: 1699-1704.

Moritani, T., and deVries, H.A. 1979. Neural factors versus hypertrophy in the time course of muscle strength gain. *American Journal of Physical Medicine* 58: 115-130.

Pruitt, L.A., Jackson, R.D., Bartels, R.L., and Lehnhard, H.J. 1992. Weight-training effects on bone mineral density in early postmenopausal women. *Journal of Bone Mineral Research* 7: 179-185.

Pruitt, L.A., Taaffe, D.R., and Marcus, R. 1995. Effects of a one-year high-intensity versus low-intensity resistance training program on bone mineral density in older women. *Journal of Bone Mineral Research* 10: 1788-1795.

Sale, D. 1988. Neural adaptation to resistance training. *Medicine and Science in Sports and Exercise* 20: S135-S145.

Schwane, J.A., Johnson, S.R., Vandenakker, C.B., and Armstrong, R.B. 1983. Delayed-onset muscular soreness and plasma CPK and LDH activities after down-hill running. *Medicine and Science in Sports and Exercise* 15: 51-56.

Sharkey, B.J. 1990. *Physiology of fitness,* 3rd ed. Champaign, IL: Human Kinetics.

Sjostrom, M., Lexell, J., Eriksson, A., and Taylor, C.C. 1992. Evidence of fiber hyperplasia in human skeletal muscles from healthy young men? *European Journal of Applied Physiology* 62: 301-304.

Smith, L.L. 1991. Acute inflammation: The underlying mechanism in delayed onset muscle soreness? *Medicine and Science in Sports and Exercise* 23: 542-551.

Staron, R.S., Karapondo, D.L., Kraemer, W.J., Fry, A.C., Gordon, S.E., Falkel, J.E., Hagerman, F.C., and Hikida, R.S. 1994. Skeletal muscle adaptations during the early phase of heavy-resistance training in men and women. *Journal of Applied Physiology* 76: 1247-1255.

Stone, M.H. 1988. Implications for connective tissue and bone alterations resulting from resistance exercise training. *Medicine and Science in Sports and Exercise* 20: S162-S168.

Stone, W.J., and Kroll, W.A. 1978. *Sports conditioning and weight training.* Boston: Allyn & Bacon.

Talag, T.S. 1973. Residual muscular soreness as influenced by concentric, eccentric, and static contractions. *Research Quarterly* 44: 458-469.

Taylor, N.A.S. and Wilkinson, J.G. 1986. Exercise-induced skeletal muscle growth: Hypertrophy or hyperplasia? *Sports Medicine* 3: 190-200.

Tesch, P.A. 1988. Skeletal muscle adaptations consequent to long-term heavy resistance exercise. *Medicine and Science in Sports and Exercise* 20: S132-S134.

Tesch, P.A. 1992. Short- and long-term histochemical and biochemical adaptations in muscle. In P. Komi, ed., *Strength and power in sports. The encyclopaedia of sports medicine,* 239-248. Oxford, England: Blackwell.

Thistle, H.G., Hislop, H.J., and Moffroid, M. 1967. Isokinetic contraction: A new concept of resistive exercise. *Archives of Physical Medicine and Rehabilitation* 48: 279-282.

Thorstensson, A., Hulten, B., vonDobeln, W., and Karlsson, J. 1976. Effect of strength training on enzyme activities and fibre characteristics in human skeletal muscle. *Acta Physiologica Scandinavica* 96: 392-398.

Tipton, C.M., Matthes, R.D., Maynard, J.A., and Carey, R.A. 1975. The influence of physical activity on ligaments and tendons. *Medicine and Science in Sports* 7: 165-175.

vanHelder, W.P., Radomski, M.W., and Goode, R.C. 1984. Growth hormone responses during intermittent weight lifting exercise in men. *European Journal of Applied Physiology* 53: 31-34.

Wathen, D. 1994. Periodization: Concepts and applications. In T. R. Baechle, ed., *Essentials of strength training and conditioning,* 459-472. Champaign, IL: Human Kinetics.

Weiss, L.W., Cureton, K.J., and Thompson, F.N. 1983. Comparison of serum testosterone and androstenedione responses to weight lifting in men and women. *European Journal of Applied Physiology* 50: 413-419.

Wilmore, J.H. 1974. Alterations in strength, body composition and anthropometric measurements consequent to a 10-week weight training program. *Medicine and Science in Sports* 6: 133-138.

Wilmore, J.H., Parr, R.B., Girandola, R.N., Ward, P., Vodak, P.A., Barstow, T.J., Pipes, T.V., Romero, G.T., and Leslie, P. 1978. Physiological alterations consequent to circuit weight training. *Medicine and Science in Sports* 10: 79-84.

Zatsiorsky, V.M. 1995. *Science and practice of strength training*. Champaign, IL: Human Kinetics.

CHAPTER 8

Assessing Body Composition

Key Questions

- Why is it important to measure body composition, and how are body composition measures used by health and fitness professionals?

- What are the standards for classifying body fat levels?

- What is the difference between two-component and multicomponent body composition models?

- What are the guidelines and limitations of the hydrostatic weighing method?

- Is dual-energy x-ray absorptiometry considered to be a "gold standard" method for measuring body composition?

- What are the guidelines, limitations, and sources of measurement error for the skinfold method?

- What is bioelectrical impedance analysis? What factors affect the accuracy of this method?

- Can circumferences and skeletal diameters be used to accurately assess body composition?

- Is near-infrared interactance a viable alternative to skinfolds and bioimpedance analysis for measuring body composition in field settings?

Body composition is a key component of an individual's health and physical fitness profile. Obesity reduces life expectancy by increasing the risks of coronary artery disease, hypertension, Type II diabetes, obstructive pulmonary disease, osteoarthritis, and certain types of cancer. Too little body fat also poses a health risk because the body needs a certain amount of fat for normal physiological functions. Essential lipids, such as phospholipids, are needed for cell membrane formation; while nonessential lipids, like triglycerides found in adipose tissue, provide thermal insulation and store metabolic fuel (free fatty acids). In addition, lipids are involved in the transport and storage of fat-soluble vitamins (A, D, E, and K); in the functioning of the nervous system, the menstrual cycle, and the reproductive system; and in growth and maturation during pubescence. Thus too little body fat, as found in individuals suffering from eating disorders (anor-

exia nervosa), exercise addiction, and certain diseases such as cystic fibrosis, can lead to serious physiological dysfunction.

This chapter describes standardized testing procedures for laboratory (hydrostatic weighing) and field (skinfold, bioimpedance, and anthropometry) methods for assessing body composition. For each method, you will learn to identify potential sources of measurement error, as well as ways to minimize these errors.

CLASSIFICATION AND USES OF BODY COMPOSITION MEASURES

To classify level of body fatness, the relative body fat (% BF) is used. Table 8.1 presents relative body fat standards for men and women. The *average % BF* is

Table 8.1 Percent Body Fat Standards for Men and Women		
	Men	**Women**
At risk[a]	≤5%	≤8%
Below average	6-14%	9-22%
Average	15%	23%
Above average	16-24%	24-31%
At risk[b]	≥25%	≥32%
[a] At risk for diseases and disorders associated with malnutrition		
[b] At risk for diseases associated with obesity		

Data from Lohman (1992) 80.

15 for men and 23 for women. The *standard for obesity* that places an individual at risk for disease is body fat ≥25% for men and ≥32% for women. *Minimal fat levels* that place an individual at risk for diseases associated with too little body fat are estimated to be ≤5% for men and ≤8% for women.

In addition to classifying your client's % BF and disease risk, body composition measures are useful for

- estimating a healthy body weight and formulating nutritional recommendations and exercise prescriptions (see chapter 9),

- estimating competitive body weight for athletes participating in sports that use body weight classifications for competition (e.g., wrestling and bodybuilding),

- monitoring the growth of children and adolescents and identifying those at risk because of under- or overfatness,

- assessing changes in body composition associated with aging, malnutrition, and certain diseases—and for assessing the effectiveness of nutrition and exercise interventions in counteracting these changes.

BODY COMPOSITION MODELS

In order to make the most valid assessment of body composition for your client, it is necessary to understand the underlying theoretical models. You may recall that the body is composed of water, protein, minerals, and fat. The two-component model of body composition (Brozek et al. 1963; Siri 1961) divides the body into a fat component and fat-free body (FFB) component. The FFB consists of all residual chemicals and tissues including water,

muscle (protein), and bone (mineral). The two-component model of body composition makes the following five assumptions:

1. The density of fat is $0.901 \text{ g} \cdot \text{cc}^{-1}$.

2. The density of the FFB is $1.100 \text{ g} \cdot \text{cc}^{-1}$.

3. The densities of fat and the FFB components (water, protein, mineral) are the same for all individuals.

4. The densities of the various tissues comprising the FFB are constant within an individual, and their proportional contribution to the lean component remains constant.

5. The individual being measured differs from the reference body only in the amount of fat; the FFB of the reference body is assumed to be 73.8% water, 19.4% protein, and 6.8% mineral.

This two-component model has served as the foundation upon which the hydrodensitometry (underwater weighing) method is based. Using the assumed proportions of water, mineral, and protein and their respective densities, equations were derived to convert the individual's total body density (Db) from hydrostatic weighing into relative body fat proportions (% BF). Two commonly used equations are the Siri (1961) equation, % BF = (4.95/Db − 4.50) × 100, and the Brozek et al. (1963) equation, % BF = (4.57/Db − 4.142) × 100. These two equations yield similar % BF estimates for body densities ranging from 1.0300 to 1.0900 g/cc. For example, if a client's measured body density is 1.0500 g/cc, the % BF estimates, obtained by plugging this value into the Siri and Brozek equations, are 21.4 and 21.0%, respectively.

Generally, *two-component model equations* provide accurate estimates of % BF as long as the basic assumptions of the model are met. However, there is no guarantee that the FFB composition of an individual within a certain population subgroup will exactly match the values assumed for the reference body. Researchers have reported that FFB density varies with age, gender, ethnicity, level of body fatness, and physical activity level, depending mainly on the relative proportion of water and mineral comprising the FFB (Baumgartner et al. 1991; Williams et al. 1993). For example, the FFB densities of black women (1.106 g/cc) and black men (1.113 g/cc) are greater than 1.10 g/cc because of their higher mineral content (~7.3% FFB) and bone density values (Cote and Adams 1993; Ortiz et al. 1992; Schutte et al. 1984). Because of this difference in FFB density, the body fat of blacks will be systematically underestimated when two-component model equations are used to estimate % BF. Likewise, the FFB density of children is estimated to be only 1.084 g/cc because of their relative lower mineral (5.2% FFB) and higher body water values (76.6% FFB) compared to the reference body (Lohman, Boileau, and Slaughter 1984). Also, the average density of the FFB of elderly men and women is 1.096 g/cc because of the relatively low

body mineral value (6.2% FFB) in this population (Heymsfield et al. 1989). Thus, the relative body fat of children and the elderly will be systematically overestimated using two-component model equations.

For certain population subgroups, therefore, scientists have applied *multicomponent models* of body composition based on measured total body water and bone mineral values. With the multicomponent approach, you can avoid systematic errors in estimating body fat by replacing the reference man with population-specific reference bodies that take into account the age (e.g. children, elderly), gender, and ethnicity of the individual. Table 8.2 provides population-specific formulas for converting Db to %BF. You will note that population-specific conversion formulas do not yet exist for all age groups within each ethnic group. You may have to use the age-specific conversion formulas developed for white males and females in these cases. Also, the population-specific conversion formulas developed for anorexic and obese females can only be used when it is obvious that your client is either obese or anorexic.

Table 8.2   Population-Specific Formulas for Conversion of Db to % BF

Population	Age	Gender	% BF	FFB$_d$ (g/cc)*
Race				
American Indian	18-60	Female	(4.81/Db)-4.34	1.108
Black	18-32	Male	(4.37/Db)-3.93	1.113
	24-79	Female	(4.85/Db)-4.39	1.106
Hispanic	20-40	Female	(4.87/Db)-4.41	1.105
Japanese Native	18-48	Male	(4.97/Db)-4.52	1.099
		Female	(4.76/Db)-4.28	1.111
	61-78	Male	(4.87/Db)-4.41	1.105
		Female	(4.95/Db)-4.50	1.100
White	7-12	Male	(5.30/Db)-4.89	1.084
		Female	(5.35/Db)-4.95	1.082
	13-16	Male	(5.07/Db)-4.64	1.094
		Female	(5.10/Db)-4.66	1.093
	17-19	Male	(4.99/Db)-4.55	1.098
		Female	(5.05/Db)-4.62	1.095
	20-80	Male	(4.95/Db)-4.50	1.100
		Female	(5.01/Db)-4.57	1.097
Levels of body fatness				
Anorexic	15-30	Female	(5.26/Db)-4.83	1.087
Obese	17-62	Female	(5.00/Db)-4.56	1.098

*FFB$_d$ = fat-free body density

Reprinted, by permission, from Heyward and Stolarczyk 1996, *Applied body composition assessment.* Champaign, IL: Human Kinetics, 12.

LABORATORY METHODS FOR ASSESSING BODY COMPOSITION

You can use a number of laboratory methods to assess body composition. The hydrostatic weighing and dual-energy x-ray absorptiometry (DXA) methods are commonly used. Other methods, such as body volume measured by air displacement, potassium 40 (K^{40}) counting, neutron activation analysis, and magnetic resonance imaging, are primarily used for research. These advanced methods require highly specialized, expensive equipment, and are impractical for most settings. Detailed information about these methods is available elsewhere (see Roche, Heymsfield, and Lohman 1996).

Hydrostatic Weighing

Hydrostatic weighing (HW) is a valid, reliable, and widely-used laboratory method for assessing total body density (Db). Hydrostatic weighing measures your client's total body volume (BV); Db is calculated by dividing body weight by body volume. The total Db is a function of the respective amounts of muscle, bone, water, and fat in the body.

Using Hydrostatic Weighing

Determine body volume by totally submerging the body in an underwater weighing tank or pool and measuring the underwater weight (UWW) of the body. To measure UWW, you can use either a chair attached to a hydrostatic weighing scale (see figure 8.1) or a platform attached to load cells (see figure 8.2). According to Archimedes' principle, the weight loss under water is directly proportional to the volume of water displaced by the BV. The BV, therefore, is equal to the body weight (BW) minus the UWW (see figure 8.3). The net UWW is the difference between the UWW and the weight of the chair or platform and its supporting equipment (i.e., tare weight). The net UWW must be corrected for the volume of air remaining in the lungs after a maximal expiration (i.e., residual volume or RV) and the volume of air in the gastrointestinal tract (GV). The GV is assumed to be 100 ml.

The RV is commonly measured using helium dilution, nitrogen washout, or oxygen dilution techniques. The RV is measured in liters and must be converted to kilograms in order to correct UWW.

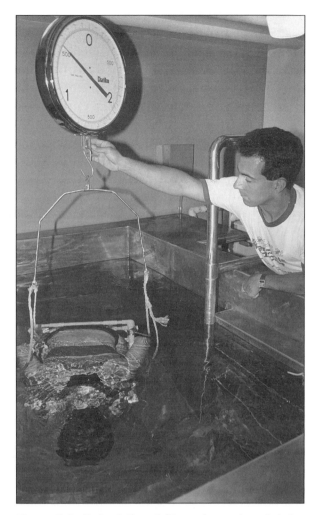

Figure 8.1 Hydrostatic weighing using scale and chair.

This is easily done because 1 L of water weighs approximately 1 kg; therefore, the water weight per liter of RV is 1 kg. The net UWW is corrected by adding the equivalent weight of the RV and the assumed GV (100 ml, or 0.1 kg). Since water density varies with the water temperature, the body volume is corrected for water density (see appendix D.1). Under normal circumstances, the water temperature of the underwater weighing tank or swimming pool will be between 34° and 36° C. The resulting equation for body volume is:

BV = [(BW – net UWW)/density of water] – (RV + GV)

Body density (Db in g/cc) is calculated by dividing body weight by body volume: Db = BW/BV. After you calculate Db, you can convert it into percent body fat by using the appropriate population-specific conversion formula (see table 8.2).

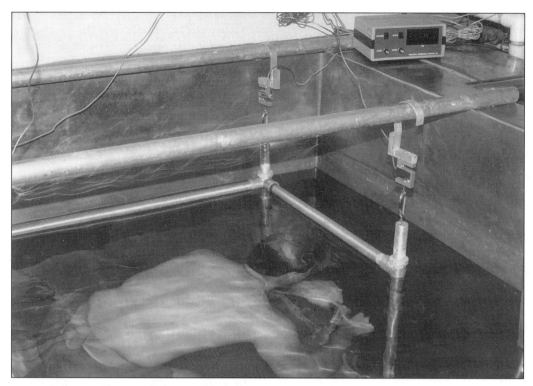

Figure 8.2   Hydrostatic weighing using load cells and platform.

Hydrostatic Weighing Data

Name _____   Date _____

Gender _____   Body weight_____ lb _____ kg   Age_____

I.   Residual volume (average 2 trials within 100 ml)

Trial 1 _____   Trial 2 _____   Trial 3 _____

Average RV = _____ L

II.   Water temperature _____ °C

Water density _____ g/cc
(see appendix D.1)

III.   Gross underwater weight (in kg)

Trial 1 _____   Trial 6 _____
Trial 2 _____   Trial 7 _____
Trial 3 _____   Trial 8 _____
Trial 4 _____   Trial 9 _____
Trial 5 _____   Trial 10 _____

Average (3 trials within 0.1 kg) = _____ kg

IV.   Tare weight (chair, platform, and
supporting equipment) _____ kg

V.   Net underwater weight gross
UWW _____ – tare weight _____
= _____ kg

VI.   Body volume

[(BW in kg – net UWW in kg)/water density]
– (RV + GV)   BV = _____ L
Note. GV assumed value = 100 ml or 0.1 L

VII.   Body density = BW (kg)/BV (L) (carry out to 5
or 6 decimal places)   Db = _____ g/cc

VIII.   % body fat (select conversion formula from
table 8.2)   BF = _____ %

IX.   Fat weight = BW × % BF (decimal)
_____ × _____   FW = _____ kg

X.   Fat-free weight = BW − FW
_____ − _____   FFW = _____ kg

Figure 8.3   Hydrostatic weighing data collection form.

Follow the guidelines below when using the hydrostatic weighing technique:

GUIDELINES FOR HYDROSTATIC WEIGHING

1. The client should wear a lightweight swimming suit.

2. The client must urinate and eliminate as much gas and feces as possible before testing.

3. Determine the accuracy of the hydrostatic weighing scale prior to use by hanging calibrated weights from the scale and checking the corresponding scale values. To calibrate a load cell system, place the weights on the platform and check the recorded values.

4. Weigh the chair or platform, as well as all of the supporting equipment underwater; this is the tare weight.

5. Check the water temperature just prior to the test; it should range between 34° and 36° C.

6. Have the client kneel on the underwater weighing platform or assume a sitting position in the chair after removing all air bubbles from swimming suit and hair. You may need to add a scuba diving belt around the client's waist to facilitate this position.

7. The client should exhale as much air as possible when totally submerged in the tank. The highest weight at the end of maximal exhalation is the gross UWW. The client should try to remain as still as possible during this procedure.

8. Administer at least 3 to 10 trials. Average the highest 3 trials within 0.1 kg, and record this figure as the gross UWW.

9. Determine the net UWW by subtracting the weight of the chair or platform, its supporting equipment, swimsuit, and scuba diving belt (if used) from the gross UWW.

Special Considerations

Some clients may have difficulty performing the hydrostatic weighing test using these standardized procedures. Accurate test results are highly dependent on the client's skill, cooperation, and motivation. The following section addresses the use of modified hydrostatic weighing testing procedures, as well as other questions and concerns about using this method.

1. What should I do when my client is unable to blow out all of the air from the lungs or remain still while underwater?

You will likely come across clients who are uncomfortable expelling all of the air from their lungs during hydrostatic weighing. In such cases, you can weigh these individuals at functional residual capacity (FRC) or total lung capacity (TLC) instead of RV. Thomas and Etheridge (1980) weighed 43 males underwater, comparing the body densities measured at FRC (taken at the end of normal expiration while submerged) and at RV (at the end of maximal expiration). Both methods yielded similar results. Similarly, Timson and Coffman (1984) reported that body density measured by hydrostatic weighing at TLC (vital capacity + RV) is similar (less than 0.3% BF difference) to that measured at RV if TLC is measured in the water. However, when the TLC was measured out of the water, the method significantly overestimated body density. When using these modifications of the hydrostatic weighing method, you must still measure RV in order to calculate the FRC or TLC of your client. Also, be certain to substitute the appropriate lung volume (FRC or TLC) for RV in the calculation of BV.

Because of their lower body density, clients with greater amounts of body fat are more buoyant than leaner individuals; therefore they have more difficulty remaining motionless under the water. To correct this problem, place a weighted scuba belt around the client's waist. Be certain to include the scuba belt when measuring the tare weight of the hydrostatic weighing system.

2. What should I do when clients are afraid to put their faces in the water or are not flexible enough to get their backs and heads completely submerged?

Occasionally you will encounter clients who are extremely fearful of being submerged, who dislike facial contact with water, or who are unable to bend forward to assume the proper body position for hydrostatic weighing. In such cases, a satisfactory alternative would be to weigh your clients at TLC while their heads remain above water level. Donnelly et al. (1988) compared this method (i.e., TLCNS or total lung capacity with head not submerged) to the criterion body density obtained from hydrostatic weighing at RV for 75 men and 67 women. Vital capacity was measured with the subject submerged in the water to shoulder level. Regression analysis yielded the following equations for predicting body density (Db) at RV, using the Db determined at TLCNS as the predictor:

Males

Db at RV = 0.5829(Db at TLCNS) + 0.4059

r = 0.88   SEE = 0.0067 g · cc^{-1}

Females

Db at RV = 0.4745 (Db at TLCNS) + 0.5173

r = 0.85   SEE = 0.0061 g · cc^{-1}

The correlations (r) between the actual Db at RV and the predicted Db at RV were high, and the standard errors of estimate (SEE) were within acceptable limits. These equations were cross-validated for an independent sample of 20 men and 20 women. The differences between the Db from hydrostatic weighing at RV and the predicted Db from weighing at TLCNS were quite small (less than 0.0014 g · cc^{-1} or 0.7% BF). This method may be especially useful for hydrostatic weighing of older adults, obese individuals with limited flexibility, and people with physical disabilities.

As an alternative to hydrostatic weighing, in research and clinical settings you can use an air displacement method to assess total body volume and body density. This method is relatively expensive, requiring the use of a whole-body plethysmograph (i.e., BOD POD™) to measure body volume. The method is quick (usually takes 5 minutes) and requires minimal compliance by the client. For this test, the client sits in the BOD POD™ and breathes normally; residual lung volume does not have to be measured. Preliminary studies show good test-retest reliability and acceptable validity (r^2 = 0.93, SEE = 1.8% BF) compared to hydrostatic weighing (McCrory et al. 1995). For detailed descriptions of test procedures and operating principles, see Dempster and Aitkens (1995).

3. Will the accuracy of the hydrostatic weighing test be affected if I estimate RV instead of measuring it?

Several prediction equations have been developed to estimate RV based on the individual's age, height, gender, and smoking status (see appendix D.2). However, these RV prediction equations have large prediction errors (SEE = 400 to 500 ml). When RV is measured, the precision of the hydrostatic weighing method is excellent (≤1% BF). However, this precision error increases substantially (±2.8 to 3.7% BF) when RV is estimated (Morrow et al. 1986).

Therefore, aways measure RV when you are using the hydrostatic weighing method.

4. When is the best time during the menstrual cycle to hydrostatically weigh my female clients?

Some women, particularly those whose body weight fluctuates widely during their menstrual cycles, may have significantly different estimates of body density and % BF when weighed hydrostatically at different times in their cycles. Bunt, Lohman, and Boileau (1989) reported that changes in total body water due to water retention can partly explain the differences in body weight and body density during a menstrual cycle. On the average, the relative body fat of the women was 24.8% BF at their lowest body weights, compared to an average of 27.6% BF at their peak body weights during their menstrual cycles. Because their low and peak body weights occurred at different times during the menstrual cycle (varied from 0 to 14 days prior to the onset of the next menses), the effect of total body water fluctuations cannot be routinely controlled by using the same day of the menstrual cycle for all women. When monitoring changes in body composition over time or establishing healthy body weight for a female client, it is recommended that you hydrostatically weigh her at the same time within her menstrual cycle and outside of the period of her perceived peak body weight.

Dual-Energy X-ray Absorptiometry

Dual-energy x-ray absorptiometry (DXA) is a relatively new technology that is gaining recognition as a reference method for body composition research (see figure 8.4). This method yields estimates of bone mineral, fat, and lean soft-tissue mass. DXA is highly reliable, and there is a high degree of agreement between % BF estimates obtained by hydrostatic weighing and by DXA (Going et al. 1993; Van Loan and Mayclin 1992). DXA is an attractive alternative to hydrostatic weighing as a reference method because it is safe, rapid (a total body scan takes 10 to 20 minutes), requires minimal subject cooperation, and most importantly, accounts for individual variability in bone mineral content. In the future, it is highly likely that body composition prediction equations will be developed and validated using DXA as a reference method. However, further research is needed before DXA can be firmly established as the best reference method (Kohrt 1995; Roubenoff et al. 1993).

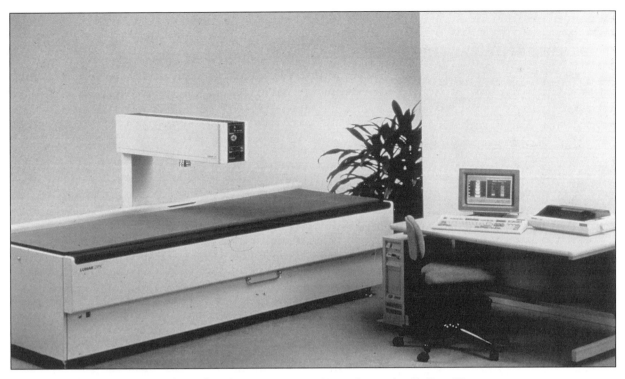

Figure 8.4 Dual-energy x-ray absorptiometer. Photo courtesy of Lunar Corporation, Madison, WI.

FIELD METHODS FOR ASSESSING BODY COMPOSITION

In field settings, you can use more practical methods to estimate your client's body composition. Your choices include bioelectrical impedance, skinfold, and other types of anthropometric prediction equations. To use these methods and equations appropriately, you need to understand the basic assumptions and principles, as well as the potential sources of measurement error, for each method. You must closely follow standardized testing procedures, and you must practice in order to perfect your measurement techniques for each method. For more detailed information about these field methods and how to apply them to various population subgroups, see Heyward and Stolarczyk (1996).

Skinfold Method

A skinfold (SKF) indirectly measures the thickness of subcutaneous adipose tissue. When you use the SKF method to estimate total body density in order to calculate relative body fat (% BF), certain basic relationships are assumed:

• *The SKF is a good measure of subcutaneous fat.* Research has demonstrated that the subcutaneous

fat, assessed by SKF measurements at 12 sites, is similar to the value obtained from magnetic resonance imaging (MRI) (Hayes et al. 1988).

• *The distribution of fat subcutaneously and internally is similar for all individuals within each gender.* The validity of this assumption is questionable. Older subjects of the same gender and body density have proportionately less subcutaneous fat than their younger counterparts. Also, lean individuals have a higher proportion of internal fat, and the proportion of fat located internally decreases as overall body fatness increases (Lohman 1981).

• *Because there is a relationship between subcutaneous fat and total body fat, the sum of several skinfolds can be used to estimate total body fat.* Research has established that SKF thicknesses at multiple sites measure a common body-fat factor (Jackson and Pollock 1976; Quatrochi et al. 1992). It is assumed that approximately one-third of the total fat is located subcutaneously in men and women (Lohman 1981). However, there is considerable biological variation in subcutaneous, intramuscular, intermuscular, and internal-organ fat deposits, as well as essential lipids in bone marrow and the central nervous system. Age, gender, and degree of fatness all affect variation in fat distribution (Lohman 1981).

• *There is a relationship between the sum of SKFs (ΣSKF) and body density (Db).* This relationship is linear for homogenous samples (population-specific SKF equations) but nonlinear over a wide range of Db (generalized SKF equations) for both men and women. A linear regression line, depicting the relationship between the SKF and Db, will fit the data well only within a narrow range of body fatness values. Thus, using a population-specific equation to estimate the Db of clients not representative of the sample originally used to develop that equation leads to an inaccurate estimate of your client's Db (Jackson 1984).

• *Age is an independent predictor of Db for both men and women.* Using age and the quadratic expression of the sum of skinfolds (SKF²) accounts for more variance in Db of a heterogeneous population than using the SKF² alone (Jackson 1984).

Using the Skinfold Method

SKF prediction equations are developed using either linear (population-specific) or quadratic (generalized) regression models. There are well over 100 population-specific equations to predict Db from various combinations of SKFs, circumferences, and bony diameters (Jackson and Pollock 1985). These equations were developed for relatively homogeneous populations and are assumed to be valid only for individuals having similar characteristics, such as age, gender, ethnicity, or level of physical activity. For example, an equation derived specifically for 18- to 21-year-old sedentary men would not be valid for predicting the Db of 35- to 45-year-old sedentary men. Population-specific equations are based on a linear relationship between skinfold fat and Db (linear model); however, research shows that there is a curvilinear relationship (quadratic model) between SKFs and Db across a large range of body fatness (see figure 8.5). Population-specific equations will tend to underestimate % BF in fatter individuals and overestimate it in leaner individuals.

Using the quadratic model, Jackson and colleagues (Jackson and Pollock 1978; Jackson, Pollock and Ward 1980) developed generalized equations applicable to individuals varying greatly in age (18 to 60 years) and body fatness (up to 45% BF). These equations also take into account the effect of age on the distribution of subcutaneous and internal fat. An advantage of the generalized equations is that one equation, instead of several, can be used to accurately estimate your clients' % BF.

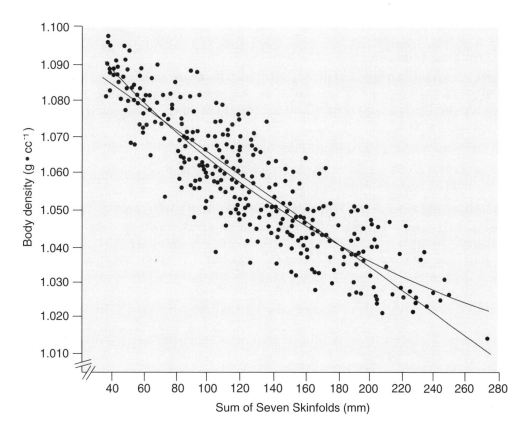

Figure 8.5 Relationship of sum of skinfolds to body density.
Reprinted, by permission, from A.S. Jackson and M.L. Pollock, 1978, "Generalized equations for predicting body density of men," *British Journal of Nutrition* 40: 502.

Most equations use two or three SKFs to predict Db. The Db is then converted to % BF using the appropriate population-specific conversion formula (see table 8.2). Table 8.3 presents commonly-used population-specific and generalized SKF prediction equations. Calculating the Db and % BF is tedious and time-consuming, especially when you are assessing the body composition of many clients. You will save time by using computer software (Ng, 1997) developed for the SKF equations included in this book. This software selects the appropriate SKF equation and population-specific conversion formula in table 8.2 to estimate % BF based on physical demographics (e.g., age, gender, ethnicity, and physical activity level) of your client. Using these equations, you can accurately estimate the % BF of your clients within ±3.5% BF.

Alternatively, nomograms exist for some SKF prediction equations. The nomogram in figure 8.6 was specifically developed for the Jackson sum of three SKF equations. To use this nomogram, plot the sum of three skinfolds (Σ3SKF) and age in the appropriate columns and use a ruler to connect these two points. The corresponding % BF is read at the point where the connecting line intersects the % BF column on the nomogram.

Although nomograms are potential time-savers, you should be aware that this nomogram is based on a two-component body composition model, using the Siri equation to convert Db to % BF. In general, use this nomogram only to calculate % BF of white males.

Skinfold Technique

It takes a great deal of time and practice to develop your skill as a SKF technician. Following standardized procedures will increase the accuracy and reliability of your measurements (Harrison et al. 1988):

STANDARDIZED PROCEDURES FOR SKINFOLD MEASUREMENTS

1. Take all SKF measurements on the right side of the body.

2. Carefully identify, measure, and mark the SKF site, especially if you are a novice SKF technician (see appendix D.3).

3. Grasp the SKF firmly between the thumb and index finger of your left hand. Lift the fold 1 cm (0.4 in) above the site to be measured.

4. Lift the fold by placing your thumb and index finger 8 cm (~3 inches) apart on a line that is perpendicular to the long axis of the skinfold. The long axis is parallel to the natural cleavage lines of the skin. For individuals with extremely large skinfolds, you will need to separate your thumb and finger more than 8 cm in order to lift the fold.

5. Keep the fold elevated while you take the measurement.

6. Place the jaws of the caliper perpendicular to the fold, approximately 1 cm below the thumb and index finger, and release the jaw pressure slowly.

7. Take the SKF measurement 4 seconds after the pressure is released.

8. Open the jaws of the caliper to remove it from the site. Close the jaws slowly to prevent damage or loss of calibration.

Table 8.3   Skinfold Prediction Equations

SKF sites[a]	Population subgroups	Gender	Age	Equation	Reference
Σ7SKF (chest + abdomen + thigh + triceps + subscapular + midaxilla)	Black or Hispanic	Women	18-55 yr	Db (g/cc)[b] = 1.0970 − 0.00046971(Σ7SKF) + 0.00000056(Σ7SKF)^2 − 0.00012828(Age)	Jackson et al. (1980)
	Black or athletes	Men	18-61 yr	Db (g/cc)[b] = 1.1120 − 0.00043499(Σ7SKF) + 0.00000055(Σ7SKF)^2 − 0.00028826(Age)	Jackson and Pollock (1978)
Σ4SKF (triceps + anterior suprailiac + abdomen + thigh)	Athletes	Women	18-29 yr	Db (g/cc)[b] = 1.096095 − 0.0006952(Σ4SKF) − 0.0000011(Σ4SKF)^2 − 0.0000714(Age)	Jackson et al. (1980)
Σ3SKF (triceps + suprailiac + thigh)	White or anorexic	Women	18-55 yr	Db (g/cc)[b] = 1.0994921 − 0.0009929(Σ3SKF) + 0.0000023(Σ3SKF)^2 − 0.0001392(Age)	Jackson et al. (1980)
(chest + abdomen + thigh)	White	Men	18-61 yr	Db (g/cc)[b] = 1.109380 − 0.0008267(Σ3SKF) + 0.0000016(Σ3SKF)^2 − 0.0002574(Age)	Jackson and Pollock (1978)
Σ2SKF (triceps + calf)	Black or White	Boys	6-17 yr	% BF = 0.735(ΣSKF) + 1.0	Slaughter et al. (1988)
	Black or White	Girls	6-17 yr	% BF = 0.610(ΣSKF) + 5.1	Slaughter et al. (1988)

[a]ΣSKF = sum of skinfolds (mm)
[b]Use population-specific conversion formulas (see table 8.2) to calculate % BF from Db.

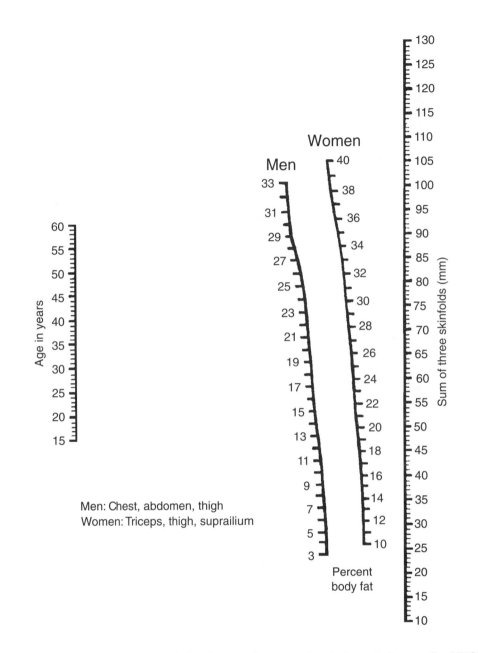

Men: Chest, abdomen, thigh
Women: Triceps, thigh, suprailium

Figure 8.6 Nomogram to estimate percent body fat of men and women using Jackson et al. generalized Σ3SKF equations.
Reprinted with permission from *Research Quarterly for Exercise and Sport,* Vol. 52, 382, Copyright 1981 by the American Alliance for Health, Physical Education, Recreation and Dance, 1900 Association Drive, Reston, VA 20191.

You also will be able to increase your skill as a SKF technician by following these recommendations made by experts in the field (Jackson and Pollock 1985; Lohman, Pollock et al. 1984; Pollock and Jackson 1984):

- Be meticulous when locating the anatomical landmarks used to identify the SKF site, when

measuring the distance, and when marking the site with a surgical marking pen.

- Read the dial of the caliper to the nearest 0.1 mm (Harpenden or Holtain), 0.5 mm (Lange), or 1 mm (plastic calipers).

- Take a minimum of two measurements at each site. If values vary from each other by more than ±10%, take additional measurements.

- When measuring SKF thicknesses at more than one site, take the measurements in a rotational order (circuits) rather than consecutive readings at each site.

- Take the measurements when the client's skin is dry and lotion-free.
- Do not measure immediately after exercise, because the shift in body fluid to the skin tends to increase the size of the SKF.
- Practice taking SKFs on 50 to 100 clients.
- Avoid using plastic calipers if you are an inexperienced SKF technician. Instead use metal calipers.
- Train with skilled SKF technicians and compare your results.
- Use a SKF training videotape that demonstrates proper SKF techniques (Lohman 1987).
- Seek additional training at workshops held at state, regional, and national conferences.

Sources of Measurement Error

The accuracy and precision of SKF measurements and the SKF method are affected by the technician's skill, type of SKF caliper, and client factors. The following questions and responses address these sources of measurement error.

1. Is there high agreement among SKF values when the measurements are taken by two different technicians?

A major source of measurement error is differences between SKF technicians. Objectivity, or between-technician reliability, is improved when SKF technicians follow standardized testing procedures, practice taking SKFs together, and mark the SKF site (Pollock and Jackson 1984). A major cause of low inter-tester reliability is improper location and measurement of the SKF sites (Lohman, Pollock, et. al. 1984).

2. Are the anatomical descriptions for specific SKF sites the same for all SKF equations?

In the past, for some SKF sites, the anatomical location and direction of the fold have varied. For example, Behnke and Wilmore (1974) recommend measuring the abdominal SKF using a horizontal fold adjacent to the umbilicus; Jackson and Pollock (1978), however, recommend measuring a vertical fold taken 2 cm (0.8 in) lateral to the umbilicus. Inconsistencies such as this have led to confusion and lack of agreement among SKF technicians. As a result, experts in the field of anthropometry have developed standardized testing procedures and

detailed descriptions for identification and measurement of SKF sites (Harrison et al. 1988). Appendix D.3 summarizes some of the most commonly used sites, as described in the *Anthropometric Standardization Reference Manual.*

Although the objective is to have all SKF technicians follow standardized procedures and recommendations for site location and SKF measurements, you may not be able to do so under all circumstances. For example, if you are using the generalized equations of Jackson and Pollock (1978) and Jackson, Pollock, and Ward (1980), the chest, midaxillary, subscapular, abdominal, and suprailiac SKFs will be located at sites which differ from those described in the reference manual. The descriptions for the sites used in the Jackson et al. equations are presented in appendix D.4.

3. How many measurements do I need to take at each SKF site?

Intra-technician reliability or consistency of measurements by the skinfold technician is another source of error for the SKF method. You will need to practice your SKF technique on 50 to 100 clients to develop a high degree of skill and proficiency (Jackson and Pollock 1985). Take a minimum of 2 measurements at each site using a rotational order. If values vary from each other by more than ±10%, take additional measurements. Average two trials within ±10% of each other for use in the prediction equation to estimate Db and % BF.

4. What types of SKF calipers are available, and how do these calipers differ?

When selecting a SKF caliper for use in the field, you should consider factors such as cost, durability, and degree of precision needed, as well as your skill and experience as a SKF technician. You can use either high-quality metal calipers or plastic calipers to measure SKF thickness (see figure 8.7). The cost of SKF calipers varies, depending on the materials used in construction (metal or plastic) and the caliper's accuracy and precision throughout the range of measurement. High-quality instruments, such as Harpenden, Lange, Holtain, and Lafayette calipers, exert constant pressure (~10 g/mm^2) throughout the range of measurement (0 mm to 60 mm). Calipers should not vary in tension more than 2.0 g/mm^2 over the range or exceed 15 g/mm^2 (Edwards et al. 1955). Excessive tension and force cause client discomfort (a pinching sensation) and significantly reduce the SKF measurement (Gruber et al. 1990). High-quality calipers also have excellent scale precision (0.2 mm and 1.0 mm for Harpenden and Lange calipers, respectively). The

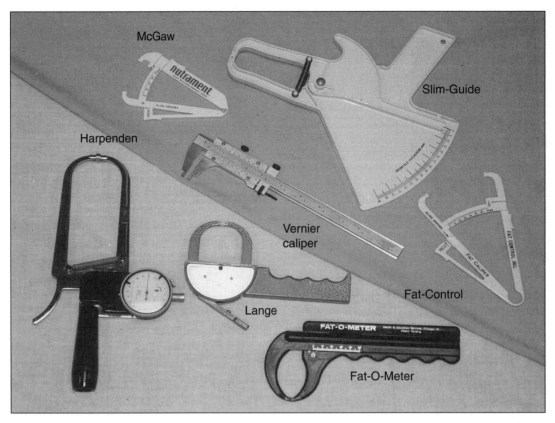

Figure 8.7   Skinfold calipers.

accuracy of your caliper should be checked periodically using a high-precision Vernier caliper or SKF calibration blocks.

Although the Harpenden and Lange SKF calipers have similar pressure characteristics, a number of researchers reported that SKFs measured with Harpenden calipers produce significantly smaller values compared to Lange calipers (Gruber et al. 1990; Lohman, Pollock, et al. 1984). Even though the pressure is similar for the Lange (9.3 g/mm²) and Harpenden (9.36 g/mm²) calipers, researchers noted that the Harpenden caliper requires three times more force to open its jaws. Therefore, it is more likely that the adipose tissue will be compressed to a greater extent, resulting in smaller SKF measurements with this type of caliper.

5. Are plastic SKF calipers as accurate as metal SKF calipers?

Compared to high-quality calipers, plastic SKF calipers have less scale precision (~2 mm), nonconstant tension throughout the range of measurement (Hawkins 1983), a smaller measurement scale (~40 mm), and less consistency when used by inexperienced SKF technicians (Lohman, Pollock, et al. 1984). Despite these differences, several researchers (Hawkins 1983; Lohman, Pollock, et al. 1984) reported no significant differences between SKFs measured with high quality calipers (Harpenden, Holtain, and Lange) and plastic calipers (McGaw caliper, Ross adipometer, and Fat-O-Meter). However, SKFs measured with Harpenden, McGaw, Slim-Guide, and Skyndex calipers are significantly smaller than those measured with Lange calipers (Burgert and Anderson 1979; Gruber et al. 1990; Hawkins 1983; Lohman, Pollock, et al. 1984; Zando and Robertson 1987). Lohman, Pollock, et al. (1984) noted that differences among instruments (Harpenden, Lange, Holtain, and Ross adipometer calipers) varied depending on the SKF technician. Differences among technicians were less for the Harpenden and Holtain calipers compared to the Lange caliper and Ross adipometer. Given that the caliper's type may be a potential source of measurement error, be sure you use the same caliper when monitoring changes in your client's SKF thicknesses.

6. Will my client's hydration level affect the skinfold measurements?

SKF measurements also may be affected by compressibility of the adipose tissue and hydration levels of your clients. Martin, Drinkwater, and Clarys

(1992) reported that variation in SKF compressibility may be an important limitation of the SKF method. In addition, an accumulation of extracellular water (edema) in the subcutaneous tissue caused by factors such as peripheral vasodilation or certain diseases may increase skinfold thicknesses (Keys and Brozek 1953). This suggests that you should not measure SKFs immediately after exercise, especially in hot environments. Also, most of the weight gain experienced by some women during their menstrual cycles is caused by water retention (Bunt et al. 1989). This theoretically could increase SKF thicknesses, particularly on the trunk and abdomen; but there are no empirical data to support or refute this hypothesis.

7. Should SKFs be measured on the right or left side of the body?

Although there are only small differences (1 to 2 mm) between SKF thicknesses on the right and left sides of the body for the typical individual, there is some disagreement about which side of the body to measure. In the United States, researchers and practitioners take SKF measurements on the right side of the body, as recommended in the *Anthropometric Standardization Reference Manual* (Lohman, Roche, and Martorell 1988). The general practice in Europe and developing countries is to measure SKFs on the left side of the body, as recommended by the International Biological Programs (Martorell et al. 1988).

8. Should I use SKFs to measure the body fat of obese clients?

It is difficult, even for highly-skilled SKF technicians, to accurately measure the SKF thickness of extremely obese individuals. Sometimes the client's SKF thickness exceeds the maximum aperture of the caliper, and the jaws of the caliper may slip off the fold during the measurement. Therefore, avoid using the SKF method to estimate body fat of extremely obese clients.

Bioelectrical Impedance Method

Bioelectrical impedance analysis (BIA) is a rapid, noninvasive, and relatively inexpensive method for evaluating body composition in field settings. With this method, a low-level electrical current is passed through the client's body, and the impedance (Z), or opposition to the flow of current, is measured with a BIA analyzer. You can estimate an individual's total body water (TBW) from the impedance measurement because the electrolytes in the body's water are excellent conductors of electrical current.

When the volume of TBW is large, the current flows more easily through the body with less resistance (R). The resistance to current flow will be greater in individuals with large amounts of body fat, since adipose tissue, with its relatively low water content, is a poor conductor of electrical current. Because the water content of the fat-free body is relatively large (73% water), you can predict fat-free mass (FFM) from TBW estimates. Individuals with large FFM and TBW have less resistance to current flowing through their bodies compared to those with a smaller FFM.

Bioelectrical impedance indirectly estimates FFM or TBW. Therefore, the following assumptions are made about the geometric shape of the body and the relationship of impedance to the length and volume of the conductor:

- *The human body is shaped like a perfect cylinder with a uniform length and cross-sectional area.* Of course, this assumption is not entirely true. Because the body segments are not uniform in length or cross-sectional area, resistance to the flow of current through these body segments will differ.

- *Assuming the body is a perfect cylinder, at a fixed signal frequency (e.g., 50 kHz), the impedance (Z) to current flow through the body is directly related to the length (L) of the conductor (height) and inversely related to its cross-sectional area* $[Z = p(L/A)$, where p is the specific resistivity of the body's tissues and is assumed to be constant]. To express this relationship in terms of Z and the body's volume, instead of its cross-sectional area, the equation is multiplied by L/L: $[Z = p(L/A)(L/L)]$. $A \times L$ is equal to volume (V), so rearranging this equation yields $V = pL^2/Z$. Thus, the volume of the FFM or TBW of the body is directly proportional to L^2, or height squared (HT^2), and indirectly proportional to Z.

- *Biological tissues act as conductors or insulators, and the flow of current through the body will follow the path of least resistance.* Because the FFM contains large amounts of water (~73%) and electrolytes, it is a better conductor of electrical current than fat. Fat is anhydrous and a poor conductor of electrical current. The total body impedance, measured at the constant frequency of 50 kHz, primarily reflects the volumes of the water and muscle compartments comprising the FFM and the extracellular water volume (Kushner 1992).

- *Impedance is a function of resistance and reactance, where* $Z = \sqrt{(R^2 + Xc^2)}$. Resistance (R) is a measure of pure opposition to current flow through the body; reactance (Xc) is the opposition to current flow caused by the capacitance of the cell membrane (Kushner 1992). R is much larger than Xc (at a 50 kHz frequency) when you measure whole body impedance; therefore R is a better predictor of FFM and TBW than Z (Lohman 1989). For these reasons, many BIA models use the resistance index (HT^2/R) instead of HT^2/Z, to predict FFM or TBW.

Using the BIA Method

BIA prediction equations are based on either population-specific or generalized models. These equations provide acceptable estimates of FFM and TBW because of theoretical and empirical relationships among FFM, TBW, and bioimpedance measures. Many population-specific BIA equations have been developed for homogenous subgroups to account for differences due to age, ethnicity, gender, physical activity level, and level of body fatness. These equations are valid only for individuals whose physical characteristics are similar to those in the specific population subgroup. For example, an equation developed for younger men will systematically overestimate the FFM of older men (Deurenberg et al. 1990).

As an alternative to population-specific equations, you can use generalized BIA equations developed for heterogeneous populations varying in age, gender, and body fatness. This approach accounts for the biological variability among population subgroups by including factors such as age and gender as predictor variables in BIA equations (Deurenberg et al. 1990; Gray et al. 1989; Kushner and Schoeller 1986; Van Loan and Mayclin 1987).

Table 8.4 presents commonly-used, population-specific and generalized BIA equations. With these equations, you can accurately estimate the FFM of your clients within ±2.8 kg for women and ±3.5 kg for men. To use these equations, obtain R and Xc directly from your BIA analyzer. Computer software exists that allows you to select an appropriate BIA equation to estimate your client's FFM based on physical characteristics (i.e., age, gender, race, physical activity level, and level of body fatness) (Ng 1997). Using this software will save time and prevent errors in calculating FFM from these equations. The % BF of your client is estimated by determining the fat mass (FM = BW – FFM) and dividing FM by the client's body weight [% BF = (FM/BW) × 100].

Experts recommend not using the FFM and % BF estimates obtained directly from your BIA analyzer (BMR, Holtain, RJL, or Valhalla) unless you know

for sure which equations are programmed into the analyzer's computer software, you obtain information from the manufacturer regarding the validity and accuracy of these equations, and you determine these equations are applicable to your clients.

Although the relative predictive accuracy of the BIA method is similar to the SKF method, BIA may be preferable in some settings for the following reasons:

- It does not require a high degree of technician skill.

- It is generally more comfortable and does not intrude as much upon the client's privacy.

- It can be used to estimate body composition of obese individuals (Gray et al. 1989; Segal et al. 1988).

BIA Technique

The tetrapolar method uses four electrodes applied to the hand, wrist, foot, and ankle (figure 8.8). An excitation current of (500 μA to 800 μA) at 50 kHz is applied at the source (distal) electrodes on the hand and foot, and the voltage drop due to impedance is detected by the sensor (proximal) electrodes on the wrist and ankle. The total resistance to current flow through the arm, trunk, and leg is measured using this type of electrode configuration.

The accuracy of the BIA method depends on controlling factors that may increase measurement error. Therefore, it is important to determine whether your client meets all BIA pretesting guidelines below.

BIA CLIENT GUIDELINES

- No eating or drinking within 4 hours of the test.
- No exercise within 12 hours of the test.
- Urinate within 30 minutes of the test.
- No alcohol consumption within 48 hours of the test.
- No diuretic medications within 7 days of the test.
- No testing of female clients who perceive they are retaining water during that stage of their menstrual cycle.

In addition, you need to closely follow the standardized testing procedures for the BIA method (see page 162).

Table 8.4   BIA Prediction Equations

Ethnicity	Gender	% BF level (Age)	Equation	Reference
American Indian, Black, Hispanic, or White	Men[b]	<20 % BF (17-62 yr)	FFM (kg) = 0.00066360(HT^2) − 0.02117(R) + 0.62854(BW) − 0.12380(Age) + 9.33285	Segal et al. (1988)
		≥20 % BF (17-62 yr)	FFM (kg) = 0.0008858(HT^2) − 0.02999(R) + 0.42688(BW) − 0.07002(Age) + 14.52435	Segal et al. (1988)
American Indian, Black, Hispanic, or White	Women[b]	<30 % BF (17-62 yr)	FFM (kg) = 0.000646(HT^2) − 0.014(R) + 0.421(BW) + 10.4	Segal et al. (1988)
		≥30 % BF (17-62 yr)	FFM (kg) = 0.00091186(HT^2) − 0.01466 (R) + 0.29990(BW) − 0.07012(Age) + 9.37938	Segal et al. (1988)
White	Boys and girls	8-15 yr	FFM (kg) = 0.62(HT^2/R) + 0.21(BW) + 0.10(Xc) + 4.2	Lohman (1992)
	Boys and girls	10-19 yr	FFM (kg) = 0.61(HT^2/R) + 0.25(BW) + 1.31	Houtkooper et al. (1992)
NR[a]	Female athletes	NR[a]	FFM (kg) = 0.73(HT^2/R) + 0.16(BW) + 2.0	Houtkooper et al. (1989)
NR[a]	Male athletes	19-40 yr	FFM (kg) = 0.186(HT^2/R) + 0.701(BW) + 1.949	Oppliger et al. (1991)

[a]NR = not reported.
[b]For clients who are obviously lean use the <20% BF (men) and <30% BF (women) equations.
For clients who are obviously obese, use the ≥20% BF (men) and ≥30% BF (women) equations.
For clients who are not obviously lean or obese, calculate their FFM using *both* the lean and obese equations and then average the two FFM estimates.

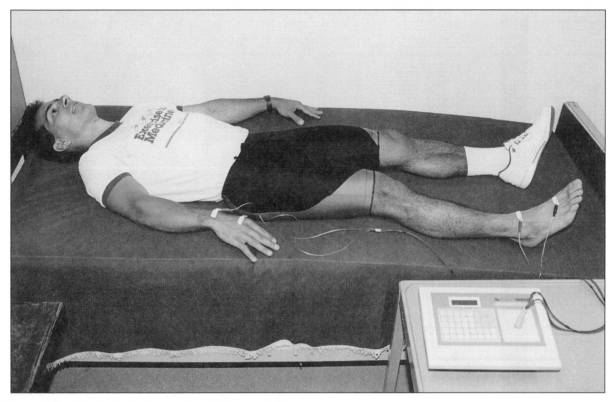

Figure 8.8 BIA electrode placement and client positioning.

STANDARDIZED TESTING PROCEDURES FOR BIA METHOD

1. Bioimpedance measures are taken on the right side of the body, with the client lying supine on a nonconductive surface, in a room with normal ambient temperature (~22° C or 72° F).

2. Clean the skin at the electrode sites with an alcohol pad.

3. Place the sensor (proximal) electrodes (see figure 8.8) on (a) the dorsal surface of the wrist so that the upper border of the electrode bisects the head of the ulna, and (b) the dorsal surface of the ankle so that the upper border of the electrode bisects the medial and lateral malleoli. You can use a measuring tape and surgical marking pen to mark these points for electrode placement.

4. Place the source (distal) electrodes at the base of the second or third metacarpal-phalangeal joints of the hand and foot (see figure 8.8). Make certain the proximal and distal electrodes are separated by at least 5 cm (2 in).

5. Attach the lead wires to the appropriate electrodes. Attach red leads to the wrist and ankle, and black leads to the hand and foot.

6. Make certain that the client's legs and arms are abducted approximately 45° to each other. There should be no contact between the thighs and between the arms and the trunk.

Sources of Measurement Error

The accuracy and precision of the BIA measurements are affected by instrumentation, technician skill, client factors, and environmental factors. The following questions and responses address these sources of measurement error.

1. Can different types of bioimpedance analyzers be used interchangeably?

Two commonly-used impedance analyzers are the RJL™ System (Detroit, MI) and Valhalla Scientific™ (San Diego, CA). Research demonstrates that the whole body resistance (hand to foot) measured by different brands of single frequency analyzers differ by as much as 36 Ω (Graves et al. 1989). For example, the average % BF estimated for men from one BIA equation differed by 6.3% BF using the Valhalla™ and Bioelectrical Sciences™ (BES, La Jolla, CA) analyzers to measure R. In general, the Valhalla analyzer produced significantly higher resistances (~16 to ~19 Ω) than the RJL analyzer for men and women, causing a systematic underestimation of FFM (Graves et al. 1989). To control for this potential source of measurement error, always use the same instrument when monitoring changes in your client's body composition.

Recently, less expensive bioimpedance analyzers have been marketed for home healthcare. The Tanita™ analyzer measures lower-body resistance between the right and left legs as the individual stands on the analyzer's electrode plates. The OMRON™ analyzer is hand-held and measures upper-body resistance between the right and left arms (see figure 8.9). The upper-body and lower-body resistances measured by these analyzers will be larger than whole-body resistance (right arm-trunk-right leg) given the relatively smaller volumes of these body segments compared to the trunk. To date there are no published reports verifying the validity and applicability of equations programmed into these newer analyzers for assessing body composition of diverse subgroups of the population.

2. Does eating or being dehydrated have any effect on bioimpedance measures?

A major source of error for the BIA method is variability due to the client's state of hydration. Eating, drinking, and dehydration alter the individual's hydration state, thereby affecting total body resistance and the estimate of FFM. Taking resistance measures 2 to 4 hours after a meal decreases R and is likely to overpredict the FFM of your client by almost 1.5 kg (Deurenberg et al. 1988). Dehydration, on the other hand, increases resistance (~40 Ω), resulting in a 5.0 kg underestimate of FFM (Lukaski 1986).

3. Will bioimpedance test results be affected if I measure my client immediately after exercise?

The degree to which test results are affected depends on intensity and duration of the exercise workout. Researchers have reported that jogging and cycling at moderate intensities (~70% $\dot{V}O_2$max) for 90 to 120 minutes substantially decrease resistance (50 to 70 Ω), resulting in a large overestimate of FFM (~12 kg) (Khaled et al. 1988; Lukaski 1986). The decrease in resistance after strenuous exercise most likely reflects the relatively greater loss of body water in the sweat and expired air, compared to the loss of electrolytes. This leads to a higher electrolyte concentration in the body's fluids, thereby lowering resistance values (Deurenberg et al. 1988). Increases in core body temperature and skin temperature also may contribute to the sharp decline in resistance after exercising, because increased skin temperature (33.4° C compared to 24° C) decreases resistance (Caton et al. 1988).

4. Are bioimpedance measures affected by the menstrual cycle?

Although the menstrual cycle alters the total body water, the ratio of extracellular to intracellular water, and body weight (Mitchell et al. 1993), there are

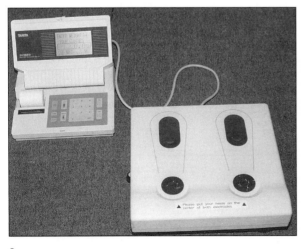

a

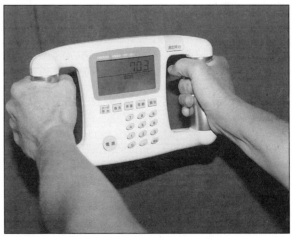

b

Figure 8.9   Tanita™ (*a*) and Omron™ (*b*) BIA analyzers.

only small changes in bioimpedance measures (Z and R) between the follicular and premenstrual stages (~5 to 8 Ω) and between menses and the follicular stage (~7 Ω) (Deurenberg et al. 1988; Gleichauf and Rose 1989). In women experiencing relatively large body weight gains (2 to 4 kg) during the menstrual cycle, a substantial part of this weight gain is due to an increase in total body water (Bunt et al. 1989). Until there are more conclusive data dealing with this issue, you should take BIA measurements at a time during the menstrual cycle when the client perceives that she is not experiencing a large weight gain. This practice should minimize error and yield a more accurate estimate of FFM for your clients.

5. Is there a high degree of agreement in bioimpedance values when measurements are taken by two different technicians?

Technician skill is not a major source of measurement error for the BIA method. There is virtually no difference in resistance measurements taken by different technicians, provided that each follows standardized procedures for electrode placement and client positioning (Jackson et al. 1988). The proximal sensor electrodes, in particular, need to be correctly positioned at the wrist and ankle. For example, a 1 cm displacement of the sensor electrodes may result in a 2% error in resistance (Elsen et al. 1987). As a standard practice, you should take bioimpedance measures on the right side of the body.

Other Anthropometric Methods

Anthropometry refers to the measurement of the size and proportion of the human body. You can use circumferences, skinfold thicknesses, skeletal breadths, and segment lengths to assess the size and proportions of body segments. In addition to measuring body size and proportions, anthropometric measures have been used to assess total body and regional body composition. Anthropometric indexes such as *body mass index (BMI)* and *waist-to-hip circumference ratio (WHR)* are used to identify individuals at risk for disease. Compared to SKF measures, these anthropometric methods are relatively simple, inexpensive, and do not require a high degree of technical skill and training.

There are basic principles associated with using anthropometric measures such as BMI, circumferences, and skeletal diameters to estimate body composition:

- *Circumferences are affected by fat mass, muscle mass, and skeletal size; therefore, these measures are related to fat mass and lean body mass.* Jackson and Pollock (1978) reported that circumference and bony diameter measures are markers of lean body mass (muscle mass and skeletal size); however, some circumferences are also highly associated with the fat component. These findings confirm that circumference measures reflect both the fat and fat-free components of body composition.

- *Skeletal size is directly related to lean body mass.* Behnke (1961) proposed that lean body mass could be accurately estimated from skeletal diameters and, subsequently, developed equations for predicting lean body mass. Cross-validation of these equations yielded a moderately high relationship (r = 0.80) and closely estimated the average lean body mass obtained from hydrodensitometry (Wilmore and Behnke 1969, 1970). Behnke's hypothesis was also supported by the observation that skeletal diameters, along with circumference measures, are strong markers of lean body mass (Jackson and Pollock 1978).

- *To estimate total body fat from weight-to-height indexes, the index should be highly related to body fat but independent of height.* Based on data from two large-scale epidemiological surveys (National Health and Nutrition Examination Surveys I and II), Micozzi et al. (1986) reported that *body mass index (body weight divided by height squared)* is not significantly related to height of men or women, but is directly related to skinfold thickness and the estimated fat area of the arm in adults. However, the relationship to body fat varies with age, gender, and ethnicity (Deurenberg, Westrate, and Seidell 1991; Wagner, Heyward, and Stolarczyk 1997). BMI is not totally independent of height, however, especially in younger children (<15 years of age).

Using Anthropometric Methods

You can use various combinations of skinfolds, circumferences, and skeletal diameters to estimate your client's body composition. This section includes only those equations using circumferences and diameters as predictors, for the following reasons:

- The predictive accuracy of anthropometric (circumference and diameter) equations is not greatly improved by adding skinfold measures.

- Anthropometric equations using only circumferences as predictors estimate the body fatness of obese individuals more accurately than skinfold prediction equations (Seip and Weltman 1991).

- Compared to skinfolds, circumferences and skeletal diameters can be measured with less error (Bray and Gray 1988a).

- Some practitioners may not have access to skinfold calipers.

Population-specific anthropometric equations are valid for and can only be applied to individuals whose physical characteristics (age, gender, and level of body fatness) are similar to those in a specific population subgroup. For example, anthropometric equations developed to estimate the body composition of obese individuals (Weltman et al. 1988; Weltman, Seip, and Tran 1987) should not be applied to nonobese individuals. On the other hand, generalized equations, applicable to individuals varying in age and body fatness, have been developed for heterogeneous populations of women (15 to 79 years of age; 13 to 63% BF) and men (20 to 78 years of age; 2 to 49% BF) (Tran and Weltman 1988, 1989). Table 8.5 provides anthropometric prediction equations that are applicable to various population subgroups. You can also use computer software to obtain body composition estimates from these equations for your clients (Ng 1997).

Anthropometric measures have other uses besides estimating body composition. For example, in epidemiological studies, BMI provides a crude index of obesity. The BMI is the ratio of body weight to height squared: BMI (kg/m^2) = WT (in kg)/HT^2 (in m). Alternatively, you can use a nomogram (see figure 8.10) to calculate and classify BMI (Bray 1978). To use this nomogram, plot your client's height and body weight in the appropriate columns and connect these two points with a straight edge. Read the corresponding BMI at the point where the connecting line intersects the BMI column on the nomogram.

Table 8.6 describes standards for classifying BMI. It is important to remember that BMI is only a crude index of obesity and should not be used to estimate body fatness of your clients because the prediction error is unacceptable ($\geq 5.0\%$ BF).

The waist-to-hip ratio (WHR) can help you distinguish between patterns of fat distribution in the upper and lower body. The WHR is strongly associated with visceral fat and appears to be an acceptable index of intra-abdominal fat (Seidell et al. 1987). Generally, young adults with WHR values in

excess of 0.94 (men) or 0.82 (women) are at high risk for adverse health consequences (Bray and Gray 1988b). However, this index is not valid for evaluating fat distribution in prepubertal children (Peters et al. 1992). The WHR norms (see table 8.7) were established using the standardized measurement procedures described in the *Anthropometric Standardization Reference Manual*. Calculate the WHR ratio by dividing waist circumference (cm) by hip circumference (cm). Alternatively, you can use a nomogram (figure 8.11) to obtain WHR. Plot the client's waist and hip circumferences in the corresponding columns of the nomogram and connect the points with a straight edge. Read the WHR at the point where this line intersects the WHR column

When you are evaluating body weight of your client using height-weight tables, you can improve their usefulness by classifying frame size according to skeletal diameters. Skeletal breadths are important estimators of the bone and muscle components of FFM; therefore, an estimate of frame size allows you to differentiate between those who weigh more because of a large musculoskeletal mass and those who are overweight because of a large fat mass. You can classify frame size by using reference data for elbow breadth (see table 8.8). The anatomical landmarks for measuring elbow breadth are described in appendix D.6.

Anthropometric Techniques

Practice is necessary to become proficient in measuring skeletal diameters and circumferences. Following the standardized procedures below will increase the accuracy and reliability of your measurements (Callaway et al. 1988; Wilmore et al. 1988).

STANDARDIZED PROCEDURES FOR ANTHROPOMETRIC MEASUREMENTS

---

1. Take all circumference and bony diameter measurements of the limbs on the right side of the body.

2. Carefully identify and measure the anthropometric site. Be meticulous about locating anatomical landmarks used to identify the measurement site (see appendix D.5 and D.6).

3. Take a minimum of three measurements at each site in rotational order.

4. To measure the breadth of smaller segments

Table 8.5   Circumference and Skeletal Diameter Prediction Equations

Ethnicity	Gender	Age	Equation	Reference
White	Women	15-79 yr	Db (g/cc)[a] = 1.168297 − 0.002824(Abdom C[b]) + 0.0000122098(Abdom C[b])^2 − 0.000733128(Hip C) + 0.000510477(HT) − 0.000216161(Age)	Tran and Weltman (1989)
	Men	18-40 yr	FFM (kg) = 39.652 + 1.0932(BW) + 0.8370 (Bi-iliac D) + 0.3297(AB$_1$ C) − 1.0008(AB$_2$ C) − 0.6478(Knee C)	Wilmore and Behnke (1969)
White	Obese women	20-60 yr	% BF = 0.11077(Abdomen C[b]) − 0.17666(HT) + 0.14354(BW) + 51.033	Weltman et al. (1988)
	Obese men	24-68 yr	% BF = 0.31457(Abdomen C[b]) − 0.10969(BW) + 10.834	Weltman et al. (1987)

[a]Use population-specific conversion formula (see table 8.2) to calculate % BF from Db.

[b]Abdom C (cm) is the average abdominal circumference measured at two sites: (1) anteriorly midway between the xiphoid process of sternum and the umbilicus and laterally between the lower end of the rib cage and iliac crests and (2) at the umbilicus level.

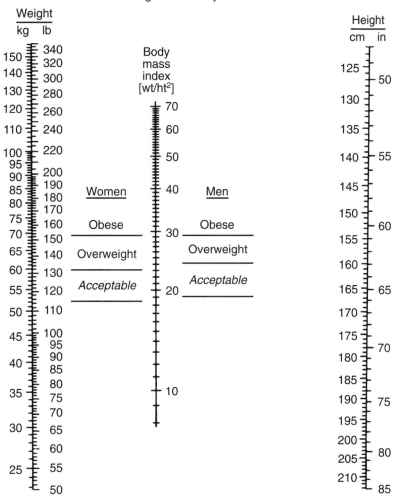

Figure 8.10 Nomogram for body mass index (BMI).
Reprinted, by permission, from G.A. Bray, 1978, "Definitions, measurements and classification of the syndromes of obesity," *International Journal of Obesity* 2(2): 99-112.

Table 8.6 Obesity Classification Based on Body Mass Index (BMI)		
Classification	**Men**	**Women**
Normal	24-27	23-26
Moderately obese	28-31	27-32
Severely obese	>31	>32

Data from *The Surgeon General's Report on Nutrition and Health* (1988) U.S. Department of Health and Human Services, 284.

Table 8.7   Waist-to-Hip Circumference Ratio (WHR) Norms for Men and Women

	Age	Risk			
		Low	Moderate	High	Very high
Men	20-29	<0.83	0.83-0.88	0.89-0.94	>0.94
	30-39	<0.84	0.84-0.91	0.92-0.96	>0.96
	40-49	<0.88	0.88-0.95	0.96-1.00	>1.00
	50-59	<0.90	0.90-0.96	0.97-1.02	>1.02
	60-69	<0.91	0.91-0.98	0.99-1.03	>1.03
Women	20-29	<0.71	0.71-0.77	0.78-0.82	>0.82
	30-39	<0.72	0.72-0.78	0.79-0.84	>0.84
	40-49	<0.73	0.73-0.79	0.80-0.87	>0.87
	50-59	<0.74	0.74-0.81	0.82-0.88	>0.88
	60-69	<0.76	0.76-0.83	0.84-0.90	>0.90

Adapted from Bray and Gray (1988b) "Obesity—Part I—Pathogenesis," *Western Journal of Medicine* 149: 432.

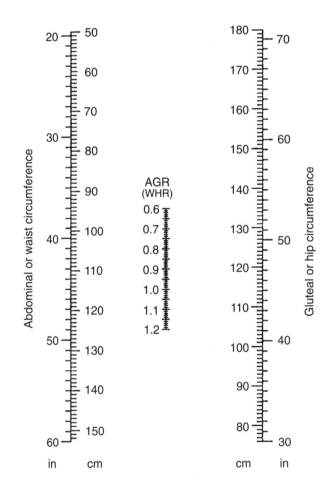

Figure 8.11   Nomogram for waist-to-hip ratio (WHR).
Reprinted by permission of *The Western Journal of Medicine*, G.A. Bray and D.S. Gray, "Obesity: Part I–Pathogenesis," 1988, 149: 432.

Table 8.8 Elbow Breadth Norms (in cm) for Men and Women in the United States

	Age (years)	Frame size		
		Small	Medium	Large
Men	18-24	≤6.6	>6.6 and <7.7	≥7.7
	25-34	≤6.7	>6.7 and <7.9	≥7.9
	35-44	≤6.7	>6.7 and <8.0	≥8.0
	45-54	≤6.7	>6.7 and <8.1	≥8.1
	55-64	≤6.7	>6.7 and <8.1	≥8.1
	65-74	≤6.7	>6.7 and <8.1	≥8.1
Women	18-24	≤5.6	>5.6 and <6.5	≥6.5
	25-34	≤5.7	>5.7 and <6.8	≥6.8
	35-44	≤5.7	>5.7 and <7.1	≥7.1
	45-54	≤5.7	>5.7 and <7.2	≥7.2
	55-64	≤5.8	>5.8 and <7.2	≥7.2
	65-74	≤5.8	>5.8 and <7.2	≥7.2

From A.R. Frisancho, 1984, "New Standards for Weight and Body Composition by Frame Size and Height for Assessment of Nutritional Status of Adults and the Elderly." *American Journal of Clinical Nutrition* 40: 810. Copyright 1984 by the *American Journal of Clinical Nutrition.* Reprinted by permission.

like the elbow or wrist, use small sliding calipers (a range of 30 cm or 11.8 in) with greater scale precision instead of larger skeletal anthropometers (a range of 60 to 80 cm or 23.6 to 31.5 in).

5. Hold the skeletal anthropometer or caliper in both hands so the tips of the index fingers are adjacent to the tips of the caliper.

6. Place the caliper on the bony landmarks and apply firm pressure to compress the underlying muscle, fat, and skin. Apply pressure until the measurement no longer continues to decrease.

7. Use an anthropometric tape to measure circumferences. Hold the zero end of the tape in your left hand, positioned below the other part of the tape which is held in your right hand.

8. Apply tension to the tape so that it fits snugly around the body part but does not indent the skin or compress the subcutaneous tissue.

9. For some circumferences (e.g., waist, hip, and thigh), you should align the tape in a horizontal plane, parallel to the floor.

Sources of Measurement Error

The accuracy and reliability of anthropometric measures are potentially affected by equipment, techni-

cian skill, and client factors (Bray et al. 1978; Callaway et al. 1988). The following questions and responses address these sources of measurement error.

1. What equipment will I need to measure bony widths?

Use skeletal anthropometers and sliding or spreading calipers to measure bony widths and body breadths (see figure 8.12). The precision characteristic (0.05 cm to 0.50 cm) and range of measurement (0 to 210 cm or 0 to 82.7 in) depends on the type of skeletal anthropometer or caliper you are using (Wilmore et al. 1988). The instruments must be carefully maintained and calibrated periodically to check their accuracy.

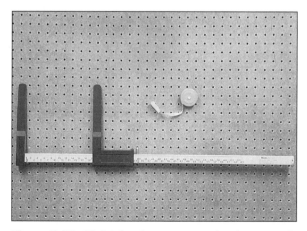

Figure 8.12 Skeletal anthropometer and anthropometric tape measure.

2. Can I use any type of tape measure to measure body circumferences?

Use an anthropometric tape measure to measure circumferences (see figure 8.12). The tape measure should be made from a flexible material that does not stretch with use. You can use a plastic-coated tape measure if an anthropometric tape measure is not available. Some anthropometric tapes have a spring-loaded handle (i.e., Gulick handle) that allows a constant tension to be applied to the end of the tape during the measurement.

3. How much skill and practice is required to ensure accurate circumference and skeletal diameter measurements?

Compared to the SKF method, technician skill is not a major source of measurement error. However, practice is needed to perfect the identification of the measurement sites and your measurement technique. Experts recommend practicing on at least 50 people and taking a minimum of three measurements for each site in rotational order (Callaway et al. 1988). Closely follow standardized testing procedures for locating measurement sites, positioning the anthropometer or tape measure, and applying tension during the measurement. Appendix D.5 and D.6 describe some of the most commonly used circumference and skeletal diameter sites.

4. Is there good agreement in circumference and skeletal diameter values when the measurements are taken by two different technicians?

Variability in circumference measurements taken by different technicians is relatively small (0.2 cm to 1.0 cm), with some sites differing more than others (Callaway et al. 1988). Skilled technicians can obtain similar values, even when measuring circumferences of obese individuals (Bray and Gray 1988a).

5. Are the circumferences of obese clients more easily measured than skinfolds?

Like the SKF method, it is more difficult to obtain consistent measurements of circumference for obese compared to lean individuals (Bray and Gray 1988a). However, circumferences are preferable to SKFs when measuring obese clients for several reasons:

- You can measure circumferences of obese individuals regardless of their size, whereas the maximum aperture of the SKF caliper may not be large enough to allow measurement.

- Circumferences require less technician skill.

- Differences between technicians are smaller for circumferences compared to SKF measurements (Bray and Gray 1988a).

6. Is it possible to accurately measure bony widths of heavily-muscled and obese clients?

Accurate measurement of bony diameters in heavily-muscled or obese individuals may be difficult because the underlying muscle and fat tissues must be firmly compressed. It may be difficult to identify and palpate bony anatomical landmarks, leading to error in locating the measurement site.

Near-Infrared Interactance Method

Near-infrared interactance (NIR) is a relatively new field method used to estimate body composition. Compared to the skinfold (SKF) and bioelectrical impedance (BIA) methods, which have been validated and refined through years of research, NIR is still in the developmental stage. Although NIR has been proposed and marketed as a viable alternative to SKF and BIA methods, much more research is needed to fully evaluate the potential of NIR for body composition assessment.

Near-infrared spectroscopy has been used since 1968 to measure the protein, fat, and water content of agricultural products. Conway, Norris, and Bodwell (1984) applied this technology to study human body composition using a high precision (6 nm), expensive, computerized spectrophotometer. Based on results from a small (N = 17) cross-validation sample, these researchers concluded that this method "successfully predicted % body fat" (p. 1129). However, their NIR prediction equation systematically overestimated relative body fat (% BF) for 10 of the 11 females in the cross-validation sample, indicating that different equations may be needed for men and women.

Shortly thereafter, less expensive, commercial NIR analyzers (Futrex-5000™ and Futrex-1000™) were marketed based on the results of Conway and Norris' (1984) work. The Futrex 5000 analyzer estimates % BF from optical density (OD) measured at the biceps site. Cross-validation of the manufacturer's equations indicates that these equations have poor validity and unacceptable prediction errors (SEE = 3.7 to 6.3% BF). Many studies show that the Futrex-5000™ equations systematically underestimate % BF of adults and overestimate the % BF of children (Eaton et al. 1993; Elia, Parkinson, and Diaz 1990; Heyward, Cook, et al. 1992; Heyward, Jenkins, et al. 1992;

Israel et al. 1989; McLean and Skinner 1992; Nielsen et al. 1992; Wilmore, McBride, and Wilmore 1994). Therefore, avoid using these equations to assess the body composition of your clients.

Key Points

- Body composition is a key component of health and physical fitness; total body fat and fat distribution are related to disease risk.
- Standards for percent body fat can be used to classify body composition.
- The average percent fat for adults is 15% for men and 23% for women.
- Obesity is defined as relative body fat equal to or exceeding 25% BF for men and 32% BF for women.
- Hydrostatic weighing is a valid and reliable laboratory method for assessing body composition.
- Population-specific conversion formulas, based on multicomponent models of body composition, should be used to convert body density into percent body fat.
- The skinfold (SKF) method is widely used in field and clinical settings
- Generalized skinfold equations for the prediction of body density are reliable and valid for a wide range of individuals.
- Bioelectrical impedance analysis (BIA) is a viable alternative for assessing body composition of diverse population subgroups.
- Circumferences and skeletal diameters can be used to estimate body composition.
- Body mass index (BMI) is a crude index of total body fatness.
- Waist-to-hip ratio (WHR) is an acceptable index of body fat distribution.
- The near-infrared interactance (NIR) method needs further validation and development.

SOURCES FOR EQUIPMENT

Product	Manufacturer's Address
Air Displacement Plethysmograph	
BOD POD Body Composition System	LMI, Inc. 1980 Olivera Rd., Ste C Concord, CA 94520 (800) 4 BOD POD
Anthropometers	
Spreading calipers Sliding calipers Standard skeletal anthropometer	Pfister Import-Export, Inc. P.O. Box 15 Ridgefield, NJ 07657 (201) 945-5400
Anthropometric Tape Measure	Country Technology, Inc. P.O. Box 87 Gays Mills, WI 54631 (608) 735-4718
Bioimpedance Analyzers	
OMRON	OMRON Healthcare, Inc. 300 Lakeview Pkwy. Vernon Hills, IL 60061 (847) 680-6200
RJL	RJL Systems 33955 Harper Ave. Clinton, TWP, MI 48035 (800) 528-4513
Tanita	Tanita Corp. 5200 Church St. Skokie, IL 60077 (847) 581-0250
Tri-frequency	Daninger Medical Technology 5160 Blazer-Memorial Pkwy. Dublin, OH 43017 (614) 718-0500
Valhalla	Valhalla Scientific Inc. 7576 Trade St. San Diego, CA 92121 (800) 395-4565
Xitron-4000	Xitron Technologies 6295 Ferris Sq. Bldg. D San Diego, CA 92121 (619) 458-9852

Calibration Instruments/Supplies

Skinfold Calibration Blocks (15 mm)	Creative Health Products 5148 Saddle Ridge Rd. Plymouth, MI 48170 (800) 742-4478
Standard Calibration Weights	Ohaus Scale Corp. 29 Hanover Rd. Florham, NJ 07932 (800) 526-0659
Vernier Caliper	L.S. Starrett Co. 121 Crescent St. Athol, MA 01331 (508) 249-3551

Dual-Energy X-ray Absorptiometers

Hologic QDR-1000	Hologic 590 Lincoln St. Waltham, MA 02154 (617) 890-2300
Norland XR-26	Norland W6340 Hackbarth Rd. Fort Atkinson, WI 53538 (800) 333-8456
Lunar DPX	Lunar Radiation Corp. 313 W. Beltline Highway Madison, WI 53713 (608) 274-2663

Scales

Chatillon underwater weighing scale Detecto balance beam scale Health-O-Meter balance beam scale Health-O-Meter digital scale Seca digital scale	Creative Health Products 5148 Saddle Ridge Rd. Plymouth, MI 48170 (800) 742-4478

Skinfold Calipers

Adipometer (plastic)	Ross Laboratories 625 Cleveland Ave. Columbus, OH 43215 (800) 227-5767
Fat-Control (plastic)	Creative Health Products 5148 Saddle Ridge Rd. Plymouth, MI 48170 (800) 742-4478
Fat-O-Meter (plastic)	Health and Education Services 2442 Irving Park Rd. Chicago, IL 60618 (773) 628-1787

Harpenden	Quinton Instruments 3303 Monte Villa Pkwy. Bothel, WA 98021 (800) 426-0538
Holtain	Pfister Import-Export, Inc. 450 Barell Ave. Carlstadt, NJ 07072 (201) 939-4606
Lafayette	Creative Health Products 5148 Saddle Ridge Rd. Plymouth, MI 48170 (800) 742-4478
Lange	Cambridge Scientific Industries 527 Poplar St. Cambridge, MD 21613 (800) 638-9566
McGaw (plastic)	McGaw Laboratories, Inc. P.O. Box 19791 Irvine, CA 92623 (714) 660-2000
Slim-guide (plastic)	Creative Health Products 5148 Saddle Ridge Rd. Plymouth, MI 48170 (800) 742-4478
Skyndex	Cramer Products P.O. Box 1001 Gardner, KS 66030 (913) 884-7511

Stadiometers

Harpenden Stadiometer Holtain Stadiometer	Pfister Import-Export, Inc. 450 Barell Ave. Carlstadt, NJ 07072 (201) 939-4606

REFERENCES

Baumgartner, R.N., Heymsfield, S.B., Lichtman, S., Wang, J., and Pierson, R.N. 1991. Body composition in elderly people: Effect of criterion estimates on predictive equations. *American Journal of Clinical Nutrition* 53: 1-9.

Baun, W.B., and Baun, M.R. 1981. A nomogram for the estimate of percent body fat from generalized equations. *Research Quarterly for Exercise and Sport* 52: 380-384.

Behnke, A.R. 1961. Quantitative assessment of body build. *Journal of Applied Physiology* 16: 960-968.

Behnke, A.R., and Wilmore, J.H. 1974. *Evaluation and regulation of body build and composition.* Englewood Cliffs, NJ: Prentice-Hall.

Bray, G.A. 1978. Definitions, measurements and classifications of the syndromes of obesity. *International Journal of Obesity* 2: 99-113.

Bray, G.A., and Gray, D.S. 1988a. Anthropometric measurements in the obese. In T.G. Lohman, A.F. Roche, and R. Martorell, eds., *Anthropometric standardization reference manual,* 131-136. Champaign, IL: Human Kinetics.

Bray, G.A., and Gray, D.S. 1988b. Obesity. Part I—Pathogenesis. *Western Journal of Medicine* 149: 429-441.

Brozek, J., Grande, F., Anderson, J.T., and Keys, A. 1963. Densiometric analysis of body composition: Revision of some quantitative assumptions. *Annals of the New York Academy of Sciences* 110: 113-140.

Bunt, J.C., Lohman, T.G., and Boileau, R.A. 1989. Impact of total body water fluctuations on estimation of body fat from body density. *Medicine and Science in Sports and Exercise* 21: 96-100.

Burgert, S.L., and Anderson, C.F. 1979. A comparison of triceps skinfold values as measured by the plastic McGaw caliper and the Lange caliper. *American Journal of Clinical Nutrition* 32: 1531-1533.

Callaway, C.W., Chumlea, W.C., Bouchard, C., Himes, J.H., Lohman, T.G., Martin, A.D., Mitchell, C.D., Mueller, W.H., Roche, A.F., and Seefeldt, V.D. 1988. Circumferences. In T.G. Lohman, A.F. Roche, and R. Martorell, eds., *Anthropometric standardization reference manual,* 39-54. Champaign, IL: Human Kinetics.

Caton, J.R., Mole, P.A., Adams, W.C., and Heustis, D.S. 1988. Body composition analysis by bioelectrical impedance: Effect of skin temperature. *Medicine and Science in Sports and Exercise* 20: 489-491.

Conway, J.M., Norris, K.H., and Bodwell, C.E. 1984. A new approach for the estimation of body composition: Infrared interactance. *American Journal of Clinical Nutrition* 40: 1123-1130.

Cote, D. K., and Adams, W.C. 1993. Effect of bone density on body composition estimates in young adult black and white women. *Medicine and Science in Sports and Exercise* 25: 290-296.

Dempster, P., and Aitkens, S. 1995. A new air displacement method for the determination of human body composition. *Medicine and Science in Sports and Exercise* 27: 1692-1697.

Deurenberg, P., van der Kooy, K., Evers, P., and Hulshof, T. 1990. Assessment of body composition by bioelectrical impedance in a population aged >60 y. *American Journal of Clinical Nutrition* 51: 3-6.

Deurenberg, P., Westrate, J.A., Paymans, I., and van der Kooy, K. 1988. Factors affecting bioelectrical impedance measurements in humans. *European Journal of Clincal Nutrition* 42: 1017-1022.

Deurenberg. P., Westrate, J.A., and Seidell, J.C. 1991. Body mass index as a measure of body fatness: Age- and sex-specific prediction formulas. *British Journal of Nutrition* 65: 105-114.

Donnelly, J.R., Brown, T.E., Israel, R.G., Smith-Sintek, S., O'Brien, K.F., and Caslavka, B. 1988. Hydrostatic weighing without head submersion: Description of a method. *Medicine and Science in Sports and Exercise* 20: 66-69.

Eaton, A.W., Israel, R.G., O'Brien, K.F., Hortobagyi, T., and McCammon, M.R. 1993. Comparison of four methods to assess body composition in women. *European Journal of Clinical Nutrition* 47: 353-360.

Edwards, D.A., Hammond, W.H., Healy, M.J., Tanner, J.M., and Whitehouse, R.H. 1955. Design and accuracy of calipers for measuring subcutaneous tissue thickness. *British Journal of Nutrition* 9: 133-143.

Elia, M., Parkinson, S.A., and Diaz, E. 1990. Evaluation of near infra-red interactance as a method for predicting body composition. *European Journal of Clinical Nutrition* 44: 113-121.

Elsen, R., Siu, M.L., Pineda, O., and Solomons, N.W. 1987. Sources of variability in bioelectrical impedance determinations in adults. In K.J. Ellis, S. Yasamura, and W.D. Morgan, eds., *In vivo body composition studies,* 184-188. London: The Institute of Physical Sciences in Medicine.

Frisancho, A.R. 1984. New standard of weight and body composition by frame size and height for assessment of nutritional status of adults and the elderly. *American Journal of Clinical Nutrition* 40: 808-819.

Gleichauf, C.N., and Rose, D.A. 1989. The menstrual cycle's effect on the reliability of bioimpedance measurements for assessing body composition. *American Journal of Clinical Nutrition* 50: 903-907.

Going, S.B., Massett, M.P., Hall, M.C., Bare, L.A., Root, P.A., Williams, D.P., and Lohman, T.G. 1993. Detection of small changes in body composition by dual-energy x-ray absorptiometry. *American Journal of Clinical Nutrition* 57: 845-850.

Graves, J.E., Pollock, M.L., Colvin, A.B., Van Loan, M., and Lohman, T.G. 1989. Comparison of different bioelectrical impedance analyzers in the prediction of body composition. *American Journal of Human Biology* 1: 603-611.

Gray, D.S., Bray, G.A., Gemayel, N., and Kaplan, K. 1989. Effect of obesity on bioelectrical impedance. *American Journal of Clinical Nutrition* 50: 255-260.

Gruber, J.J., Pollock, M.L., Graves, J.E., Colvin, A.B., and Braith, R.W. 1990. Comparison of Harpenden and Lange calipers in predicting body composition. *Research Quarterly for Exercise and Sport* 61: 184-190.

Harrison, G.G., Buskirk, E.R., Carter Lindsay, J.E., Johnston, F.E., Lohman, T.G., Pollock, M.L., Roche, A.F., and Wilmore, J.H. 1988. Skinfold thicknesses and measurement technique. In T.G. Lohman, A.F. Roche, and R. Martorell, eds., *Anthropometric standardization reference manual*, 55-70. Champaign, IL: Human Kinetics.

Hawkins, J.D. 1983. An analysis of selected skinfold measuring instruments. *Journal of Health, Physical Education, Recreation, and Dance* 54 (1): 25-27.

Hayes, P.A., Sowood, P.J., Belyavin, A., Cohen, J.B., and Smith, F.W. 1988. Subcutaneous fat thickness measured by magnetic resonance imaging, ultrasound, and calipers. *Medicine and Science in Sports and Exercise* 20: 303-309.

Heymsfield, S.B., Wang, J., Lichtman, S., Kamen, Y., Kehayias, J., and Pierson, R.N. 1989. Body composition in elderly subjects: A critical appraisal of clinical methodology. *American Journal of Clinical Nutrition* 50: 1167-1175.

Heyward, V.H., Cook, K.L., Hicks, V.L., Jenkins, K.A., Quatrochi, J.A., and Wilson, W. 1992. Predictive accuracy of three field methods for estimating relative body fatness of nonobese and obese women. *International Journal of Sport Nutrition* 2: 75-86.

Heyward, V.H., Jenkins, K.A., Cook, K.L., Hicks, V.L., Quatrochi, J.A., Wilson, W., and Going, S. 1992. Validity of single-site and multi-site models of estimating body composition of women using near-infrared interactance. *American Journal of Human Biology* 4: 579-593.

Heyward, V.H., and Stolarczyk, L.M. 1996. *Applied body composition assessment.* Champaign, IL: Human Kinetics.

Houtkooper, L.B., Going, S.B., Lohman, T.G., Roche, A.F., and Van Loan, M. 1992. Bioelectrical impedance estimation of fat-free body mass in children and youth: A cross-validation study. *Journal of Applied Physiology* 72: 366-373.

Houtkooper, L.B., Lohman, T.G., Going, S.B., and Hall, M.C. 1989. Validity of bioelectric impedance for body composition assessment in children. *Journal of Applied Physiology* 66: 814-821.

Israel, R.G., Houmard, J.A., O'Brien, K.F., McCammon, M.R., Zamora, B.S., and Eaton, A.W. 1989. Validity of near-infrared spectrophotometry device for estimating human body composition. *Research Quarterly for Exercise and Sport* 60: 379-383.

Jackson, A.S. 1984. Research design and analysis of data procedures for predicting body density. *Medicine and Science in Sports and Exercise* 16: 616-620.

Jackson, A.S., and Pollock, M.L. 1976. Factor analysis and multivariate scaling of anthropometric variables for the assessment of body composition. *Medicine and Science in Sports and Exercise* 8: 196-203.

Jackson, A.S., and Pollock, M.L. 1978. Generalized equations for predicting body density of men. *British Journal of Nutrition* 40: 497-504.

Jackson, A.S., and Pollock, M.L. 1985. Practical Assessment of body composition. *The Physician and Sportsmedicine* 13: 76-90.

Jackson, A.S., Pollock, M.L., Graves, J.E., and Mahar, M.T. 1988. Reliability and validity of bioelectrical impedance in determining body composition. *Journal of Applied Physiology* 64: 529-534.

Jackson, A.S., Pollock, M.L., and Ward, A. 1980. Generalized equations for predicting body density of women. *Medicine and Science in Sports and Exercise* 12: 175-182.

Keys, A., and Brozek, J. 1953. Body fat in adult man. *Physiological Reviews* 33: 245-325.

Khaled, M.A., McCutcheon, M.J., Reddy, S., Pearman, P.L., Hunter, G.R., and Weinsier, R.L. 1988. Electrical impedance in assessing human body composition: The BIA method. *American Journal of Clinical Nutrition* 47: 789-792.

Kohrt, W. 1995. Body composition by DXA: Tried and true? *Medicine and Science in Sports and Exercise* 27: 1349-1353.

Kushner, R.F. 1992. Bioelectrical impedance analysis: A review of principles and applications. *Journal of the American College of Nutrition* 11: 199-209.

Kushner, R.F., and Schoeller, D.A. 1986. Estimation of total body water in bioelectrical impedance analysis. *American Journal of Clinical Nutrition* 44: 417-424.

Lohman, T.G. 1981. Skinfolds and body density and their relation to body fatness: A review. *Human Biology* 53: 181-225.

Lohman, T.G. 1987. *Measuring body fat using skinfolds* [videotape]. Champaign, IL: Human Kinetics.

Lohman, T.G. 1989. Bioelectrical impedance. In *Applying new technology to nutrition: Report of the ninth roundtable on medical issues*, 22-25. Columbus, OH: Ross Laboratories.

Lohman, T.G. 1992. *Advances in body composition assessment. Current issues in exercise science series.* Monograph No.3. Champaign, IL: Human Kinetics.

Lohman, T.G., Boileau, R.A., and Slaughter, M.H. 1984. Body composition in children and youth. In R.A. Boileau, ed., *Advances in pediatric sport sciences*, 29-57. Champaign, IL: Human Kinetics.

Lohman, T.G., Pollock, M.L., Slaughter, M.H., Brandon, L.J., and Boileau, R.A. 1984. Methodological factors and the prediction of body fat in female athletes. *Medicine and Science in Sports and Exercise* 16: 92-96.

Lohman, T.G., Roche, A.F., and Martorell, R., eds., 1988. *Anthropometric standardization reference manual.* Champaign, IL: Human Kinetics.

Lukaski, H.C. 1986. Use of the tetrapolar bioelectrical impedance method to assess human body composition. In N.G. Norgan, ed., *Human body composition and fat distribution*, 143-158. Wageningen, Netherlands: Euronut.

Martin, A.D., Drinkwater, D.T., and Clarys, J.P. 1992. Effects of skin thickness and skinfold compressibility on skinfold thickness measurements. *American Journal of Human Biology* 4: 453-460.

Martorell, R., Mendoza, F., Mueller, W.H., and Pawson, I.G. 1988. Which side to measure: Right or left? In T.G. Lohman, A.F. Roche, and R. Martorell, eds., *Anthropometric standardization reference manual*, 87-91. Champaign, IL: Human Kinetics.

McCrory, M.A., Gomez, T.D., Bernauer, E.M., and Mole, P.A. 1995. Evaluation of a new displacement plethysmograph for measuring human body composition. *Medicine and Science in Sports and Exercise* 27: 1686-1691.

McLean, K.P., and Skinner, J.S. 1992. Validity of Futrex-5000 for body composition determination. *Medicine and Science in Sports and Exercise* 24: 253-258.

Micozzi, M.S., Albanes, D., Jones, Y., and Chumlea, W.C. 1986. Correlations of body mass indices with weight, stature, and body composition in men and women in NHANES I and II. *American Journal of Clinical Nutrition* 44: 725-731.

Mitchell, C.O., Rose, J.F., Familoni, B., Winders, S.E., and Lancaster, E. 1993. The use of multifrequency bioelectrical impedance analysis to estimate fluid volume changes as a function of the menstrual cycle. In K.J. Ellis and J.D. Eastman, eds., *Human body composition: In vivo methods, models and assessment*, 189-191. New York, NY: Plenum Press.

Morrow, J.R., Jackson, A.S., Bradley, P.W., and Hartung, G.H. 1986. Accuracy of measured and predicted residual lung volume on body density measurement. *Medicine and Science in Sport and Exercise* 18: 647-652.

Ng, N. 1997. Comprehensive body composition software. Champaign, IL: Human Kinetics.

Nielsen, D.H., Cassady, S.L., Wacker, L.M., Wessels, A.K., Wheelock, B.J., and Oppliger, R.A. 1992. Validation of the Futrex-5000 near-infrared spectrophotometer analyzer for assessment of body composition. *Journal of Orthopaedic and Sports Physical Therapy* 16: 281-287.

Oppliger, R.A., Nielsen, D.H., and Vance, C.G. 1991. Wrestlers' minimal weight: Anthropometry, bioimpedance, and hydrostatic weighing compared. *Medicine and Science in Sports and Exercise* 23: 247-253.

Ortiz, O., Russell, M., Daley, T.L., Baumgartner, R.N., Waki, M., Lichtman, S., Wang, S., Pierson, R.N., and Heymsfield, S.B. 1992. Differences in skeletal muscle and bone mineral mass between black and white females and their relevance to estimates of body composition. *American Journal of Clinical Nutrition* 55: 8-13.

Peters, D., Fox, K., Armstrong, N., Sharpe, P., and Bell, M. 1992. Assessment of children's abdominal fat distribution by magnetic resonance imaging and anthropometry. *International Journal of Obesity* 16 (Suppl. 2): S35 (Abstract).

Pollock, M.. and Jackson, A.S. 1984. Research progress in validation of clinical methods of assessing body composition. *Medicine and Science in Sports and Exercise* 16: 606-613.

Quatrochi, J.A., Hicks, V.L., Heyward, V.H., Colville, B.C., Cook, K.L., Jenkins, K.A., and Wilson, W. 1992. Relationship of optical density and skinfold measurements: Effects of age and level of body fatness. *Research Quarterly for Exercise and Sport* 63: 402-409.

Roche, A.F., Heymsfield, S.B., and Lohman, T.G. 1996. *Human body composition*. Champaign, IL: Human Kinetics.

Roubenoff, R., Kehayias, J.J., Dawson-Hughes, B., and Heymsfield, S.B. 1993. Use of dual-energy x-ray absorptiometry in body-composition studies: Not yet a "gold standard." *American Journal of Clinical Nutrition* 58: 589-591.

Schutte, J.E., Townsend, E.J., Hugg, J., Shoup, R.F., Malina, R.M., and Blomqvist, C.G. 1984. Density of lean body mass is greater in Blacks than in Whites. *Journal of Applied Physiology* 56: 1647-1649.

Segal, K.R., Van Loan, M., Fitzgerald, P.I., Hodgdon, J.A., and Van Itallie, T.B. 1988. Lean body mass estimation by bioelectrical impedance analysis: A four-site cross-validation study. *American Journal of Clinical Nutrition* 47: 7-14.

Seidell, J.C., Oosterlee, A., Thijssen, M., Burema, J., Deurenberg, P., Hautvast, J., and Ruijs, J. 1987. Assessment of intra-abdominal and subcutaneous abdominal fat: Relation between anthropometry and computed tomography. *American Journal of Clinical Nutrition* 45: 7-13.

Seip, R., and Weltman, A. 1991. Validity of skinfold and girth based regression equations for the prediction of body composition in obese adults. *American Journal of Human Biology* 3: 91-95.

Siri, W.E. 1961. Body composition from fluid space and density. In J. Brozek and A. Henschel, eds., *Techniques for measuring body composition*, 223-224. Washington, DC: National Academy of Sciences.

Slaughter, M.H., Lohman, T.G., Boileau, R.A., Horswill, C.A., Stillman, R.J., Van Loan, M.D., and Bemben, D.A. 1988. Skinfold equations for estimation of body fatness in children and youth. *Human Biology* 60: 709-723.

Thomas, T.R., and Etheridge, G.L. 1980. Hydrostatic weighing at residual volume and functional residual capacity. *Journal of Applied Physiology* 49: 157-159.

Timson, B.F., and Coffman, J.L. 1984. Body composition by hydrostatic weighing at total lung capacity and residual volume. *Medicine and Science in Sports and Exercise* 16: 411-414.

Tran, Z.V., and Weltman, A. 1988. Predicting body composition of men from girth measurements. *Human Biology* 60: 167-175.

Tran, Z.V., and Weltman, A. 1989. Generalized equation for predicting body density of women from girth measurements. *Medicine and Science in Sports and Exercise* 21: 101-104.

U.S. Department of Health and Human Services. 1988. *The Surgeon General's report on nutrition and health.* DHHS [PHS] Publication No. 88-50210. Washington, DC: U.S. Government Printing Office.

Van Loan, M.D., and Mayclin, P.L. 1987. Bioelectrical impedance analysis: Is it a reliable estimator of lean body mass and total body water? *Human Biology* 59: 299-309.

Van Loan, M.D., and Mayclin, P.L. 1992. Body composition assessment: Dual-energy x-ray absorptiometry (DEXA) compared to reference methods. *European Journal of Clinical Nutrition* 46: 125-130.

Wagner, D., Heyward, V., and Stolarczyk, L. 1997. Body mass index as a measure of body fatness: Influence of gender, age, and ethnicity. *Sports Medicine, Training, and Rehabilitation* 81: in press [abstract]

Weltman, A., Levine, S., Seip, R.L., and Tran, Z.V. 1988. Accurate assessment of body composition in obese females. *American Journal of Clinical Nutrition* 48: 1179-1183.

Weltman, A., Seip, R.L., and Tran, Z.V. 1987. Practical assessment of body composition in adult obese males. *Human Biology* 59: 523-535.

Williams, D.P., Going, S.B., Massett, M.P., Lohman, T.G., Bare, L.A., and Hewitt, M.J. 1993. Aqueous and mineral fractions of the fat-free body and their relation to body fat estimates in men and women aged 49-82 years. In K.J. Ellis, and J.D. Eastman, eds., *Human body composition: In vivo methods, models and assessment,* 109-113. New York: Plenum Press.

Wilmore, J.H., and Behnke, A.R. 1969. An anthropometric estimation of body density and lean body weight in young men. *Journal of Applied Physiology* 27: 25-31.

Wilmore, J.H., and Behnke, A.R. 1970. An anthropometric estimation of body density and lean body weight in young women. *American Journal of Clinical Nutrition* 23: 267-274.

Wilmore, J.H., Frisancho, R.A., Gordon, C.C., Himes, J.H., Martin, A.D., Martorell, R., and Seefeldt, R.D. 1988. Body breadth equipment and measurement techniques. In T.G. Lohman, A.F. Roche, and R. Martorell, eds., *Anthropometric standardization reference manual,* 27-38. Champaign, IL: Human Kinetics.

Wilmore, K.M., McBride, P.J., and Wilmore, J.H. 1994. Comparison of bioelectric impedance and near-infrared interactance for human body composition assessment in a population of self-perceived overweight adults. *International Journal of Obesity* 18: 375-381.

Zando, K.A., and Robertson, R.J. 1987. The validity and reliability of the Cramer skyndex caliper in the estimation of percent body fat. *Athletic Training* 22: 23-25, 79.

CHAPTER 9

Designing Weight Management and Body Composition Programs

Key Questions

- What is obesity, and how prevalent is it in the U.S. population?
- What are the health risks associated with having high and low levels of body fat?
- What are the primary causes of overweight and obesity?
- How is healthy body weight determined?
- What are the guidelines for a well-balanced diet? Are vitamin and mineral supplements necessary for most clients?
- What steps are followed in planning a weight management program?
- What are the recommended guidelines for weight-loss and weight-gain programs?
- Why is exercise important for weight management?
- What types of exercise are best for weight loss?
- Does exercising without dieting improve body composition?

Obesity is a serious health problem that reduces life expectancy and threatens the quality of one's life. Obese individuals have a higher risk of cardiovascular disease, hypercholesterolemia, hypertension, diabetes mellitus, obstructive pulmonary disease, osteoarthritis, and certain cancers. The prevalences of hypercholesterolemia, hypertension, and Type II diabetes are, respectively, 2.9, 2.1, and 2.9 times greater in overweight than in nonoverweight persons (National Institutes of Health 1985). Obesity also increases the risk of developing CHD, independent of other standard CHD risk factors (Hubert et al. 1983).

Obesity is on the rise in the American population. Approximately one out of every three adults and one of every four children and adolescents are overweight (Kuczmarski et al. 1994; Troiano et al. 1995). These proportions have risen at an alarming rate over the past 15 years. In light of this trend, it is highly unlikely that the Healthy People 2000 goal of reducing the prevalence of overweight among U.S. adults to no more than 20% of the population will be reached. Russell, Williamson, and Byers (1995) projected that to reach this goal, overweight persons need to lose 6.6 kg (14.5 lb) on average, while nonoverweight persons maintain their present body weight.

Obesity is an excessive amount of body fat relative to body weight and is not synonymous with overweight. In epidemiological studies, *overweight* is defined as excess weight relative to a desirable body weight (>120% of desirable weight), or as a body mass index (BMI) in excess of 29.3 for women and 29.8 for men. Because these overweight criteria do not take into account the composition of the excess weight, they are limited as indexes of obesity and may result in misclassifications of obesity. There is considerable variability in body composition for any given BMI. Some individuals with low BMIs have as much fat as those with higher BMIs. Older people have more body fat at any given BMI than younger people (Baumgartner, Heymsfield, and Roche 1995). Thus, the prevalence of obesity could even be worse than currently thought.

At the opposite extreme, individuals with too little body fat tend to be malnourished. These people have a relatively higher risk of fluid-electrolyte imbalances, osteoporosis and osteopenia, bone fractures, muscle wasting, cardiac arrhythmias and sudden death, edema, and renal and reproductive disorders (Fohlin 1977; Mazess, Barden, and Ohlrich 1990; Vaisman, Corey, et al. 1988).

One disease associated with extremely low body fat levels is anorexia nervosa. *Anorexia nervosa* is an eating disorder found primarily in females and is characterized by excessive weight loss. Anorexia nervosa is estimated to afflict 1% of the female population (American Psychiatric Association 1994). Compared to normal women, anorexics have extremely low body fat (8 to 13% BF), signs of muscle wasting, and less bone mineral content and bone density (Mazess, Barden, and Ohlrich 1990; Vaisman, Rossi et al. 1988).

Combating obesity and eating disorders is not an easy task. Many overweight and obese individuals have incorporated patterns of overeating and physical inactivity into their lifestyles, while others have developed food and/or exercise addictions. In an effort to lose weight quickly and to prevent weight gain, many are lured by fad diets and exercise gimmicks, and some resort to extreme behaviors such as avoiding food, bingeing and purging, and exercising compulsively. In a survey of weight control practices of adults in the United States, Serdula et al. (1994) reported that 38% of women and 24% of men were trying to lose weight by counting calories, participating in organized weight loss programs, taking special supplements or diet pills, or fasting. Only 50% of those trying to lose weight reported using the recommended method of restricting caloric intake and increasing physical activity. Thus,

as a health/fitness professional, you have an enormous challenge and responsibility to educate and provide scientifically sound weight control programs for your clients.

This chapter presents techniques for determining healthy body weight based on a client's body composition. You will learn about weight control principles and practices, as well as guidelines for designing exercise programs for weight loss, weight gain, and body composition change.

TYPES OF OBESITY

The way in which fat is distributed in the body may be more important than total body fat for determining one's risk of disease. The waist-to-hip ratio (WHR) is strongly associated with visceral fat, and the impact of regional fat distribution on health is related to the amount of visceral fat located in the abdominal cavity. Abdominal fat is strongly associated with diseases such as CHD, diabetes, hypertension, and hyperlipidemia (Bjorntorp 1988; Blair et al. 1984; Ducimetier, Richard, and Cambien 1989).

The terms *android obesity* and *gynoid obesity* describe individuals who localize excess body fat mainly in the upper body (android) or lower body (gynoid). Android obesity (apple-shaped) is more typical of males; gynoid obesity (pear-shaped) is more characteristic of females. However, obese men and women can be, and often are, classified into either group. There are other terms used to describe types of obesity and regional fat distribution. Android obesity is frequently called *upper-body obesity*, and gynoid obesity is often described as *lower-body obesity.*

In field settings, you can assess regional fat distribution using the waist-to-hip ratio (WHR). Chapter 8 presents measurement procedures and WHR norms. Generally, young adults with WHR values in excess of 0.94 for men and 0.82 for women are at very high risk for adverse health consequences (Bray and Gray 1988).

CAUSES OF OVERWEIGHT AND OBESITY

Many questions may arise in regard to overweight and obesity. This section addresses common questions relating to these conditions.

Why Do People Gain or Lose Weight?

An energy imbalance in the body results in a weight gain or loss. There is energy balance when caloric intake equals energy expenditure. A *positive energy balance* is created when the input (food intake) exceeds the expenditure (resting metabolism plus activity level). For every 3500 kcal of excess energy accumulated, 1 pound (0.45 kg) of fat is stored in the body. A *negative energy balance* is produced when the energy expenditure exceeds the energy input. This can be accomplished by reducing the food intake or increasing the physical activity level. A caloric deficit of approximately 3500 kcal produces a loss of 1 pound of fat.

How Are Energy Needs and Energy Expenditure Measured?

Energy need and expenditure are measured in kilocalories (kcal). A kilocalorie is defined as the amount of heat needed to raise the temperature of 1 kg (2.2 lb) of water 1° C. Direct calorimetry is used to measure the energy yield and caloric equivalent of various foods. The foods are burned in a closed chamber in the presence of oxygen, and the amount of heat liberated is measured precisely in kilocalories. Table 9.1 gives the energy yield and caloric equivalents for carbohydrate, protein, and fat.

The energy or caloric need is a function of the individual's metabolic rate and physical activity level. The *basal metabolic rate (BMR)* is a measure of the minimal amount of energy (kcal) needed to maintain basic and essential physiological functions. BMR varies according to age, gender, body size, and body composition. To assess BMR, the individual must be rested and fasted, and should be in a controlled environment. Since this is not always practical, we use the term, *resting metabolic rate (RMR)* to indicate the energy required to maintain essential physiological processes in a relaxed, awake, and reclined state.

You can measure energy expenditure during basal, resting, or activity states using indirect calorimetry. In this case, you estimate the body's energy expenditure from the oxygen utilization. Every liter of oxygen consumed per minute yields approximately 5 kcal (see table 9.1). Intense physical activity can increase the rate of energy expenditure more than 10 times above the resting level.

How Is Resting Metabolic Rate Regulated?

Thyroxine is extremely important in regulating RMR. Inadequate levels of this hormone can be produced by thyroid tumors or lack of iodine in the diet. Underproduction of thyroxine can reduce RMR 30 to 50%. If energy input and expenditure are not adjusted accordingly, the positive energy balance that is created results in a weight gain.

Growth hormone, epinephrine, norepinephrine, and various sex hormones may elevate RMR as much as 15 to 20%. These hormones increase during exercise and may be responsible for the elevation in resting metabolic rate after cessation of exercise.

What Causes Weight Gain?

Improper diet, overeating, hormonal disturbances, and physical inactivity may create a positive energy balance, which leads to excessive weight gain and obesity. Lack of physical activity rather than overeating is a more common cause of obesity in children and adults (Corbin and Fletcher 1968; Mayer 1968). In a small percentage of cases (1 per 1000), obesity is caused by metabolic disorders due to hormonal imbalances (Sharkey 1990).

Does Weight Gain Increase Both the Number and Size of Fat Cells?

Obesity is associated with increases in the both the number and size of fat cells. A normal-weight individual has 25 to 30 billion fat cells, whereas an obese person may have as many as 42 to 106 billion fat cells. Also, the adipose cell size of obese individuals is on average 40% larger than that of nonobese persons (Hirsh 1971). An increase in fat cell number (hyperplasia) occurs rapidly during the first year of life and again during adolescence, but remains

Table 9.1	Energy Yield and Caloric Equivalents for Macronutrients	
Nutrient	Energy yield (kcal/g)	Caloric equivalents (kcal/L O_2)
Carbohydrate	4.1	5.1
Protein	4.3	4.4
Fat	9.3	4.7

fairly stable in adulthood except in cases of morbid obesity. Fat cells increase in size (hypertrophy) during the adolescent growth spurt and continue to grow when excess fat is stored in the cells as triglycerides. Weight gain in adults is typically characterized by the enlargement of existing fat cells, rather than the creation of new fat cells. Similarly, caloric restriction and exercise are effective in reducing fat cell size but not the number of fat cells in adults (Hirsh 1971). Perhaps the key to preventing obesity is to closely monitor the dietary intake and energy expenditure, especially during the adolescent growth spurt and puberty. This could potentially retard the development of new fat cells and control the size of existing fat cells.

What Is the Relative Importance of Genetics and Environment in Developing Obesity?

Scientists have debated the relative contributions of genetics and environment to obesity. Mayer (1968) observed that only 10% of children who had normal-weight parents were obese. The probability of being obese is increased to 40% and 80%, respectively, if one parent or both parents are obese. Although these data suggest a strong genetic influence, they do not rule out environmental influences such as eating and exercise habits.

In a controlled study of long-term (100 days) overfeeding in identical twins, Bouchard et al. (1990) observed large individual differences in the tendency towards obesity and distribution of body fat, even within each pair of twins. Increases in body weight due to overfeeding of twins were moderately correlated (r = 0.55). Overall, increases in body weight, fat mass, trunk fat, and visceral fat were three times greater in high-weight gainers compared to low-weight gainers. These data suggest that genotype explains some, but not all, of a person's adaptation to a sustained energy surplus. Approximately 25% of the variability among individuals in absolute and relative body fat is attributed to genetic factors and 30% is associated with cultural (environmental) factors (Bouchard et al. 1988).

Do Psychological Factors Play an Important Role in Obesity?

Overweight and obesity may be caused by psychological factors. Some overweight and obese individuals use food and eating as a coping mechanism

or defense mechanism. Compulsive eaters may eat to cope with feelings of insecurity, anxiety, depression, loneliness, stress, and tension rather than to satisfy hunger (terHeun 1981). In this case, the individual needs to recognize the fact that he or she is eating compulsively, identify the underlying reasons for this behavior, and take steps to modify these behaviors. Encourage clients with eating disorders to seek psychological counseling.

What Is the Best Way to Combat Overweight and Obesity?

The battle of controlling body weight and obesity may be won by understanding why we eat, monitoring food intake closely, and incorporating more physical activity into the lifestyle. The physically active lifestyle is characterized by

- daily aerobic exercise,
- increased participation in recreational activities such as bowling, golf, tennis, and dancing, and
- increased physical activity in the daily routine at home and work by restricting use of labor-saving devices such as escalators, power tools, automobiles, and home and garden appliances.

In addition to these suggestions, you should encourage your clients to follow the *Dietary Guidelines for Americans* (U.S. Department of Health and Human Services 1995):

- Eat a variety of foods.
- Balance the food you eat with physical activity—maintain or improve your weight.
- Choose a diet with plenty of grain products, vegetables, and fruits.
- Choose a diet low in fat, saturated fat, and cholesterol.
- Choose a diet moderate in sugars.
- Choose a diet moderate in salt and sodium.
- If you drink alcoholic beverages, do so in moderation.

What Is the Most Effective Technique for Implementing Lifestyle Changes?

Behavior modification techniques can help people make these lifestyle changes. In the case of weight control, the individual identifies the unwanted behavior and establishes rewards to reinforce the new eating or exercise behavior. Exercise specialists, nutritionists, and psychologists need to work together to help their clients, especially obesity-prone individuals, modify their physical activity and eating attitudes and behaviors.

WEIGHT MANAGEMENT PRINCIPLES AND PRACTICES

Proper nutrition (eating a well-balanced diet) and daily physical activity are key components of a weight management program. In weight management programs, most clients are interested in losing body weight and body fat, but some need to gain body weight. The basic principle underlying safe and effective weight-loss programs is that weight can only be lost through a negative energy balance, which is produced when the caloric expenditure exceeds the caloric intake. The most effective way of creating a caloric deficit is through a combination of diet (restricting caloric intake) and exercise (increasing caloric expenditure). On the other hand, for weight-gain programs, the caloric intake must exceed the caloric expenditure in order to create a positive energy balance. Principles and practices underlying the design of a weight management programs are summarized below.

Weight Management Principles

Weight Loss	*Weight Gain*	*Exercise*
• A well-balanced diet for good nutrition contains carbohydrate, protein, fat, vitamins, minerals, and water.	• The dietary protein intake should be increased to 1.2 to 1.6 g · kg^{-1} body weight.	• The major cause of obesity is lack of physical activity, not overeating.
• The weight loss should be gradual—no more than 2 pounds (0.90 kg) a week.	• The weight gain should be gradual—no more than 2 pounds a week.	• For fat-weight loss, aerobic exercise should be performed daily or twice daily.
• The caloric intake should be at least 1200 kcal/day, and the caloric deficit should not exceed 1000 kcal/day.	• The daily caloric intake should exceed caloric needs by 400 to 500 kcal/day.	• Resistance exercise training is an excellent way to maintain fat-free mass (for weight-loss programs) and increase FFM (for weight-gain programs).
• A caloric deficit of 3,500 kcal is needed to lose 1 pound (0.45 kg) of fat.	• A positive energy balance of 2,800 to 3,500 kcal is needed to gain 1 pound of muscle tissue.	• For weight-loss programs, exercise helps create a caloric deficit by increasing caloric expenditure.
• Weight loss should be due to loss of fat rather than lean body tissue.	• Weight gain should be due to increased fat-free mass rather than fat mass.	• Exercise is more effective than dieting for maximizing fat loss and minimizing lean tissue loss.
• On the same diet, a taller, heavier person—who has a higher RMR—will lose weight at a faster rate than a shorter, lighter person.	• The individual should eat 3 meals and 2 to 3 healthy snacks per day. Dried fruits, nuts, seeds, and some liquid meals are good snack foods.	• For increased caloric expenditure, avoid using labor-saving devices around the home and workplace.
• The rate of weight loss will decrease over time because the difference between the caloric intake and caloric needs gets smaller as one loses weight.	• Protein powders are no more effective than natural protein sources (e.g., lean meats, skim milk, and egg whites).	• Low-intensity, longer duration exercise is more effective than high-intensity, shorter duration exercise for maximizing total energy expenditure.

(continued)

Weight Management Principles *(continued)*

Weight Loss	*Weight Gain*	*Exercise*
• Men lose weight faster than women because men have a higher RMR.	• Protein and amino acid supplements do not promote muscle growth.	• RMR remains elevated 30 minutes or longer after vigorous exercise.
• The individual should eat at least 3 meals a day.	• Vitamin B12, boron, and chromium supplementation do not increase fat-free mass.	• At a given heart rate, the more physically fit individual expends calories at a faster rate than the less fit individual.
• Quick weight-loss diets, diet pills, and appetite suppressants should be avoided.		• Exercise does not increase appetite.
• Carnitine supplementation does not promote body fat loss.		• Passive exercise devices, such as vibrators and sauna belts, do not massage away excess fatty tissues.
• Compulsive eating behaviors should be identified and modified.		• Spot-reduction exercises do not preferentially mobilize subcutaneous fat stored near the exercising muscles.

WELL-BALANCED DIET

A well-balanced diet should contain adequate amounts of protein, fat, carbohydrate, vitamins, minerals, and water. Figure 9.1 compares the typical American diet to the dietary goals established by the U.S. Senate Select Committee on Nutrition and Human Needs (1977). A 1985 survey of food intakes of 658 men and 1,459 women between the ages of 19 and 50 years indicated that the average percentage of total energy intake from carbohydrate (46%), fat (37%), and protein (16%) did not comply with U.S. dietary goals. Also, the average dietary cholesterol (435 mg · dl^{-1}) and sodium intake of men exceeded the recommended levels. Women, on the average, only took in 78% of the estimated safe and adequate daily dietary intake for calcium, 61% of iron, 60% of zinc, and 72% of magnesium (U.S. Department of Health and Human Services 1988).

Carbohydrates

The largest proportion (58% to 65%) of the daily caloric intake should be in the form of carbohydrates. Three kinds of carbohydrates are sugars, starches, and cellulose. The ingestion of refined and processed sugars should be limited to 10% of the daily caloric intake (see figure 9.1). Complex carbohydrates (i.e., starches and fiber) and naturally occurring sugars should be consumed to meet the carbohydrate requirements of a well-balanced diet. Diets with a high fiber content are less likely to produce colon cancer and hemorrhoids.

Carbohydrates are stored in the liver and muscle as glycogen. However, the amount of glucose that can be stored in the body as muscle and liver glycogen is limited. If the glycogen storage capability of the body is exceeded, a positive energy balance is created. These excess calories in the form of carbohydrate provide the building blocks for the synthesis of trigyclerides, which eventually are stored in adipose tissue and in the muscles as intramuscular fat.

Protein

Approximately 12% to 15% of the daily caloric intake should be protein. The diet should include sources of the essential amino acids needed for protein synthesis. Lack of these essential amino acids may produce a loss of muscle tissue or prevent the synthesis of hormones, enzymes, and cellular structures. The average individual needs 0.8 g of protein per kilogram of body weight to meet the daily protein needs of the body. Protein supplementation beyond the average level is usually not

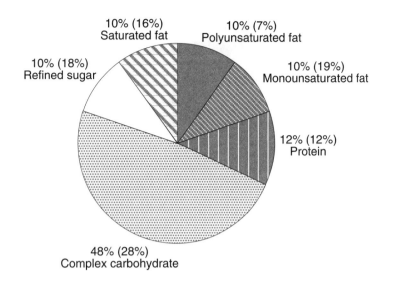

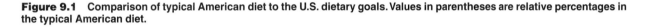

Figure 9.1   Comparison of typical American diet to the U.S. dietary goals. Values in parentheses are relative percentages in the typical American diet.

necessary unless the individual is participating in a strenuous training program. In such cases, the individual may increase daily protein intake to 1.2 to 2.0 g · kg^{-1} of body weight in the early stages of training. This amount represents about 150% to 250% of the current RDA for adults (Lemon 1989).

Excess protein cannot be stored in the body and is broken down into amino acids. Amino acids also cannot be stored and, therefore, will be used as fuel for energy. Too much protein in the diet causes dehydration due to excessive production of urea, which must be eliminated in the urine.

Fats

In the typical American diet, approximately 34% of the daily caloric intake is in the form of fats (Lenfant and Ernst 1994). Because of a possible link between serum triglyceride and cholesterol levels with atherosclerosis, hypertension, and coronary heart disease (CHD), individuals should restrict dietary fat intake, especially saturated fats and cholesterol.

Some dietary fat is needed to supply essential fatty acids and to absorb the fat-soluble vitamins. In addition, free fatty acids are an important energy source during aerobic exercise. In the *Dietary Guidelines for Americans* (U.S. Department of Health and Human Services 1995), it is recommended that total fat intake should not exceed 30% of the daily caloric intake. Saturated fat intake should not be greater than 1/3 of the total fat intake or 10% of the total daily caloric intake. The remaining fat intake should

be evenly divided between polyunsaturated (10% of total daily kcal) and monounsaturated (10% of total daily kcal) fats. Excess fat in the diet cannot be used to synthesize glucose; instead, the free fatty acids are resynthesized and stored as triglyceride in the muscle and adipose tissue.

Vitamins-Minerals-Water

A well-balanced diet usually does not need to be supplemented to meet the minimum daily vitamin and mineral requirements of the body. Table 9.2 gives recommended dietary allowances (RDA) and food sources for vitamins and minerals.

Vitamins

Eating a well-balanced diet typically provides an individual's vitamin requirements. The body does not store the water-soluble vitamins (B complex and C), and an excess amount of most of these vitamins is excreted in the urine. The excess accumulation of fat-soluble vitamins (A, D, E, and K) may produce decalcification of bones, headaches, nausea, diarrhea, and other toxic effects (Williams 1992).

Antioxidant vitamins (C, E, and beta-carotene) may protect against muscle damage following intense, eccentric exercise by counteracting the negative effects of free radicals and lipid peroxidation on muscle tissue (Singh 1992). However, additional research is needed before recommending antioxidant vitamin supplementation as a means

Table 9.2 Recommended Dietary Allowances for Adults, and Food Sources for Selected Vitamins and Minerals

Vitamins	Daily requirements		Food sources
	Men	Women	
A (µg RE)[a]	1000	800	Beef liver, fish liver oils, egg yolks, milk, butter, cheese, carrots, sweet potatoes, spinach, collards
B$_1$ (thiamin) (mg)	5	5	Pork, dried peas and beans, milk, nuts, whole grain bread, vegetables, fruits
Niacin (mg)	19	15	Lean meats, organ meats, poultry, legumes, peanuts, whole grain, and enriched cereals
B$_6$ (mg)	2.0	1.6	Meat, poultry, fish, whole grain cereals, seeds, vegetables
Pantothenic acid (mg)	4-7	4-7	Meat, poultry, fish, milk, cheese, legumes, whole grain products
Folacin (µg)	200	180	Meats, liver, eggs, milk, legumes, whole wheat products, green leafy vegetables
B$_{12}$ (µg)	2.0	2.0	Meat, poultry, fish, eggs, milk, cheese, butter
C (mg)	60	60	Citrus fruits, tomatoes, broccoli, brussels sprouts, cabbage, salad greens, cauliflower
D (µg)	5	5	Liver, tuna, salmon, cod liver oil, eggs, fortified milk, and margarine
E (mg α-TE)[b]	10	8	Legumes, nuts, seeds, margarine, salad oils, wheat germ oil, green leafy vegetables
K (µg)	80	65	Pork, liver, meats, green leafy vegetables, spinach, cauliflower, cabbage
Minerals			
Calcium (mg)	800	800[c]	Milk, cheese, ice cream, yogurt, dried beans and peas, sardines
Iron (mg)	10	15	Meat, fish, poultry, liver, shellfish, dried beans and peas, whole grain products, leafy green vegetables, dried fruits
Sodium (mg)	2400	2400	Milk, cheese, pickles, cereals, pretzels, luncheon meats, tuna (in oil), canned foods, prepared foods, condiments
Zinc (mg)	15	12	Meat, fish, poultry, liver, shellfish, milk, cheese, nuts, whole grain products, asparagus, spinach

[a] µg RE = Retinol equivalents

[b] mg α-TE = α-tocopheral

[c] The National Academy of Sciences recommends 800 mg per day. The National Institutes of Health suggest 1000 to 1,500 mg per day for adults, especially postmenopausal women.

Data from Subcommittee on the 10th Edition of the RDAs, Food and Nutrition Board, Commission on Life Sciences, National Research Council (1989). *Recommended Dietary Allowances*, p. 284. Washington, DC: National Academy Press.

to prevent exercise-induced muscle damage (Goldfarb 1993).

Minerals

The most common mineral deficiencies are iron, zinc, and calcium. Physically active individuals, particularly those who choose to exclude meat from their diets, need to carefully plan their diets so that adequate amounts of iron and zinc are available. In some cases, it may be appropriate for you to recommend daily supplementation of iron, zinc and calcium at 100% RDA in order to ensure adequate intake of these nutrients.

Iron is found in hemoglobin (in the red blood cells) which transports oxygen to exercising muscles. Iron deficiency has been frequently reported for both male and female athletes, but is more common among women (Clarkson 1990). Thus, iron supplementation may be warranted for some exercising individuals (Rajaram et al. 1995)

Zinc plays an important role in energy metabolism (as a cofactor for enzymes), hormonal function, and the immune system. The average zinc intake of sedentary and athletic women in the U.S. is below the RDA (12 mg/day); for men, it typically exceeds the RDA (Clarkson and Haymes 1994). Zinc deficiency may result in decreased strength and endurance (Krotkiewski et al. 1982).

The RDA for calcium is 1200 mg per day up to age 25. Calcium RDAs for adults and elderly are controversial. The National Academy of Sciences recommends 800 mg/day, but the National Institutes of Health suggest 1000 to 1500 mg/day for adults and postmenopausal women (Sanborn 1990). Most people can meet their calcium requirements by eating a well-balanced diet that contains milk products. When this is not possible, they should use calcium supplements.

Adequate dietary calcium intake and exercise are essential for bone mineralization and skeletal growth. Inadequate bone mineralization or excessive bone resorption results in bone loss and osteoporosis (Sanborn 1990). In early menopausal women, a high calcium intake (1500 mg/day), in combination with estrogen therapy, deterred bone loss. Calcium supplementation alone did not prevent bone loss in this group (Ettinger, Genault, and Cann 1987).

The typical American diet contains more sodium than the recommended daily amount of 2400 mg per day. The *Dietary Guidelines for Americans* (U.S. Dept. Health and Human Services 1995) recommend limiting salt intake to less than 6,000 mg per day (approximately one level teaspoon of salt). Excess salt (sodium chloride) intake may disrupt the electrolyte balance of the body and lead to increased fluid retention, hypertension, and calcium excretion. Thus, the amount of sodium in the diet should be restricted, especially for hypertensive or coronary-prone individuals.

Fraudulent claims sway many physically active individuals, particularly bodybuilders and strength-trained athletes, into believing that multivitamin and mineral supplements enhance muscle growth and exercise performance. Research suggests that long-term use of vitamin-mineral supplements does not increase strength or sport performance (Telford et al. 1992). Scientific studies demonstrate that (Williams 1993)

- vitamin B12 supplementation does not increase muscle growth or strength;

- carnitine (a vitamin-like compound) supplementation does not facilitate loss of body fat;

- chromium supplementation does not increase fat-free mass or decrease body fat;

- boron supplementation does not increase serum testosterone or fat-free mass; and

- magnesium supplementation does not improve muscle strength.

Water

The major sources of water for the body are fluid intake, food intake, and oxidation of foodstuffs by the body. Water is lost in the urine, feces, perspiration, and expired air. During strenuous exercise, as much as 3 liters of water may be lost through sweating. This water loss should be replenished immediately to prevent dehydration and electrolyte imbalances. Fluid replacement should not be restricted during exercise. Although plain water is effective for this purpose much of the time, carbohydrate sport drinks also may be used to maintain blood glucose levels and replace fluids lost during exercise. These beverages are effective in replenishing muscle glycogen stores after exercise. The ideal fluid replacement beverage contains some sodium and glucose or sucrose. Follow these guidelines for fluid replacement, especially for individuals who are competing or engaging in intense, long-duration (>1 hour) activities (Nadel 1988):

- Drink 2 1/2 cups, 2 hours prior to exercise.

- Drink 1 1/2 cups, 15 minutes before competition.

- Do not restrict fluids during exercise; drink at least 1 cup every 15 to 20 minutes during exercise.

- When exercising in a hot environment, the beverage should contain small amounts of sodium.

- If training is intense, the beverage should contain 6 to 8% carbohydrate (glucose or sucrose).

DESIGNING WEIGHT MANAGEMENT PROGRAMS: PRELIMINARY STEPS

In planning and designing weight management programs for weight loss or weight gain, you need to set body weight goals and assess the caloric intake and expenditure for your clients.

Setting Body Weight Goals

To set healthy body weight goals for your clients, you must first assess their present body weight and body fat levels. You can easily measure the client's weight by using a calibrated bathroom or doctor's scale. Clients should wear indoor clothing but not shoes.

When you are evaluating your client's body weight, do not use height-weight tables established by the Metropolitan Life Insurance Company (Society of Actuaries and Association of Life Insurance Medical Directors of America 1980). These tables are limited for the following reasons:

- The values represent height and weight with shoes and clothing; whether individuals were measured with shoes and clothing was not standardized.

- Data were obtained from individuals who could afford life insurance; the data represent predominantly young and middle-aged white males and females, and therefore are not representative of other population groups.

Determining a healthy body weight from height-weight tables alone may lead to invalid conclusions regarding your client's level of body fatness. Even though these tables include average body weights for varying skeletal frames, they do not take into account the body composition of the individual. For example, according to these tables, many mesomorphs having a large fat-free mass are over-

weight; yet their body fat content may be lower than average. Similarly, individuals may be overfat or obese even though they are underweight according to the standard tables. Therefore, you should use the body composition technique to estimate healthy body weights and body fat levels for your clients.

When you use the body composition technique for estimating healthy body weight and body fat levels, assess the fat-free mass (FFM) and percent fat (% BF) using one of the methods described in chapter 8. A healthy body weight is based on the client's present FFM and % BF goal. Because some fat is needed for good health and nutrition, individuals should attempt to achieve a % BF somewhere between minimal and maximal values for disease risk (see table 8.1). Remember, minimal % BF for adults is estimated to be 5% BF for men and 8% BF for women. Cut-off values for obesity are 25% BF and 32% BF for men and women, respectively. Figure 9.2 illustrates a sample calculation of healthy body weight using the body composition technique.

With aging, there is a gradual tendency to accumulate body weight and excess fat. Typically, one may expect a 1% gain in fat per decade of life between the ages of 20 and 60 years (Wilmore 1986). This weight gain is primarily characterized by an increase in body fat and a decrease in muscle mass and is associated with declining physical activity levels with age. Height-weight tables allow for increments in body weight with age. However, these average population values may not be desirable in terms of one's health and physical fitness. We should not necessarily accept getting fatter as we grow older. Each individual should attempt to maintain body weight and fatness at healthy levels.

Assessing Caloric Intake and Expenditure

The second step in planning weight management programs is to assess the client's energy (calorie) intake and expenditure. You will use these baseline data to estimate the rate of weight loss or weight gain and the amount of time needed to achieve long-term goals of body composition and body weight.

Energy Intake

A food record (see appendix E.1) details the daily caloric intake of the individual. The client keeps a record of the type and quantity of foods eaten each day for 3 to 7 days. Use computer software to assess the average daily caloric intake and to compare average nutrient intakes to recommended amounts

Demographic Data

Client: 31-year-old male

Current body composition:
Body weight = 185 lb (84.1 kg)
Body fat = 20% BF
Fat-free mass (FFM) = 148 lb (67.3 kg)

Goals: 12% BF and 88% FFM

Steps:

1. Determine the client's present % BF using one of the body composition methods (see chapter 8).

2. Calculate the client's present FFM (in lb): 185 lb × 0.80 (current % FFM) = 148 lb.

3. Set reasonable body composition goals for client: 12% BF and 88% FFM.

4. Divide the present FFM (in lb) by the % FFM goal to obtain target body weight: 148 lb/0.88 = 168 lb (76.4 kg).

5. Calculate weight loss by subtracting target body weight from present body weight: 185 − 168 = 17 lb (7.7 kg). Assuming that FFM is maintained, this client must lose 17 lb of fat to achieve his target body weight and body fat level.

Figure 9.2   Sample calculation of healthy body weight using body composition method.

for each nutrient (see appendix E.2 for sample output). The food record also can help analyze dietary patterns such as types of foods consumed, frequency of eating, and the caloric content of each meal.

Energy Expenditure

Assess the calorie needs of an individual by estimating the resting metabolic rate (RMR) and the additional calories expended during work, exercise, household chores, and personal daily activities. See page 189 for a summary of various methods used to estimate RMR

Estimation of RMR

The RMR is the minimum amount of calories needed to sustain the vital functions of the body during a relaxed, reclined, and waking state. Since RMR is proportional to the body size and surface area of the individual, taller and heavier persons have a higher RMR than shorter and lighter persons. You can estimate body surface area (BSA) from height and weight using the nomogram in figure 9.3.

The average male or female between 20 and 40 years of age burns 38 kcal and 35 kcal per hour, respectively, for each square meter of body surface area. For example, according to method I for finding RMR (page 189), a 5 ft 2 in (157.5 cm), 120-pound

(54.5 kg) female would have an estimated surface area of 1.54 m² and a daily resting metabolic need of 1294 kcal (1.54 m² × 35 kcal · hr⁻¹ × 24 hr).

A simpler but less accurate estimate of RMR can be determined by multiplying the body weight in pounds by a factor of 10 or 11 for women or men, respectively (see Method IV, page 189). With this method, the resting metabolic need for the woman in our example is 1200 kcal (120 lb × 10).

RMR gradually decreases with age, because the number of metabolically active cells is reduced. RMR declines 2% to 5% during each decade of life after age 25 (Sharkey 1990). To prevent gradual weight gain with aging, people must appropriately reduce caloric intake or increase physical activity. The Harris-Benedict (1919) equations (Method II on page 189) are widely used to estimate RMR. These equations are gender-specific and take into account not only height and weight, but also age.

In addition to body size and age, body composition affects RMR. Muscular individuals have a higher RMR than fatter individuals of the same weight, because fat tissue is less metabolically active than muscle tissue. RMRs of women are 5% to 10% lower than those of men (McArdle et al. 1996). This lower rate may be due to a greater relative fat content and lower fat-free mass for women. To use Method III, you must measure the fat-free body mass of your

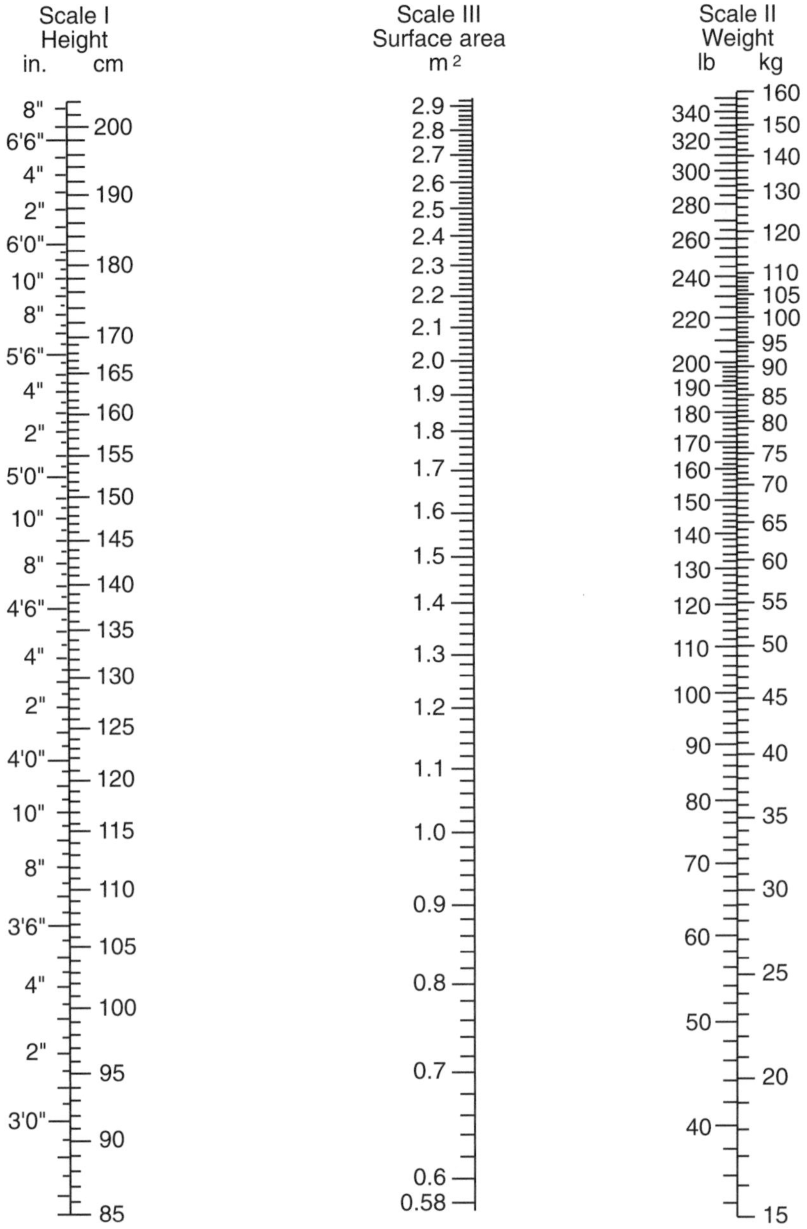

Scale I Height in. cm	Scale III Surface area m^2	Scale II Weight lb kg

Directions

To find body surface of a patient, locate the height in inches (or centimeters) on Scale I and the weight in pounds (or kilograms) on Scale II. Place a straight edge (ruler) between these two points which will intersect Scale III at the patient's surface area.

Figure 9.3   Nomogram to predict body surface area (BSA).
Reprinted, by permission, W.E. Collins, 1967, *Clinical Spirometry*, Braintree, MA: Warren E. Collins. Copyright 1967 by Warren E. Collins, 33.

Methods of Estimating Resting Metabolic Rate (RMR)

Method	*Equation*
I. Body surface area (BSA)[a]	
Men	$RMR = BSA\ (m^2) \times 38\ kcal \cdot hr^{-1}/m^2 \times 24\ hr$
Women	$RMR = BSA\ (m^2) \times 35\ kcal \cdot hr^{-1}/m^2 \times 24\ hr$
II. Harris-Benedict equations[b]	
Men	$RMR = 66.473 + 13.751(BW) + 5.0033(HT) - 6.755(Age)$
Women	$RMR = 655.0955 + 9.463(BW) + 1.8496(HT) - 4.6756(Age)$
III. Fat-free mass (FFM)	
Men and women	$RMR = 1.3\ kcal \cdot hr^{-1} \cdot kg^{-1}\ FFM \times 24\ hr$
IV. Quick estimate—lb BW	
Men	$RMR = BW\ (in\ lb) \times 11\ kcal \cdot lb^{-1}$
Women	$RMR = BW\ (in\ lb) \times 10\ kcal \cdot lb^{-1}$
V. Quick estimate—kg BW	
Men	$BW\ (in\ kg) \times 24.2\ kcal \cdot kg^{-1}$
Women	$BW\ (in\ kg) \times 22.0\ kcal \cdot kg^{-1}$

[a] Adjust RMR for age. RMR decreases 2 to 5% per decade after age 40.

[b] BW in kg; HT in cm; Age in yr

client using one of the body composition methods suggested in chapter 8. The constant, $1.3\ kcal \cdot hr^{-1} \cdot kg^{-1}$ FFM, is the same for men and women, and you need not correct for age if your client is between 20 and 60 years old (Grande and Keys 1980).

Estimation of Additional Caloric Requirements

RMR accounts for 50% to 70% of total daily caloric needs, but this value depends on the activity level of the person. The percentage is greater for less active individuals who require fewer calories above the resting level. For example, if a sedentary male office worker has a resting metabolic need of 1680 kcal, the additional caloric need due to the nature of his work is approximately 40% above resting level, or 672 kcal. Provided he performs no additional physical activities, his total daily caloric need is 2352 kcal. In this case, RMR accounts for 71% of his total daily caloric requirements. Table 9.3 presents additional caloric requirements for selected activity levels.

Alternatively, you can estimate your client's additional energy expenditure by using a physical activity log (appendix E.3). The individual records every activity performed and the total amount of time spent in each activity. This includes activities such as sleeping, eating, showering, watching television, talking, working, and exercising. The estimated energy expenditures in METs for a variety of personal, work, recreational, and sport activities are listed in appendix E.4. You can calculate the total caloric expenditure for each activity by converting the METs to $kcal \cdot kg^{-1} \cdot hr^{-1}$ ($1\ MET = 1\ kcal \cdot kg^{-1} \cdot hr^{-1}$) and multiplying this value by the client's body weight (in kg). This yields the total amount of kilocalories that the client expends per hour of that activity.

Keeping a physical activity log is a very time-consuming process for both you and your client; and it may not increase the accuracy of your estimate of additional caloric expenditure, because many clients tend to overestimate the actual duration of their physical activity. It is best to just estimate additional energy requirements based on your client's occupation (see table 9.3)

DESIGNING WEIGHT-LOSS PROGRAMS

When caloric expenditure exceeds caloric intake, a negative energy balance or caloric deficit is created. The most effective way to produce this deficit is to use a combination of caloric restriction and exercise. The daily caloric deficit should not exceed 1,000 kcal per day. This produces a gradual weight loss of 2 pounds (0.90 kg) a week given that a deficit of 3,500 kcal is needed to lose 1 pound (0.45 kg) of fat (1000 kcal $\times$ 7 days, or 2 lb).

To ensure that the weight loss is due to the loss of body fat rather than lean body tissue, you should

Table 9.3   Additional Energy Requirements for Selected Activity Levels

Occupational activity level*	Percentage above basal metabolism	
	Men	Women
Sedentary	15	15
Lightly active	40	35
Moderately active	50	45
Very active	85	70
Exceptionally active	110	100

*Examples for each occupational activity level are as follows:

Sedentary = inactive

Lightly active = most professionals, office workers, shop workers, teachers, homemakers

Moderately active = workers in light industry, most farm workers, active students, department store workers, soldiers not in active service, commerical fishing workers

Very active = full-time athletes and dancers, unskilled laborers, forestry workers, military recruits and soldiers in active service, mine workers, steel workers

Exceptionally active = lumberjacks, blacksmiths, female construction workers

- use the body composition method to estimate your client's healthy body weight and fat loss,

- encourage participation in an aerobic exercise program on a daily basis to enhance the loss of fat and to conserve fat-free mass, and

- prescribe a high-carbohydrate, low-fat diet to prevent depletion of muscle glycogen stores and to maximize the protein-sparing effect of carbohydrate.

When you design weight-loss programs of diet and exercise, use descriptive data to help you set reasonable goals for your clients. These data include age, gender, height, body weight, relative body fat (% BF), % BF goal, average caloric intake, cardiorespiratory fitness level, and occupation. Figure 9.4 illustrates the steps to follow in designing a weight-loss program.

Dietary Analysis and Planning

It is strongly recommended that you consult and work closely with a licensed nutritionist or registered dietitian when modifying and planning diets for your clients. When comparing your client's typical nutrient intakes to RDAs, you should focus on the following questions:

1. How does the average caloric intake compare with the caloric needs and expenditure of the individual?

2. What is the relative percentage of carbohydrate, protein, and fat in the diet?

3. How much of the total fat intake is saturated fat?

4. Is the minimum daily protein requirement being met?

5. What is the dietary cholesterol level?

6. What is the sodium intake?

7. Are the vitamin and mineral requirements being met through the food intake?

8. How many meals per day are eaten? What is the average caloric content of each meal? At what meal are most of the kilocalories consumed?

9. What types of snack foods are eaten? If the diet contains a lot of junk food, suggest more nutritious snack foods.

10. At what time of day does eating appear to be a problem?

A high-carbohydrate, low-fat diet provides an excellent source of energy and typically contains as much as 58 to 70% carbohydrate (i.e., 48 to 60% complex carbohydrate and no more than 10% refined sugars), 12 to 15% protein, and 20 to 30% fat. In planning a well-balanced diet with these relative amounts of macronutrients, refer to the *Food Guide Pyramid* (see figure 9.5) to determine the number of servings from each of the food groups. Table 9.4 lists common sources for protein, carbohydrate (starches and sugars), and fat. Be sure to consult with your clients when selecting food choices within each group for their diets. Computerized software programs are available to help you plan nutritious and well-balanced meals for your clients.

Summary of Client's Demographic Data

1. Client's age and gender (35 yr female)
2. Height (62 in. or 157.5 cm)
3. Body weight (131 lb or 59.55 kg)
4. Percent fat (26% BF); relative FFM (74%)
5. Percent fat goal (20% BF); relative FFM goal (80%)
6. Average daily caloric intake (2000 kcal)
7. Cardiorespiratory fitness level (below average)
8. Occupation (secretary)

Steps:

1. Assess the body weight and body composition of the client.
2. Assess the daily caloric intake of the subject (use 3- or 7-day food records).
3. Estimate a healthy, target body weight based on the client's percent fat goal.
   Present FFM = 96.9 lb (131 lb × 0.74) (relative FFM)
   Target body weight = 121 lb (96.9 lb/0.80) (relative FFM goal)
4. Calculate the weight loss and total caloric deficit needed to achieve that weight loss.
   a. Weight loss = 10 lb (131 lb − 121 lb)
   b. Caloric deficit = 35,000 kcal (10 lb × 3,500 kcal · lb^{-1})
5. Estimate the daily energy expenditure of the client from the equation: Energy expenditure = RMR + daily activity level.
   a. RMR = 655.0955 + 9.463 (59.55 kg) + 1.8496 (157.5 cm) − 4.6756 (35 yr) = 1346 kcal
   b. Daily occupational activity level: lightly active 35% above basal level (see table 9.3).
      Additional kcal = 1346 × 0.35 = 471 kcal
   c. Total energy expenditure = 1346 + 471 = 1817 kcal
6. Plan to produce a caloric deficit of 700 to 800 kcal per day by reducing the caloric intake by 500 kcal per day and increasing the caloric expenditure by 200 to 300 kcal per day through exercise. To calculate caloric expenditure during exercise refer to appendix E.4. Multiply the calories burned per minute per kilogram of body weight by the duration of the activity and the client's body weight. Continue this program until the total caloric deficit of 35,000 kcal is reached.

Week 1	exercise = 100 kcal · day^{-1} × 7 days	=	700 kcal
	diet = 500 kcal · day^{-1} × 7 days	=	3,500 kcal
	Total	=	4,200 kcal
Week 2	exercise = 150 kcal · day^{-1} × 7 days	=	1,050 kcal
	diet = 500 kcal · day^{-1} × 7 days	=	3,500 kcal
	Total	=	4,550 kcal
Week 3-4	exercise = 200 kcal · day^{-1} × 14 days	=	2,800 kcal
	diet = 500 kcal · day^{-1} × 14 days	=	7,000 kcal
	Total	=	9,800 kcal
Week 5-6	exercise = 250 kcal · day^{-1} × 14 days	=	3,500 kcal
	diet = 500 kcal · day^{-1} × 14 days	=	7,000 kcal
	Total	=	10,500 kcal
Week 7	exercise = 300 kcal · day^{-1} × 7 days	=	2,100 kcal
	diet = 500 kcal · day^{-1} × 7 days	=	3,500 kcal
	Total	=	5,600 kcal
	Total Weeks 1-7	=	34,650 kcal

   In a little over 7 weeks the client will lose approximately 10 lb. This is a gradual average weight loss of 1 1/2 lb per week. Reassess the body composition to see if the percent fat goal was reached.
7. Put the client on a maintenance diet and exercise program.
   a. Calculate the total energy expenditure using an estimate of RMR based on the new body weight.
      RMR + activity level + exercise = total energy expenditure where:
      RMR = 1303 kcal (use Harris-Benedict formula substituting a body weight of 55 kg)
      Activity level = 456 kcal (1303 × 0.35)
      Exercise = 300 kcal
      Total energy expenditure = 1303 + 456 + 300 = 2059 kcal
   b. Advise the client that if she continues to exercise daily, expending approximately 300 kcal per workout, she may increase her caloric intake to 2050 kcal per day. However, for days in which she cannot exercise, the caloric intake must be restricted to 1750 kcal.

Figure 9.4   **Steps for designing a weight-loss program.**

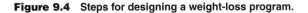

Table 9.4 Common Sources of Carbohydrate, Protein, and Fat	
Macronutrient	**Food sources**
Carbohydrate	
Starches	Pasta, rice, grains, breads, cereals, potatoes, dried beans and peas
Sugars	Fruits, candy, cookies, cakes, jelly, sugar, honey, syrup, molasses, soda pop
Protein	Meats, fish, poultry, eggs, milk, yogurt, cheese, nuts, dried beans
Fat	
Saturated	Animal fats, butter, cheese, whole milk, mayonnaise, egg yolks, ice cream, chocolate, lard, hydrogenated oils, coconut and palm oils
Polyunsaturated	Some margarines, nuts, and oils (i.e., corn, safflower, soybean, cottonseed, sesame, and sunflower oils)
Monounsaturated	Olive, canola, and peanut oils

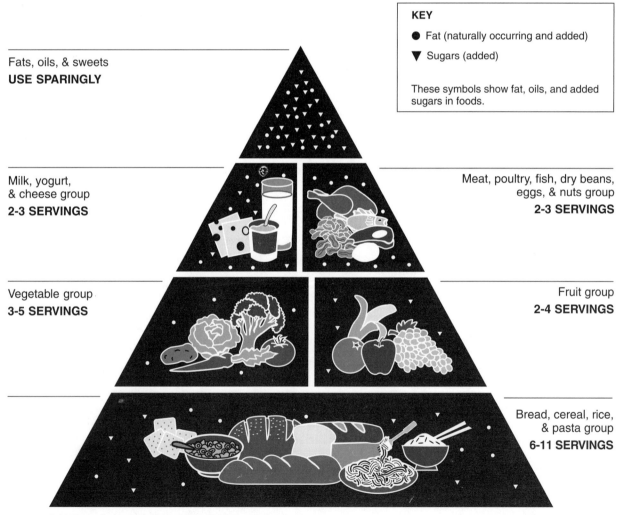

United States Department of Agriculture and Health and Human Services

Figure 9.5   The food guide pyramid.
Note. From "The Food Guide Pyramid" by U.S. Department of Agriculture, Human Nutrition Information Service, 1992, Leaflet No. 572, U.S. Government Printing Office, Washington, D.C.

Exercise Prescription for Weight Loss

Physical activity and exercise are just as important as restricting calories to create a negative energy balance for weight loss. The exercise program is designed to produce a weight loss by increasing the caloric expenditure. To maximize the total energy expenditure, select a mode of activity that can be performed at a low-to-moderate intensity for a long duration. See the guidelines below for developing an exercise prescription for weight loss.

GUIDELINES FOR EXERCISE PRESCRIPTION FOR WEIGHT LOSS

Mode: Group I or II aerobic activities (see p. 85)

Intensity: 60 to 70% $\dot{V}O_2$max or heart rate range

Duration: 30 minutes or longer

Frequency: Once or twice a day

Length of program: Dependent on desired weight loss

Benefits of Exercise

This section highlights some common questions about the benefits of exercise in a weight-loss program.

Why Is Exercise an Essential Part of Weight-Loss Programs?

In addition to increasing energy expenditure and helping to create a negative energy balance for weight loss, daily exercise ensures that the weight loss is due to loss of fat rather than muscle tissue. Pavlou et al. (1985) studied the contribution of exercise to the preservation of fat-free mass in mildly obese males on a rapid weight-loss diet. The exercise group dieted and participated in an 8-week walking-jogging program, 3 days a week. The nonexercising group dieted only. Although the total weight loss of the exercise (–11.8 kg) and nonexercise (–9.2 kg) groups was similar, the composition of the weight loss differed significantly. The exercise group maintained FFM (–0.6 kg) while the nonexercise group lost a significant amount of FFM (–3.3 kg). Also, the exercise group lost more fat (11.2 kg) than the nonexercise group (5.9 kg). In other words, for the nonexercising subjects, only 64% of the total weight loss was fat weight compared to 95% for the exercising subjects. The researchers concluded that

the addition of aerobic exercise to the dietary regimen preserves existing FFM, increases fat utilization for energy production, and is more effective in reducing fat stores than diet alone.

How Does Exercise Promote Fat Loss and the Preservation of Lean Body Mass?

In response to aerobic and resistance exercise, levels of growth hormone, epinephrine, and norepinephrine increase. These hormones stimulate the mobilization of fat from storage and activate the enzyme lipase, which breaks down triglycerides into free fatty acids. Free fatty acids are then metabolized and serve as an important energy source, especially during aerobic exercise. Heavy resistance exercise also stimulates the release of anabolic hormones such as testosterone and growth hormone, resulting in increased protein synthesis, muscle growth, and fat-free mass (Kraemer et al. 1991).

How Does Improved Cardiorespiratory Fitness Help Control Body Weight?

As the individual's cardiorespiratory fitness level increases through training, the amount of work that can be accomplished at a given submaximal heart rate increases. Thus, the more fit individual expends calories at a faster rate than the less fit individual at a given exercise heart rate. For example, at a heart rate of 150 beats per minute, the rate of energy expenditure is approximately 10 and 15 kcal · min^{-1} for fair and superior fitness levels, respectively (Sharkey 1990).

During high-intensity aerobic exercise, lactate production increases and inhibits fatty acid metabolism. However, endurance training increases the lactate threshold (point at which lactate accumulates in the blood during the exercise). In aerobically trained individuals, the percentage of the energy derived from the oxidation of free fatty acids during submaximal exercise is greater than that derived from glucose oxidation (Coyle 1995; Mole, Oscai, and Holloszy 1971). The reduction in muscle glycogen utilization is also associated with a greater oxidation rate of intramuscular triglycerides (Coyle 1995).

What Effect Does Exercise Have on the Resting Metabolic Rate?

Another reason for including exercise as a part of the weight-loss program is its positive effect on resting metabolic rate. Research indicates that exercise may counter the reduction in RMR that usually occurs as a result of dieting. It is well known that the rate of weight loss declines in the later stages of dieting because of a decrease in RMR. The lowered RMR is an energy-conserving metabolic adaptation to prolonged periods of caloric restriction (Donahue et al. 1984). In a study of 12 overweight females, Donahue et al. (1984) reported that diet alone caused a 4.4% reduction in the relative RMR (RMR/BW). After adding 8 weeks of aerobic exercise to the program, the relative RMR increased by 5%. The net effect of exercise was to offset the diet-induced metabolic adaptation, returning the RMR to the normal, prediet level.

Exercise may also facilitate weight loss by causing an increase in postexercise RMR. Moderate- to high-intensity aerobic exercise increases the postexercise RMR by 5 to 16%, and the elevated RMR may persist for 12 to 39 hours postexercise (Bahr et al. 1987; Bielinski, Schultz, and Jequier 1985; Sjodin et al. 1996). The postexercise elevation in RMR appears to be related to the exercise intensity and duration (Brehm 1988). Cycling at 70% $\dot{V}O_2$max for 20 minutes produced a 5 to 14% elevation in RMR for 12 hours in young, healthy men (Bahr et al. 1987). Although it is tempting to apply these findings to elderly and obese clients, it is not known whether the postexercise metabolic response of these individuals is similar to that of young men.

Types of Exercise

This section addresses common concerns regarding the types of exercise suitable for weight-loss programs.

Is Aerobic Exercise Better Than Resistance Exercise for Weight Loss?

A recent study evaluated the effects of aerobic and/or resistance training, in combination with a moderate calorie-restricted diet, in moderately overweight women (Marks et al. 1995). All of the exercise intervention groups (cycling only, resistance training only, and combination of the two) maintained FFM. The diet-only group lost only a minimal amount of FFM, suggesting that FFM can be maintained provided that the daily caloric intake is at least 1200 kcal a day. Compared to a control group, all diet and exercise intervention groups lost greater amounts of body weight (–3.7 to –5.4 kg) and fat mass; but there were no differences in weight loss and fat loss among the intervention groups. These data suggest that resistance training may be as effective as aerobic training in weight-loss programs.

Is High-Intensity Exercise Better Than Low-Intensity Exercise for Weight Loss?

An important reason for including exercise as part of a weight-loss program is to maximize energy expenditure, thereby creating a larger negative energy balance. Close examination of energy expenditure during selected physical activities (appendix E.4) reveals that increases in speed (intensity) of exercise produce only small increases in the rate of energy expenditure (METs). For example, if a 123-pound (56-kg) woman increases the speed of running from a slow (5.0 mph or 12 min per mile) to a faster speed (7.0 mph or 8.5 min per mile), the rate of expenditure increases only 3.2 kcal · min⁻¹. At the 8.5 minute per mile pace, the woman expends 11.5 METs (11.5 kcal · kg⁻¹ · hr⁻¹ or 10.7 kcal · min⁻¹) and is able to run a maximum distance of 3 miles (4.8 km). The duration of the workout is 25.5 minutes (8.5 min · mi⁻¹ × 3 mi), and the total caloric expenditure is 274 kcal (25.5 min × 10.7 kcal · min⁻¹). When she reduces the exercise intensity by decreasing her speed to a 12-minute per mile pace, her relative energy expenditure decreases (8 METs or 8 kcal · kg⁻¹ · hr⁻¹ or 7.5 kcal · min⁻¹), and she is able to run a distance of 4 miles (6.4 km). The duration of the workout increases to 48 minutes (12 min · mi⁻¹ × 4 mi), and the total caloric expenditure is increased (48 min × 7.5 kcal · min⁻¹ = 360 kcal). Thus, the duration of the exercise and total distance is much more important than the speed (intensity) of exercise for maximizing the energy expenditure.

Are Spot Reduction Exercises Effective for Decreasing Body Fat in Localized Regions of the Body?

Specific spot reduction exercises are no more effective than general aerobic exercise for changing limb and body girth measurements or for altering total body composition (Carns et al. 1960; Noland and Kearney 1978; Roby 1962; Schade et al. 1962). Katch et al. (1984) assessed changes in the diameter of adipose cells from the abdomen, gluteal, and subscapular sites resulting from a 27-day training program in which each subject performed 5,004 sit-ups. Although the training significantly reduced fat cell diameter, the effect was similar at all three sites: abdomen (–6.4%), gluteal (–5.0%), and subscapular (–3.7%). It appears that a sit-up exercise program does not preferentially reduce the fat in the abdominal region.

Despres et al. (1985) reported that a 20-week cycling program significantly reduced % BF and body weight. Cycling affected trunk SKFs (–22%) more than extremity SKFs (–12.5%). If fat was mobilized preferentially from subcutaneous stores near the exercising muscle mass, one would expect the lower extremity SKFs to be more affected by cycling than the trunk SKFs. Yet, Despres et al. noted an 18% reduction in the suprailiac SKF compared to a 13% reduction in the thigh SKF. This suggests that subcutaneous fat cells in the abdomen are more sensitive to the lipolytic effect of catecholamines than subcutaneous fat cells in the thighs (Smith et al. 1979).

The enzyme lipoprotein lipase (LPL) is responsible for lipid accumulation. In women LPL activity is higher in the gluteofemoral region than in the abdominal region (Litchell and Boberg 1978). Estrogen and progesterone appear to enhance the LPL activity in women. Also, lipolytic response to catecholamines is lower in the femoral than in the abdominal depots for both men and women (Rebuffe-Scrive 1985).

Thus, the regional distribution and mobilization of adipose tissue appears to follow a biologically selective pattern regardless of type of exercise. Even with weight reduction, the relative fat distribution remains stable as measured by the waist-to-hip ratio; however, the waist-to-thigh ratio decreases, suggesting that the thigh region is slightly more resistant to fat mobilization in women (Ashwell et al. 1985).

QUICK WEIGHT-LOSS DIETS AND PRECAUTIONS

The desire to lose weight quickly and easily makes clients vulnerable to fad diets that may be unsafe and nutritionally unsound. Teach them that the safest way to lose weight is to limit caloric intake while eating a well-balanced diet and increasing exercise. Some diets ignore the importance of well-balanced meals for adequate nutrition by excluding or restricting the carbohydrate, fat, or protein intake. The following questions address concerns about quick weight-loss diets.

Why Should a Weight-Loss Diet Include at Least 58 to 70% Carbohydrate?

Carbohydrate, in the form of glucose, helps maintain normal function of the nervous system because nerve tissue relies solely on glucose as a fuel for energy. Consuming adequate amounts of carbohydrate on a daily basis prevents the depletion of glycogen stores and the need to synthesize glucose from the body's protein (protein-sparing effect). When glycogen stores are depleted, the glucose needs of the body are met through the breakdown of muscle protein. This leads to a loss of lean tissue rather than fat.

Carbohydrate is also essential for fat metabolism. When carbohydrates are restricted or carbohydrate stores are depleted, more free fatty acids are mobilized from adipose tissue than can be metabolized by the body. This results in the incomplete breakdown of lipids and the formation of ketone bodies that may cause ketosis.

In addition, muscle glycogen and glucose are the primary fuels used during intense, short-term exercise and prolonged, submaximal exercise. Inclusion of adequate amounts of carbohydrate in the diet prevents depletion of muscle glycogen and the consequent reduction in endurance performance.

Why Do Low-Carbohydrate Diets Produce Such a Rapid Weight Loss?

Diets that limit or totally exclude carbohydrates produce a rapid weight loss. When the carbohydrate intake is low, muscle glycogen stores are depleted rapidly. For every gram of carbohydrate, 3 grams of water are stored in the body. Thus, when glycogen stores are depleted, the loss of water leads to a dramatic weight loss because each liter of water weighs approximately 2 pounds (0.90 kg). The weight is regained rapidly, however, when carbohydrate intake returns to normal.

Why Are Low-Carbohydrate Diets Unsafe?

Low carbohydrate intake may lead to fatigue, hypoglycemia, and ketosis. As mentioned earlier, in an attempt to remedy low blood glucose levels, more free fatty acids are mobilized from adipose tissue than can be metabolized, resulting in incomplete breakdown of fat and the formation of ketone bodies by the liver. The production of ketone bodies may exceed the body's ability to metabolize them (ketosis). The excess ketone bodies normally are excreted in the urine and expired air. In this condition, however, the blood pH may be lowered to dangerous levels. Examples of popular diets that are low in carbohydrates or totally eliminate intake of carbohydrates are the Atkins, Yudkin, Stillman, Cooper, Mayo Clinic, and Scarsdale diets.

Are High-Protein Diets Safe?

High-protein diets that limit carbohydrate intake promote muscle tissue loss. When carbohydrate intake is restricted, the glucose needs of the body are met by breaking down muscle proteins. The average exercising individual needs no more than 1.2 to 1.6 g of protein per kilogram of body weight each day to meet the additional protein requirements of the body (Lemon et al. 1992; Tarnopolsky et al. 1992). Excess protein intake beyond this level does not promote protein synthesis. Instead, the excess protein is metabolized. The amino acids are deaminated, the excess nitrogen is excreted in the urine as urea, and the remaining carbon skeleton is converted to glucose or used as an energy fuel.

Some high-protein diets require drinking large quantities of water to prevent the dehydration caused by excess urea production and to wash away ketone bodies. Dehydration and the additional stress placed on the kidneys may be potentially dangerous, especially for individuals with kidney problems or gout. Examples of popular diets that are high in protein are the Pennington, Stillman, Cooper, Mayo Clinic, and Scarsdale diets.

Why Are High-Fat Diets Unsafe?

Diets that allow unlimited consumption of fats produce high levels of serum cholesterol and triglycerides. This is potentially unhealthy, because cholesterol in the form of low-density lipoproteins is associated with atherosclerosis and CHD. Typically, high-fat diets are high in calories. Each gram of fat yields 9.3 kcal, while protein and carbohydrate yield 4.3 and 4.1 kcal $\cdot$ g^{-1}, respectively (see table 9.1). Thus, the total quantity of food that can be consumed on a high-fat diet is less than that of a high-carbohydrate or high-protein diet when the calorie intake is the same. Because there are no metabolic pathways in the body for converting fatty acids to glucose, excess fat is stored in adipose tissue. The Atkins diet is an example of a high-fat diet that restricts carbohydrate intake and allows unlimited consumption of meat and fat.

What Is the Danger of Fasting or Skipping Meals to Promote Weight Loss?

For some people, abstaining from food completely may be easier than limiting the amount of food eaten. Fasting, however, may produce serious problems such as kidney malfunction, hyperuricemia, loss of hair, dizziness, fainting, and muscle cramping. When the body is deprived of food, it responds by increasing the fat-depositing enzymes and storing more fat. Also, because carbohydrate and fat are not readily available as a source of energy, the body metabolizes protein to meet its energy needs.

Skipping meals to restrict caloric intake also leads to an increase in the deposition and storage of fat. When we eat just one meal per day, the body is subjected to a fasting condition (23-hour fast) that increases the fat-depositing enzymes. The body quickly adapts to this condition by increasing the percentage of food absorbed by the small intestine. For this reason, nutrition experts advise eating at least three, and as many as six, small meals a day.

DESIGNING WEIGHT-GAIN PROGRAMS

Because genetics plays an important role in weight gain, some clients may have difficulty gaining weight—especially if they have inherited a high resting metabolic rate. Before prescribing weight-gain programs, you should rule out the possibility that diseases and psychological disorders associated with malnutrition (e.g., anorexia nervosa) are not causing your client to be underweight.

The amount of additional calories needed to gain 1 pound (0.45 kg) of muscle tissue has not yet been firmly established. However, research suggests it takes an excess of 2800 to 3500 kcal in order to do so. Thus, adding 400 to 500 kcal to the estimated daily caloric needs (RMR + activity level) of an individual should produce a gradual weight gain of 1 pound per week (Williams 1992). The caloric intake must also be adjusted for additional calories expended during exercise.

To ensure that your client's weight gain is due to increases in lean tissues rather than body fat, you should

- use the body composition method to estimate a healthy target body weight and gain in fat-free mass;

- prescribe a resistance training program designed to maximize muscle size;

- plan a high-calorie, well-balanced diet in which 60 to 70% of the total kcal intake is derived from carbohydrate, 12 to 15% from protein, and less than 30% from fat;

- increase daily protein intake to 1.2 to 1.6 g per kg of body weight to increase muscle size; and

- monitor body composition regularly throughout the weight-gain program using methods described in chapter 8.

Dietary Analysis and Planning

Again, it is highly recommended that you consult with a trained nutrition professional when planning weight-gain diets. When comparing your client's typical nutrient intakes to RDAs, focus on the same questions outlined for weight-loss programs (see Dietary Analysis and Planning, page 190). If your clients' caloric intakes are low, it is highly likely that their vitamin and mineral intakes also will be deficient.

Exercise Prescription for Weight Gain

A high-volume resistance training program is the best approach to maximize the development of muscle size (see table 7.3). Because some clients may not be able to tolerate this volume of training at first, novice weightlifters should start slowly, performing only three sets of each exercise at the prescribed intensity and reducing the number of exercises for each muscle group. Depending on your client's goal, this may be sufficient to increase FFM. For some clients, however, you may need to progressively increase the training volume in order to elicit further improvements in muscle size and FFM. Recommended guidelines for developing an exercise prescription for weight gain are as follows:

GUIDELINES FOR EXERCISE PRESCRIPTION FOR WEIGHT GAIN

Mode: Resistance training

Intensity: 70 to 75% 1-RM or 10- to 12-RM

Sets: 3 for novice, 5 to 6 for advanced weightlifters

Number of exercises: 1 to 2 per muscle group for novice, 3 to 4 per muscle group for advanced weightlifters

Duration: 60 minutes or longer

Frequency: 3 days a week for novice, 5 to 6 days a week for advanced weightlifters

Length of program: Dependent on desired weight gain

DESIGNING PROGRAMS TO IMPROVE BODY COMPOSITION

Some clients may wish to improve their body composition without changing their body weight. For these individuals, you can design exercise programs to either decrease body fat, increase fat-free mass, or both. Research has shown that regular participation in an exercise program may alter an individual's body composition. Aerobic exercise and resistance training are effective modes for decreasing skinfold thicknesses, fat weight, and % BF of both women and men. The following sections address questions about exercise and body composition changes.

What Is the Effect of Aerobic Exercise Training on Body Fat?

Numerous studies have addressed the effect of aerobic exercise training on body composition. The modes of exercise include cycling, walking, jogging, running, and swimming. Wilmore et al. (1970) reported that a 10-week jogging program (3 times per week) produced a significant increase in body density of sedentary men. Because total body weight decreased and fat-free mass remained stable, the increase in body density was attributed almost entirely to fat loss. Pollock et al. (1971) also noted that a 20-week (4 times a week) walking program produced a decrease in % BF and total body weight of men.

Which Aerobic Exercise Mode Is Best for Maximizing Fat Loss?

One study compared cycling, running, and walking of equal frequency, duration, and intensity (Pollock, Dimmick et al. 1975). All three programs produced significant reductions in % BF and body weight. Despres et al. (1985) reported that a 20-week cycling program (4 to 5 times a week) resulted in significant reductions in body weight, % BF, and fat cell weight in a group of sedentary men. These studies suggest that aerobic exercise modes are equally effective in altering body composition.

How Many Times a Week Should I Exercise to Maximize the Loss of Body Fat?

The frequency of the training program may affect the magnitude of the changes in body composition.

Pollock, Miller, et al. (1975) compared aerobic exercise programs consisting of 2, 3, or 4 days a week. Even though the total mileage and caloric expenditure were the same, exercising 2 days a week was not sufficient to produce significant alterations in body composition. They concluded that a 3- or 4-days a week program produces significant body composition changes, with four days a week being superior to three.

Is High-Intensity Better Than Low-Intensity Aerobic Exercise for Promoting Fat Loss?

The intensity of aerobic exercise leads to alterations in body composition. Girandola (1976) compared the effects of a low- and high-intensity cycling program (three days a week) on the body composition of college-age women. Although the body weight and lean body weight for both groups did not change significantly, relative body fat decreased significantly only in the low-intensity group.

What Effect Does Resistance Training Have on Body Fat and Lean Body Mass?

Dynamic resistance training is effective for decreasing % BF and increasing fat-free mass of men and women (Brown and Wilmore 1974; Mayhew and Gross 1974; Wilmore 1974). In Wilmore's study (1974), subjects trained 2 days a week for 10 weeks. At each training session, they performed two sets of 7- to 9-RM for eight different weight training exercises. Men and women exhibited similar alterations in body composition. Although the total body weight remained stable, the fat-free mass increased significantly for both sexes. As a result of resistance training, the relative body fat decreased 9.6% and 10.0% for women and men, respectively.

How Does Exercise Promote Body Composition Changes?

The significant loss of fat weight and % BF with aerobic exercise and resistance training is a function of hormonal responses to the exercise. Exercise increases the circulatory levels of growth hormone (GH), and the levels remain elevated for 1 to 2 hours after exercise (Hartley et al. 1972; Hartley 1975).

Exercise also stimulates the release of catecholamines from the adrenal medulla. Both GH and catecholamines increase the mobilization of free fatty acids from storage (Hartley 1975). Eventually, the muscle may metabolize these free fatty acids during rest and low-intensity exercise.

While low-intensity aerobic exercise is more beneficial for fat loss, high-intensity resistance training is better for fat-free mass gain. The increase in fat-free mass with resistance training may be due to muscle hypertrophy, increased protein content in the muscle, or increased bone density. Muscle hypertrophy and increased protein are mediated by changes in serum testosterone and GH levels in response to weightlifting. Immediately following heavy resistance weightlifting, serum testosterone levels are significantly elevated for men but not for women (Fahey et al. 1976; Weiss, Cureton, and Thompson 1983). GH levels in men are increased significantly for 15 minutes following a 21-minute bout of high-intensity (85% of 1-RM) leg press exercises. However, low-intensity, high-repetition (28% of 1-RM, 21 reps per set) leg presses produced no significant change in GH even though the total amount of work and duration of exercise were equal. Thus, the intensity and number of repetitions play a role in GH release in response to weightlifting exercise (Vanhelder, Radomski, and Goode 1984).

Exercise Prescription for Body Composition Change

When designing exercise programs to promote changes in body composition, follow the guidelines below. Prescribe aerobic exercises to reduce body fat and dynamic resistance exercise to increase fat-free mass.

GUIDELINES FOR EXERCISE PRESCRIPTION FOR FAT LOSS

Goal: Fat loss

Mode: Type I or II aerobic activities (see page 85)

Intensity: $\leq 70\%$ $\dot{V}O_2max$

Duration: >30 minutes

Frequency: Minimum of 3 days a week

Length: Minimum of 8 weeks

GUIDELINES FOR EXERCISE PRESCRIPTION FOR FFM GAIN

Goal: Increase fat-free mass and reduce body fat

Mode: Dynamic resistance training

Intensity: 70 to 85% 1-RM

Repetitions: 6 to 12

Sets: 3 sets

Frequency: Minimum of 3 days per week

Length: Minimum of 8 weeks

Key Points

- Obesity is an excess of body fat that increases health risks.
- Overweight is defined as body weight in excess of 120% of desired body weight or a body mass index in excess of 29.3 for women and 29.8 for men.
- Two types of obesity are upper-body (android) and lower-body (gynoid) obesity.
- The number of fat cells in the body is determined primarily during childhood and adolescence.
- Weight gain in adults is associated with an increase in the size of existing fat cells (hypertrophy), rather than an increase in the number of fat cells (hyperplasia).
- Physical inactivity rather than overeating is a more common cause of obesity.
- The body composition method provides a useful estimate of a healthy body weight.
- A well-balanced diet includes adequate amounts of carbohydrate, protein, fat, minerals, vitamins, and water.
- A high-carbohydrate, low-fat diet provides an excellent source of energy and complies with the recommended *Dietary Guidelines for Americans*.
- Effective weight-loss programs create a negative energy balance by restricting caloric intake and increasing exercise; weight-gain programs create a positive energy balance by increasing caloric intake.
- For weight-loss programs, the combined daily caloric deficit due to calorie restriction and extra exercise should not exceed 1000 kcal; for weight-gain programs, the daily caloric intake should exceed the energy need by no more than 400 to 500 kcal.
- Aerobic exercise maximizes fat loss in weight-loss programs.
- For weight-gain programs, resistance training will ensure that most of the weight gain is due to increases in lean body tissues.
- Aerobic exercise and resistance training are effective ways to improve body composition without changing body weight.

REFERENCES

American Psychiatric Association. 1994. *Diagnostic and statistical manual of mental disorders*: IV, 4th ed. Washington, DC: Author.

Ashwell, M., McCall, S.A., Cole T.J., and Dixon, A.K. 1985. Fat distribution and its metabolic complications: Interpretations. In N.G. Norgan, ed., *Human body composition and fat distribution*, 227-242. Wageningen, Netherlands: Euronut.

Bahr, R., Ingnes, I., Vaage, O., Sjersted, O.M., and Newsholme, E.A. 1987. Effect of duration of exercise on excess post-exercise O_2 consumption. *Journal of Applied Physiology* 62: 485-490.

Baumgartner, R.N., Heymsfield, S.B., and Roche, A.F. 1995. Human body composition and the epidemiology of chronic disease. *Obesity Research* 3: 73-95.

Bielinski, R., Schultz, Y., and Jequier, E. 1985. Energy metabolism during the postexercise recovery in man. *American Journal of Clinical Nutrition* 42: 69-82.

Bjorntorp, P. 1988. Abdominal obesity and the development of non-insulin diabetes mellitus. *Diabetes and Metabolism Reviews* 4: 615-622.

Blair, D., Habricht, J.P., Sims, E.A., Sylwester, D., and Abraham, S. 1984. Evidence of an increased risk for hypertension with centrally located body fat, and the effect of race and sex on this risk. *American Journal of Epidemiology* 119: 526-540.

Bouchard, C., Perusse, L., Leblanc, C., Tremblay, A., and Theriault, G. 1988. Inheritance of the amount and distribution of human body fat. *International Journal of Obesity* 12: 205-215.

Bouchard, C., Tremblay, A., Despres, J.P., Nadeau, A., Lupien, P.J., Theriault, G., Dussault, J., Moorjani, S., Pianist, S., and Fournier, G. 1990. The response of long-term overfeeding in identical twins. *New England Journal of Medicine* 322: 1477-1482.

Bray, G.A., and Gray, D.S. 1988. Obesity. Part I—Pathogenesis. *Western Journal of Medicine* 149: 429-441.

Brehm, B.A. 1988. Elevation of metabolic rate following exercise—implications for weight loss. *Sports Medicine* 6: 72-78.

Brown, C.H., and Wilmore, J.H. 1974. The effects of maximal resistance training on the strength and body composition of women athletes. *Medicine and Science in Sports* 6: 174-177.

Carns, M.L., Schade, M.L., Liba, M.R., Hellebrandt, F.A., and Harris, C.W. 1960. Segmented volume reduction by localized versus generalized exercise. *Human Biology* 32: 370-376.

Clarkson, P.M. 1990. Tired blood: Iron deficiency in athletes and effects of iron supplementation. *Sports Science Exchange* 3, no. 28. Gatorade Sports Science Institute: Quaker Oats Co.

Clarkson, P.M., and Haymes, E.M. 1994. Trace mineral requirements for athletes. *International Journal of Sport Nutrition* 4: 104-119.

Collins, W.E. 1967. *Clinical spirometry*. Braintree, MA: Author.

Corbin, C.A., and Fletcher, P. 1968. Diet and physical activity patterns of obese and nonobese elementary school children. *Research Quarterly* 39: 922-928.

Coyle, E.F. 1995. Fat metabolism during exercise. *Sports Science Exchange* 8, no. 6. Gatorade Sports Science Insitute: Quaker Oats Co.

Despres, J.P., Bouchard, C., Tremblay, A., Savard, R., and Marcotte, M. 1985. Effects of aerobic training on fat distribution in male subjects. *Medicine and Science in Sports and Exercise* 17: 113-118.

Donahue, C.P., Lin, D.H., Kirschenbaum, D.S., and Keesey, R.E. 1984. Metabolic consequence of dieting and exercise in the treatment of obesity. *Journal of Counseling and Clinical Psychology* 52: 827-836.

Ducimetier, P., Richard, J., and Cambien, F. 1989. The pattern of subcutaneous fat distribution in middle-aged men and the risk of coronary heart disease: The Paris prospective study. *International Journal of Obesity* 10: 229-240.

Ettinger, B., Genault, H.K., and Cann, C.E. 1987. Postmenopausal bone loss is prevented by treatment with low-dosage estrogen with calcium. *Annals of Internal Medicine* 106: 40-45.

Fahey, T.D., Rolph, R., Moungmee, P., Nagel, J., and Mortara, S. 1976. Serum testosterone, body composition, and strength of young adults. *Medicine and Science in Sports* 8: 31-34.

Fohlin, L. 1977. Body composition, cardiovascular and renal function in adolescent patients with anorexia nervosa. *Acta Paediatrica Scandinavica* 268(Suppl.): 7-20.

Girandola, R.N. 1976. Body composition changes in women: Effect of high and low exercise intensity. *Archives of Physical Medicine and Rehabilitation* 57: 297-300.

Goldfarb, A. 1993. Antioxidants: Role of supplementation to prevent exercise-induced oxidative stress. *Medicine and Science in Sports and Exercise* 25: 232-236.

Grande, F. and Keys, A. 1980. Body weight, body composition, and calorie status. In R.S. Goodhart and M.E. Shils, eds., *Modern nutrition in health and disease*, 27. Philadelphia: Lea & Febiger.

Harris, J.A. and Benedict, F.G. 1919. *A biometric study of basal metabolism in man* (Publication No.279). Washington, DC: Carnegie Institute.

Hartley, L.H. 1975. Growth hormone and catecholamine response to exercise in relation to physical training. *Medicine and Science in Sports* 7: 34-36.

Hartley, L.H., Mason, J.W., Hogan, R.P., Jones, L.G., Kotchen, T.A., Mougey, E.H., Wherry, R., Pennington, L., and Ricketts, P. 1972. Multiple hormonal responses to graded exercise in relation to physical conditioning. *Journal of Applied Physiology* 33: 602-606.

Hirsh, J. 1971. Adipose cellularity in relation to human obesity. *Advances in Internal Medicine* 17: 289-300.

Hubert, H.B., Feinleib, M., McNamara, P.M., and Castelli, W.P. 1983. Obesity as an independent risk factor for cardiovascular disease: A 26-yr follow-up of participants in the Framingham study. *Circulation* 67: 968-979.

Katch, F.I., Clarkson, P.M., Kroll, W., McBride, T., and Wilcox, A. 1984. Effects of sit-up exercise training on adipose cell size and adiposity. *Research Quarterly for Exercise and Sport* 55: 242-247.

Kraemer, W.J., Gordon, S.E., Fleck, S.J., Marchitelli, L.J., Mello, R., Dziados, J.E., Friedl, K., Harman, E., Maresh, C., and Fry, A.C. 1991. Endogenous anabolic hormonal and growth factor responses to heavy resistance exercise in males and females. *International Journal of Sports Medicine* 12: 228-235.

Krotkiewski, M., Gudmundsson, M., Backstrom, P., and Mandroukas, K., 1982. Zinc and muscle strength and endurance. *Acta Physiologica Scandinavica* 116: 309-311.

Kuczmarski, R.J., Flegal, K.M., Campbell, S.M., and Johnson, C.L. 1994. Increasing prevalence of overweight among U.S. adults: The National Health and Nutrition Examination Surveys, 1960 to 1991. *Journal of the American Medical Association* 272: 205-211.

Lemon, P.W. 1989. Influence of dietary protein and total energy intake on strength improvement. *Sports Science Exchange* 2, no. 14. Gatorade Sports Science Institute: Quaker Oats Co.

Lemon, P.W., Tarnopolsky, M.A., MacDougall, J.D., and Atkinson, S.A. 1992. Protein requirements and muscle mass/strength changes during intensive training in novice bodybuilders. *Journal of Applied Physiology* 73: 767-775.

Lenfant, C., and Ernst, N. 1994. Daily dietary fat and total food-energy intakes: Third National Health and Nutrition Examination Survey, Phase I, 1988-91. *Morbidity and Mortality Weekly Report* 43: 116-117.

Litchell, H., and Boberg, J. 1978. The lipoprotein lipase activity of adipose tissue from different sites in obese women and relationship to cell size. *International Journal of Obesity* 2: 47-52.

Marks, B.L., Ward, A., Morris, D.H., Castellani, J., and Rippe, J.M. 1995. Fat-free mass is maintained in women following a moderate diet and exercise program. *Medicine and Science in Sports and Exercise* 27: 1243-1251.

Mayer, J. 1968. *Overweight: Causes, costs and control.* Englewood Cliffs, NJ: Prentice-Hall.

Mayhew, J.L., and Gross, P.M. 1974. Body composition changes in young women with high resistance weight training. *Research Quarterly* 45: 433-440.

Mazess, R.B., Barden, H.S., and Ohlrich, E.S. 1990. Skeletal and body-composition effects of anorexia nervosa. *American Journal of Clinical Nutrition* 52: 438-441.

McArdle, W.D., Katch, F.I., and Katch, V.L. 1996. *Exercise physiology.* Baltimore: Williams & Wilkins.

Mole, P.A., Oscai, L.B., and Holloszy, J.O. 1971. Adaptation of muscle to exercise: Increase in levels of palmityl CoA synthetase, carnitine palmityl-transferase, and palmityl CoA dehydrogenase and the capacity to oxidize fatty acids. *Journal of Clinical Investigation* 50: 2323-2329.

Nadel, E.R. 1988. New ideas for rehydration during and after exercise in hot weather. *Sports Science Exchange* 1, no. 3. Gatorade Sports Science Institute: Quaker Oats Co.

National Institutes of Health Consensus Development Panel 1985. Health implications of obesity: National Institutes of Health consensus development statement. *Annals of Internal Medicine* 103: 1073-1079.

Noland, M., and Kearney, J.T. 1978. Anthropometric and densitometric responses of women to specific and general exercise. *Research Quarterly* 49: 322-328.

Pavlou, K.N., Steffee, W.P., Lerman, R.H., and Burrows, B.A. 1985. Effects of dieting and exercise on lean body mass, oxygen uptake, and strength. *Medicine and Science in Sports and Exercise* 17: 466-471.

Pollock, M.L., Dimmick, J., Miller, H.S., Kendrick, Z., and Linnerud, A.C. 1975. Effects of mode of training on cardiovascular function and body composition of middle-aged men. *Medicine and Science in Sports* 7: 139-145.

Pollock, M.L., Miller, H.S., Janeway, R., Linnerud, A.C., Robertson, B., and Valentino, R. 1971. Effects of walking on body composition and cardiovascular function of middle-aged men. *Journal of Applied Physiology* 30: 126-130.

Pollock, M.L., Miller, H.S., Linnerud, A.C., and Cooper, K.H. 1975. Frequency of training as a determinant for improvement in cardiovascular function and body composition of middle-aged men. *Archives of Physical Medicine and Rehabilitation* 56: 141-145.

Rajaram, S., Weaver, C.M., Lyle, R.M., Sedlock, D.A., Martin, B., Templin, T.J., Beard, J.L., and Percival, S.S. 1995. Effects of long-term moderate exercise on iron status in young women. *Medicine and Science in Sports and Exercise* 27: 1105-1110.

Rebuffe-Scrive, M. 1985. Adipose tissue metabolism and fat distribution. In N.G. Norgan, ed., *Human body composition and fat distribution,* 212-217. Wageningen, Netherlands: Euronut.

Roby, R.B. 1962. Effect of exercise on regional subcutaneous fat accumulations. *Research Quarterly* 33: 273-278.

Russell, C.M., Williamson, D.F., and Byers, T. 1995. Can the Year 2000 objective for reducing overweight in the United States be reached? A simulation study of the required changes in body weight. *International Journal of Obesity and Related Metabolic Disorders* 19: 149-153.

Sanborn, C.F. 1990. Exercise, calcium, and bone density. *Sports Science Exchange* 2, no. 14. Gatorade Sports Science Institute: Quaker Oats Co.

Schade, M., Hellebrandt, F.A., Waterland, J.C., and Carns, M.L. 1962. Spot reducing in overweight college women: Its influence on fat distribution as determined by photography. *Research Quarterly.* 33: 461-471.

Serdula, M.K., Williamson, D.F., Anda, R.F., Levy, A., Heaton, A., and Byers, T. 1994. Weight control practices in adults: Results of a multistate telephone survey. *American Journal of Public Health* 84: 1821-1824.

Sharkey, B.J. 1990. *Physiology of fitness,* 3rd ed. Champaign, IL: Human Kinetics.

Singh, V. 1992. A current perspective on nutrition and exercise. *Journal of Nutrition* 122: 760-765.

Sjodin, A.M., Forslund, A.H., Westerterp, K.R., Andersson, A.B., Forslund, J.M., and Hambraeus, L.M. 1996. The influence of physical activity on BMR. *Medicine and Science in Sports and Exercise* 28: 85-91.

Smith, U., Hammerstein, J., Bjorntorp, P., and Kral, J.G. 1979. Regional differences and effect of weight reduction on human fat cell metabolism. *EuropeanJournal of Clinical Investigation* 9: 327-332.

Society of Actuaries and Association of Life Insurance Medical Directors of America. 1980. *1979 build study*. New York: Metropolitan Life Insurance.

Subcommittee on the 10th Edition of the RDAs, Food and Nutrition Board, Commission on Life Sciences, National Research Council. 1989. *Recommended dietary allowances*. Washington DC: National Academy Press.

Tarnopolsky, M.A., Atkinson, S.A., MacDougall, J.D., Chesley, A., Phillips, S., and Schwarcz, H.P. 1992. Evaluation of protein requirements for trained strength athletes. *Journal of Applied Physiology* 73: 1986-1995.

Telford, R., Catchpole, E., Deakin, V., Hahn, A., and Plank, A. 1992. The effect of 7 to 8 months of vitamin/mineral supplementation on athletic performance. *International Journal of Sport Nutrition* 2: 135-153.

terHeun, P. 1981. *Being fat has nothing to do with food*. Millbrae, CA: Celestial Arts.

Troiano, R.P., Flegal, K.M., Kuczmarski, R.J., Campbell, S.M., and Johnson, C.L. 1995. Overweight prevalence and trends for children and adolescents. The National Health and Nutrition Examination Surveys 1963-1991. *Archives of Pediatric and Adolescent Medicine* 149: 1085-1091.

U.S. Department of Agriculture. 1992. *The food guide pyramid*. Hyattsville, MD: Human Nutrition Information Service.

U.S. Department of Health and Human Services. 1988. *The Surgeon General's report on nutrition and health*. DHHS [PHS] Publication No. 88-50210. Washington, DC: U.S. Government Printing Office.

U.S. Department of Health and Human Services 1995. *Dietary guidelines for Americans*. Washington, DC: U.S. Government Printing Office.

U.S. Senate Select Committee on Nutrition and Human Needs. 1977. *Dietary goals for the United States*, 1-56. Washington, DC: U.S. Government Printing Office.

Vaisman, N., Corey, M., Rossi, M.F., Goldberg, E., and Pencharz, P. 1988. Changes in body composition during refeeding of patients with anorexia nervosa. *Journal of Pediatrics* 113: 925-929.

Vaisman, N., Rossi, M.F., Goldberg, E., Dibden, L.J., Wykes, L.J., and Pencharz, P.B. 1988. Energy expenditures and body composition in patients with anorexia nervosa. *Journal of Pediatrics* 113: 919-924.

Vanhelder, W.P., Radomski, M.W., and Goode, R.C. 1984. Growth hormone responses during intermittent weight lifting exercise in men. *European Journal of Applied Physiology* 53: 31-34.

Weiss, L.W., Cureton, K.J., and Thompson, F.N. 1983. Comparison of serum testosterone and androstenedione responses to weight lifting in men and women. *European Journal of Applied Physiology* 50: 413-419.

Williams, M.H. 1993. Nutritional supplements for strength trained athletes. *Sports Science Exchange* 6, no. 6. Gatorade Sports Science Institute: Quaker Oats Co.

Williams, M.H. 1992. *Nutrition for fitness and sport*. Dubuque, IA: Brown and Benchmark.

Wilmore, J.H. 1974. Alterations in strength, body composition, and anthropometric measurements consequent to a 10-week weight training program. *Medicine and Science in Sports* 6: 133-138.

Wilmore, J.H. 1986. Body composition: A roundtable. *The Physician and Sportsmedicine* 14: 144-162.

Wilmore, J.H., Royce, J., Girandola, R.N., Katch, F.I., and Katch, V.L. 1970. Body composition changes with a 10-week program of jogging. *Medicine and Science in Sports* 2: 113-119.

CHAPTER 10

Assessing Flexibility and Designing Stretching Programs

Key Questions

- What are static and dynamic flexibility?
- What factors affect flexibility?
- How is flexibility assessed?
- Are all types of stretching exercises safe and effective for improving flexibility?
- What are the recommended guidelines for designing a stretching program?
- Can low back syndrome be prevented?
- What exercises are specifically recommended for low back care programs?

Flexibility is an important, yet often neglected, component of physical fitness. As an exercise specialist, you will encounter many clients who experience musculoskeletal injuries and low back problems. In many cases, the combination of poor muscle strength and lack of flexibility is the cause of these problems, particularly in sedentary, middle-aged, and older populations. Adequate flexibility in all joints of the body is important, especially in older adults, to prevent musculoskeletal injury and to maintain functional independence with aging.

This chapter describes direct and indirect methods for assessing flexibility. It presents guidelines for designing flexibility programs, as well as recommendations for prescribing exercises suitable for low back care programs.

DEFINITION AND NATURE OF FLEXIBILITY

Flexibility is the ability of a joint, or series of joints, to move fluidly through a full range of motion (ROM). *Static flexibility* is a measure of the total ROM at the joint; *dynamic flexibility* is a measure of the torque or resistance to movement. Both types of flexibility are important in performance of sport skills as well as activities of daily living, such as bending to pick up the newspaper or getting out of the back seat of a two-door car.

The ROM is highly specific to the joint and depends on morphological factors such as the joint geometry, joint capsule, ligaments, tendons, and

203

Table 10.1 Joint Classification by Structure and Function

Type of joint	Axes of rotation	Movements	Examples
Gliding	Nonaxial	Gliding, sliding, twisting	Intercarpal, intertarsal, tarsometatarsal
Hinge	Uni-axial	Flexion, extension	Knee, elbow, ankle, interphalangeal
Pivot	Uni-axial	Medial and lateral rotation	Proximal radioulnar, atlantoaxial
Condyloid and saddle	Bi-axial	Flexion, extension, abduction, adduction, circumduction	Wrist, atlanto-occipital, metacarpophalangeal, first carpometacarpal
Ball and socket	Tri-axial	Flexion, extension, abduction, adduction, circumduction, rotation	Hip, shoulder

muscles spanning the joint. The joint structure determines the planes of motion and may limit the ROM at a given joint. *Triaxial joints* (e.g., ball and socket joints of the hip and shoulder) afford a greater degree of movement in more directions than either the *uniaxial* or *biaxial joints* (see table 10.1).

The tension within the muscle-tendon unit affects both static flexibility (ROM) and dynamic flexibility (resistance to motion). The tension within this unit is attributed to the viscoelastic properties of connective tissues, as well as the degree of muscular contraction resulting from the stretch reflex (McHugh et al. 1992). Individuals with less flexibility and tighter muscles and tendons have a greater contractile response during stretching exercises and resistance to stretching. The elastic deformation of the muscle-tendon unit during stretching is proportional to the load or tension applied, whereas the viscous deformation is proportional to the speed at which the tension is applied. When the muscle and tendon are stretched and held at a fixed length (e.g., during static stretching), the tension within the unit, or tensile stress, decreases over time (McHugh et al. 1992). This is called *stress relaxation*. Thus, static stretching exercises are an excellent way to induce viscoelastic stress relaxation.

The tightness of soft tissue structures such as muscle, tendons, and ligaments is a major limitation to both static and dynamic flexibility. Johns and Wright (1962) determined the relative contribution of soft tissues to the total resistance encountered by the joint during movement:

- Joint capsule—47%
- Muscle and its fascia—41%
- Tendons and ligaments—10%
- Skin—2%

The joint capsule and ligaments consist predominantly of collagen, a nonelastic connective tissue.

The muscle and its fascia are composed of more elastic tissue; therefore, they are the most important and modifiable structures in terms of reducing resistance to movement and increasing dynamic flexibility.

FACTORS AFFECTING FLEXIBILITY

Flexibility is related to body type, age, gender, and physical activity. This section addresses some commonly asked questions about flexibility.

Does Body Type Limit Flexibility?

Individuals with large hypertrophied muscles or excessive amounts of subcutaneous fat may score poorly on ROM tests, because adjacent body segments in these people contact each other sooner compared to those with smaller limb and trunk girths. However, this does not necessarily mean that all heavily-muscled or obese individuals have poor flexibility. Many bodybuilders and obese individuals who routinely stretch their muscles have adequate levels of flexibility.

Why Do Older Individuals Tend to Be Less Flexible Than Younger People?

Flexibility progressively decreases with aging because of changes in the elasticity of the soft tissues and a decrease in the physical activity level. In a recent study, however, Girouard and Hurley (1995) reported significant improvements in shoulder and hip ROM of older men (50 to 69 years) following 10 weeks of flexibility training. Thus, older persons can benefit from flexibility training and should be encouraged to perform stretching exercises at least three times a week to counteract age-related decreases in ROM.

Are Females More Flexible Than Males?

Some evidence suggests that females generally are more flexible than males at all ages (Alter 1996). The greater flexibility of women is usually attributed to gender differences in pelvic structure and to hormones that may affect the laxity of connective tissue (Alter 1996). However, the effect of gender on ROM appears to be joint- and motion-specific. Females tend to have more hip flexion and spinal lateral flexion compared to males of the same age. On the other hand, males have greater ROM in hip extension and spinal flexion and extension in the thoracolumbar region (Norkin and White 1995).

How Do Physical Activity and Inactivity Affect Flexibility?

Habitual movement patterns and physical activity levels apparently are more important determinants of flexibility than gender, age, and body type (Harris 1969; Kirby et al. 1981). Lack of physical activity is a major cause of inflexibility. It is well documented that inactive persons tend to be less flexible than active persons (McCue 1953) and that exercise increases flexibility (Chapman, deVries, and Swezey 1972; deVries 1962; Hartley-O'Brien 1980). Disuse, due to lack of physical activity or immobilization, produces contracture and shortening of the connective tissue which, in turn, restrict joint mobility.

Moving the joints and muscles in a repetitive pattern or maintaining habitual body postures also may restrict ROM because of the tightening and shortening of the muscle tissue. For example, joggers and people who sit behind a desk for long periods need to stretch the hamstrings and low back muscles to counteract the tautness developed in these muscle groups.

Does Warm-Up Affect Flexibility?

Wright and Johns (1960) reported that warming the joint (113° F) produces a 20% increase in ROM, whereas cooling the joint (65° F) results in a 10 to 20% decrease in flexibility. When you administer flexibility tests, make certain that (a) your client performs some type of warm-up activity to increase circulation and internal body temperature and (b) you administer multiple trials of each test item.

Can You Develop Too Much Flexibility?

It is important to recognize that excessive amounts of stretching and flexibility training may result in hypermobility, or an increased ROM of joints beyond normal, acceptable values. Hypermobility leads to joint laxity (looseness or instability) and may increase the risk of musculoskeletal injuries. For example, it is not uncommon for gymnasts and swimmers to experience shoulder dislocations because of joint laxity and hypermobility. As an exercise specialist, you need to be able to accurately assess ROM and to design stretching programs that improve your clients' flexibility without compromising joint stability.

ASSESSMENT OF FLEXIBILITY

Field and clinical tests are available for assessing static flexibility. Although ROM data are important, measures of joint stiffness and resistance to movement may be more meaningful in terms of physical performance. However, little research has focused on the assessment of dynamic flexibility. Typically, static flexibility is assessed in field and clinical settings by measuring the ROM directly or indirectly.

GENERAL GUIDELINES FOR FLEXIBILITY TESTING

To assess a client's flexibility, you should select a number of test items because of the highly specific nature of flexibility (Dickinson 1968; Harris 1969). Direct tests that measure the range of joint rotation in degrees are usually more useful than indirect tests that measure static flexibility in linear units. When administering these tests,

- have the client perform a short warm-up prior to the test and avoid fast, jerky movements and stretching beyond the pain-free range of joint motion;

- administer three trials of each test item;

- compare the client's best score to norms in order to obtain a flexibility rating for each test item; and

- use the test results to identify joints and muscle groups in need of improvement.

Direct Methods of Measuring Static Flexibility

To assess static flexibility directly, measure the amount of joint rotation in degrees using a goniometer, flexometer, or inclinometer. The following sections describe the procedures for these tests.

Universal Goniometer Test Procedures

The universal goniometer is a protractor-like device with two steel or plastic arms that measure the joint angle at the extremes of the ROM (see figure 10.1). The stationary arm of the goniometer is attached at the zero line of the protractor and the other arm is moveable. To use the goniometer, place the center of

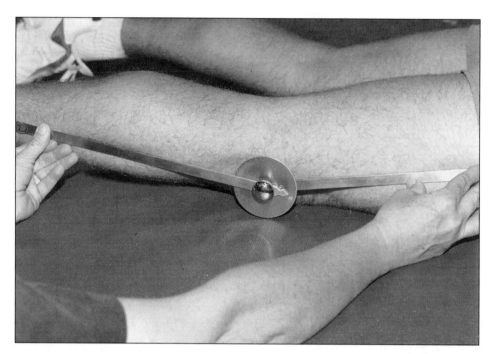

a

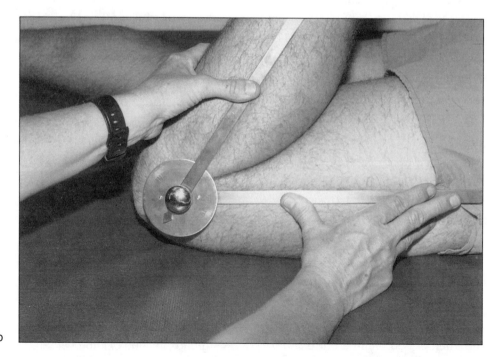

b

Figure 10.1 Measuring ROM at knee joint using universal goniometer: (*a*) starting position and (*b*) ending position.

the instrument so it coincides with the fulcrum, or axis of rotation, of the joint. Align the arms of the goniometer with bony landmarks along the longitudinal axis of each moving body segment. Measure the ROM as the difference between the joint angles (degrees) at the extremes of the movement.

Table 10.2 summarizes the procedures for measuring ROM for various joints using a universal goniometer. For more detailed descriptions of these procedures, see Greene and Heckman (1994) and Norkin and White (1995). Table 10.3 presents average ROM values for healthy adults.

Flexometer Test Procedures

Another tool that can be used to measure ROM is the Leighton flexometer (see figure 10.2). This device consists of a weighted 360-degree dial and weighted pointer. The ROM is measured in relation to the downward pull of gravity on the dial and pointer. To use this device, strap the instrument to the body segment and lock the dial at 0° at one extreme of the ROM. After the client executes the movement, lock the pointer at the other extreme of the ROM. The degree of arc through which the movement takes place is read directly from the dial. Tests have been devised to measure the ROM at the neck, trunk, shoulder, elbow, radioulnar, wrist, hip, knee, and ankle joints using the Leighton flexometer (Hubley-Kozey 1991; Leighton 1955).

Inclinometer Test Procedures

The inclinometer is another type of gravity-dependent goniometer (see figure 10.3). To use this device, hold it on the distal end of the moving body segment. The inclinometer measures the angle between the long axis of the moving segment and the line of gravity. This device is easier to use than the flexometer and universal goniometer because it is hand-held on the moving body segment during the measurement and does not have to be aligned with specific bony landmarks. Also, the American Medical Association (1988) recommends the double inclinometer technique, using two inclinometers, to measure spinal mobility (see figure 10.3).

Validity and Reliability of Direct Measures

The validity and reliability of these devices for directly measuring ROM is highly dependent on the joint being measured and technician skill. Radiography is considered to be the best reference method for establishing validity of goniometric measurements. Research shows high agreement between ROM measured by radiographs and universal goniometers for the hip and knee joints (Ahlback and Lindahl 1964; Enwemeka 1986). Mayer, Tencer, and Kristoferson (1984) reported no difference between radiography and the double-inclinometer technique for assessing spinal ROM in patients with low back pain.

The intratester and intertester reliability of goniometric measurements is affected by difficulty in identifying the axis of rotation and in palpating bony landmarks. Measurements of upper-extremity joints are generally more reliable than ROM measurements of the lower extremity joints (Norkin and White 1995). The intertester reliability of inclinometer measurements is variable and joint-specific. Studies reported reliability coefficients ranging from 0.48 for lumbar extension (Williams et al. 1993) to 0.96 for subtalar joint position (Sell et al. 1994). In order to obtain accurate and reliable ROM measurements, you need knowledge of anatomy and standardized testing procedures, as well as training and practice to develop your measurement techniques.

Indirect Methods of Measuring Static Flexibility

You also can assess static flexibility indirectly using linear measurements of the ROM. For this purpose, you use a tape measure, yardstick, and sit-and-reach box to measure flexibility in inches or centimeters rather than degrees of joint motion. A major weakness of some flexibility field tests is that the length or width of the body segments may affect the performance (Wear 1963). For example, an individual with short legs relative to the trunk will have an advantage when taking the standard sit-and-reach test. Some commonly used indirect tests for assessing spinal mobility and low back flexibility are the standard and modified sit-and-reach tests and the skin distraction test.

Standard Sit-and-Reach Test

The ACSM (1995) recommends using the standard sit-and-reach test to evaluate low back and hip flexibility. You can use either a sit-and-reach box or a yardstick. Secure the yardstick to the floor by placing tape at a right angle to the 15-inch (38 cm) mark of the yardstick. The client sits, straddling the yardstick, with the knees extended (but not locked) and legs spread 10 to 12 inches (25.4 to 30.5 cm)

Table 10.2   Universal Goniometer Measurement Procedures

Joint	Body position	Axis of rotation	Goniometer position		Stabilization	Special considerations
			Stationary arm	Moving arm		
Shoulder						
Extension	Prone	Acromion process	Midaxillary line	Lateral epicondyle of humerus	Scapula and thorax	Elbow is slightly flexed and palm of hand faces body.
Flexion	Supine	Same as extension	Same as extension	Same as extension	Scapula and thorax	Palm of hand faces body
Abduction	Supine	Anterior axis of acromion process	Midline of anterior aspect of sternum	Medial midline of humerus	Scapula and thorax	Palm of hand faces anteriorly; humerus is laterally rotated; elbow is extended.
Medial/ lateral rotation	Supine	Olecranon process	Perpendicular to floor	Styloid process of ulna	Distal end of humerus and scapula	Arm is abducted 90°; forearm is perpendicular to supporting surface in mid-pronated-supinated position; humerus rests on pad so that it is level with acromion process.
Elbow						
Flexion	Supine	Lateral epicondyle of humerus	Lateral midline of humerus	Lateral midline of radial head and styloid process	Distal end of humerus	Arm is close to body; pad is placed under distal end of humerus; forearm is fully supinated.
Forearm						
Pronation	Sitting	Lateral to ulna styloid process	Parallel to anterior midline of humerus	Lies across dorsal aspect of forearm, just proximal to styloid processes of radius and ulna	Distal end of humerus	Arm is close to body, elbow flexed 90°; forearm is midway between supination and pronation (thumb towards ceiling).
Supination	Sitting	Medial to ulna styloid process	Parallel to anterior midline of humerus	Lies across the ventral aspect of forearm, just proximal to styloid processes of radius and ulna	Distal end of humerus	Testing position is same as for pronation of forearm

Joint and motion	Position	Axis	Stationary arm	Moving arm	Stabilize	Instructions
Wrist						
Flexion and extension	Sitting	Lateral aspect of wrist over the triquetrum	Lateral midline of ulna, using olecranon and ulnar styloid processes for reference.	Lateral midline of fifth metacarpal	Radius and ulna	Client sits next to supporting surface, abducts shoulder 90°, and flexes elbow 90°; forearm is in mid-supinated-pronated position; palm of hand faces ground; forearm rests on supporting surface; hand is free to move.
Radial or ulna deviation	Sitting	Middle of dorsal aspect of wrist over capitate	Dorsal midline of forearm, using lateral humeral epicondyle as reference	Dorsal midline of third metacarpal	Distal ends of radius and ulna	Same as for wrist flexion
Hip						
Flexion and extension	Supine Prone	Lateral aspect of hip joint, using greater trochanter as reference	Lateral midline of pelvis	Lateral midline of femur, using lateral epicondyle for reference	Pelvis	Knee is allowed to flex as range of hip flexion is completed; knee is flexed during hip extension.
Abduction and adduction	Supine	Centered over anterior superior iliac spine	Horizontally align arm with imaginary line between anterior superior iliac spines	Anterior midline of femur, using midline of patella for reference	Pelvis	Knee is extended during abduction. Contralateral hip is abducted to allow hip being adducted to complete its ROM.
Medial/lateral rotation	Sitting	Centered over anterior aspect of patella	Perpendicular to floor	Anterior midline of lower leg, using crest of tibia and point midway between malleoli for reference	Distal end of femur. Avoid rotation and lateral tilt of pelvis.	Client sits on supporting surface, knees flexed 90°, hip flexed 90°; place towel roll under distal end of femur; contralateral knee may need to be flexed so that hip being measured can complete full range of lateral rotation.
Knee						
Flexion	Supine	Over the lateral epicondyle of femur	Lateral midline of femur, using greater trochanter for reference	Lateral midline of fibula, using lateral malleolus and fibular head for reference	Femur to prevent rotation, abduction, and adduction	As knee flexes, the hip also flexes.
Ankle						
Dorsiflexion and plantar flexion	Sitting	Over the lateral aspect of lateral malleolus	Lateral midline of fibula, using head of fibula for reference	Parallel to lateral aspect of fifth metatarsal	Tibia and fibula	Client sits on end of table with knee flexed and ankle positioned at 90°.

(continued)

Table 10.2 *(Continued)*

| Joint | Body position | Goniometer position | | | Stabilization | Special considerations |
		Axis of rotation	Stationary arm	Moving arm		
Subtalar						
Inversion and eversion	Sitting	Centered over anterior aspect of ankle midway between malleoli	Anterior midline of lower leg, using the tibial tuberosity for reference	Anterior midline of second metatarsal	Tibia and fibula	Client sits with knee flexed 90° and lower leg over edge of supporting surface.
Lumbar spine						
Lateral flexion	Standing	Centered over posterior aspect of spinous process of S1	Perpendicular to ground	Posterior aspect of spinous process of C7	Pelvis to prevent lateral tilt	Client stands erect with 0° of spinal flexion, extension, and rotation.
Rotation	Sitting	Centered over superior aspect of client's head	Parallel to imaginary line between tubercles of iliac crests	Imaginary line between two acromion processes	Pelvis to prevent rotation	Keep feet flat on floor to stabilize pelvis.

Table 10.3   Average ROM Values (in Degrees) for Healthy Adults

Joint	ROM	Joint	ROM
Shoulder		Thoracic-lumbar spine	
Flexion	150-180	Flexion	60-80
Extension	50-60	Extension	20-30
Abduction	180	Lateral flexion	25-35
Medial rotation	70-90	Rotation	30-45
Lateral rotation	90		
		Hip	
Elbow		Flexion	100-120
Flexion	140-150	Extension	30
Extension	0	Abduction	40-45
		Adduction	20-30
Radio-ulnar		Medial rotation	40-45
Pronation	80	Lateral rotation	45-50
Supination	80		
		Knee	
Wrist		Flexion	135-150
Flexion	60-80	Extension	0-10
Extension	60-70		
Radial deviation	20	Ankle	
Ulnar deviation	30	Dorsiflexion	20
		Plantar flexion	40-50
Cervical spine			
Flexion	45-60	Subtalar	
Extension	45-75	Inversion	30-35
Lateral flexion	45	Eversion	15-20
Rotation	60-80		

Data from the American Academy of Orthopaedic Surgeons (Greene and Heckman 1994) and the American Medical Association (1988).

apart. The heels of the feet touch the tape at the 15-inch mark. If a sit-and-reach box is available, the heels are placed against the edge of the box (see figure 10.4). Instruct the client to reach forward slowly and as far as possible along the yardstick or box while keeping both hands parallel (fingertips may overlap), and to hold this position momentarily. Make certain that the knees do not flex and that the client avoids leading with one hand. The score (in inches) is the most distant point on the yardstick or box contacted by the fingertips.

Although most exercise specialists assume the standard sit-and-reach test to be a valid measure of low back and hip flexibility, Jackson and Baker (1986) reported that the sit-and-reach scores of 13- to 15-year-old girls were only moderately correlated with hamstring flexibility (r = 0.64) and poorly correlated with criterion measures of total back (r = 0.07), upper back (r = –0.16), and lower back (r = 0.28) flexibility. They concluded that the sit-and-reach test does not validly assess lower back flexibility of teenage girls. Jackson and Langford (1989) examined the validity of the standard sit-and-reach test as a field test for hamstring and low back flexibility in adult women and men, ages 20 to 45 years. They reported that the sit-and-reach test had excellent criterion-related validity as a test of hamstring flexibility (r = 0.89) but was only moderately related to low back flexibility (r = 0.59) in men. For women, the sit-and-reach test had moderate criterion-related validity as a test of hamstring flexibility (r = 0.70) but was poorly related to low back flexibility (r = 0.12).

Modified Sit-and-Reach Test

As mentioned previously, individuals having short legs relative to the trunk have a definite advantage when performing the standard sit-and-reach test. Hoeger (1989) developed a modified sit-and-reach test which takes into account the distance between the end of the fingers and the sit-and-reach box and uses the finger-to-box distance as the relative zero point. For this test, a 12-inch high box or a sit-and-reach box is used (see figure 10.4). The client sits on the floor with buttocks, shoulders, and head in contact with the wall; extends (but does not lock) his knees; and places the soles of the feet against the box. A yardstick is placed on top of the box with the zero end toward the client. Keeping the head and

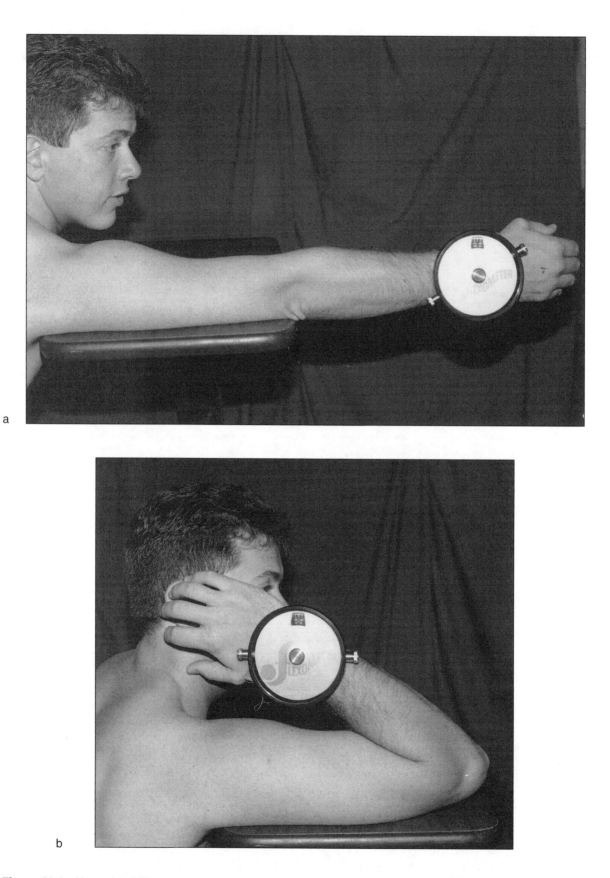

Figure 10.2   Measuring ROM at elbow joint using Leighton flexometer: (*a*) starting position and (*b*) ending position.

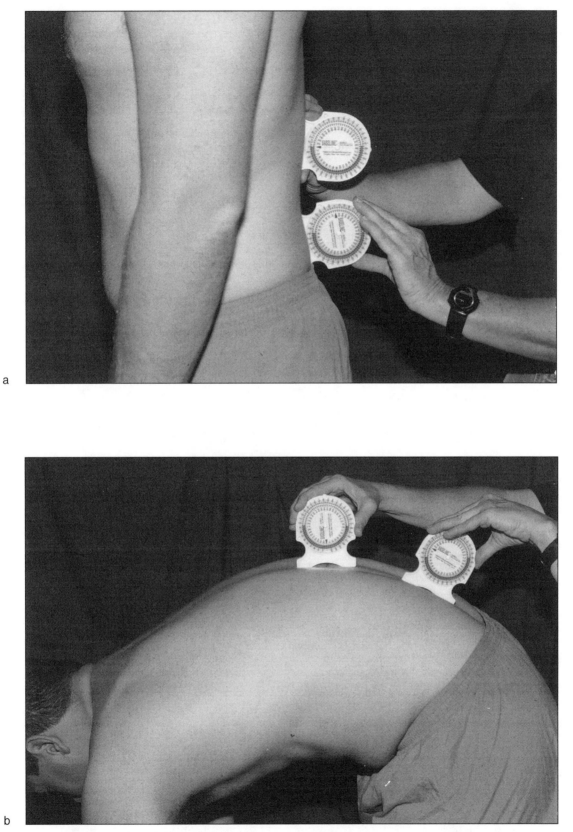

a

b

Figure 10.3   Measuring lumbosacral flexion using the double inclinometer technique: (*a*) starting position and (*b*) ending position.

shoulders in contact with the wall, the client reaches forward with one hand on top of the other, and the yardstick is then positioned so that it touches his fingertips. This procedure establishes the relative zero point for each client. As you firmly hold the yardstick in place, the client reaches forward slowly, sliding his fingers along the top of the yardstick. The score (in inches) is the most distant point on the yardstick contacted by the fingertips. Table 10.4 provides age-gender percentile norms for the modified sit-and-reach test. Clients scoring less than the 50th percentile have below-average flexibility.

Research comparing the standard and modified sit-and-reach test scores indicated that individuals with proportionally longer arms than legs (lower finger-to-box distance) had significantly better scores on the standard sit-and-reach test than those with moderate or high finger-to-box distances, whereas the modified sit-and-reach test scores did not differ significantly among the three groups (Hoeger et al. 1990; Hoeger and Hopkins 1992). However, Minkler and Patterson (1994) reported that the modified sit-and-reach test was only moderately related to criterion measures of hamstring flexibility for

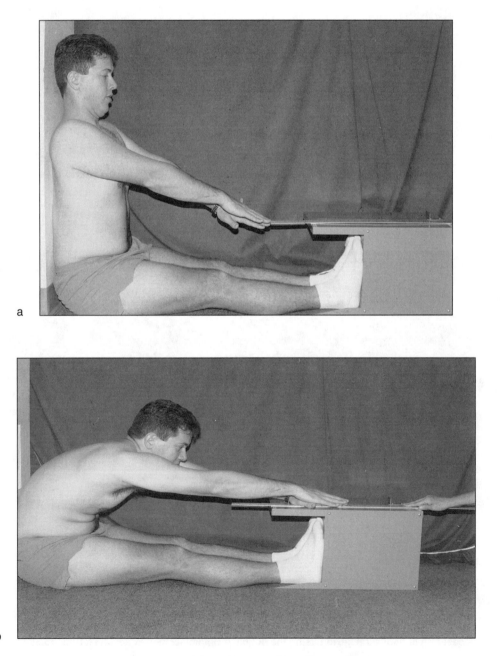

a

b

Figure 10.4   Modified sit-and-reach test: (a) starting position and (b) ending position.

Table 10.4   Percentile Ranks for the Modified Sit-and-Reach Test*

Percentile rank	Women			Men		
	≤35 yr	36-49 yr	≥50 yr	≤35 yr	36-49 yr	≥50 yr
99	19.8	19.8	17.2	24.7	18.9	16.2
95	18.7	19.2	15.7	19.5	18.2	15.8
90	17.9	17.4	15.0	17.9	16.1	15.0
80	16.7	16.2	14.2	17.0	14.6	13.3
70	16.2	15.2	13.6	15.8	13.9	12.3
60	15.8	14.5	12.3	15.0	13.4	11.5
50	14.8	13.5	11.1	14.4	12.6	10.2
40	14.5	12.8	10.1	13.5	11.6	9.7
30	13.7	12.2	9.2	13.0	10.8	9.3
20	12.6	11.0	8.3	11.6	9.9	8.8
10	10.1	9.7	7.5	9.2	8.3	7.8
05	8.1	8.5	3.7	7.9	7.0	7.2
01	2.6	2.0	1.5	7.0	5.1	4.0

*Sit-and-reach scores measured to nearest 0.25 inch

©Morton Publishing Company, *Lifetime Physical Fitness & Wellness* (1989) by Werner W.K. Hoeger.

women (r = 0.66) and men (r = 0.75) and poorly related to low back flexibility of women (r = 0.25) and men (r = 0.40). It appears that neither the standard nor modified sit-and-reach tests is very good for assessing low back flexibility.

Skin Distraction Test

The modified Schober test (Mcrae and Wright 1969) and the simplified skin distraction test (VanAdrichem and van der Korst 1973) are useful in assessing low back flexibility. These field tests are reliable and have good agreement with radiographic measurements of spinal flexion and extension (Williams et al. 1993). For the simplified skin distraction test, place a 0-cm mark on the midline of the lumbar spine at the intersection of a horizontal line connecting the left and right posterior superior iliac spines while the client is standing erect. Place a second mark 15 cm (5.9 in) superior to the 0-cm mark (see figure 10.5). As the client flexes the lumbar spine, these marks move away from each other; use an anthropometric tape measure to measure the new distance between the two marks. The lumbar flexion score is the difference between this measurement and the initial length between the skin markings (15 cm). In a group of 15- to 18-year-old subjects, the simplified skin distraction scores averaged 6.7 ± 1.0 cm in males and 5.8 ± 0.9 cm in females. Normal values for other

age groups are not yet available. You also can use this technique to measure lumbar spinal extension (simplified skin attraction test) by having the client extend backward and measuring the difference between the initial length and the new distance between the superior and inferior skin markings.

DESIGNING FLEXIBILITY PROGRAMS

After assessing your client's flexibility, you must identify those joints and muscle groups which are in need of improvement and select an appropriate exercise mode and specific exercises for the flexibility program. The specificity and progressive overload principles apply to the design of flexibility programs. Flexibility is highly joint-specific (Cotten 1972; Harris 1969; Munroe and Romance 1975); therefore, to increase flexibility of a particular joint, select exercises that stretch the appropriate muscle groups. To improve ROM at the joint, your client must overload the muscle group by stretching the muscles beyond their normal resting length—but never beyond the pain-free range of motion. Periodically your client will need to increase both the amount of time the stretched position is maintained and the number of repetitions of the exercise to

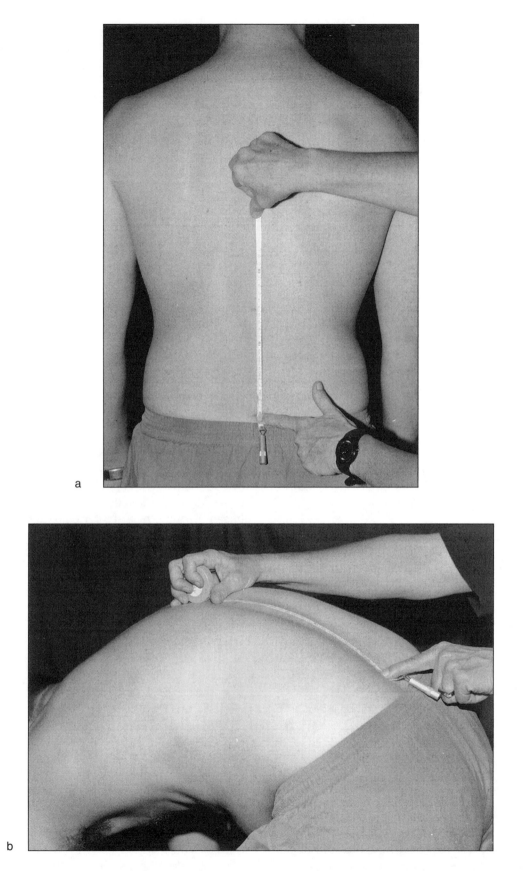

Figure 10.5   Measuring lumbosacral flexion using the simplified skin distraction test: (*a*) starting position and (*b*) ending position.

ensure the overload required for further improvement. The following questions address issues and concerns that you should consider when designing flexibility programs.

Modes of Stretching

Three types of stretching techniques are ballistic stretching, slow and static stretching, and proprioceptive neuromuscular facilitation (PNF) stretching. Table 10.5 summarizes the advantages and disadvantages of these stretching techniques.

What Mode of Stretching Is Best for Improving Flexibility?

All three types of stretching are effective in increasing the ROM (deVries 1962; Hartley-O'Brien 1980, Holt, Travis, and Okita 1970; Worrell, Smith, and Winegardner 1994). However, Wallin et al. (1985) reported significantly better improvement in the flexibility of the plantar flexors and hip adductors and extensors for subjects who trained using the PNF (11 to 25% increase) technique compared to ballistic stretching (3 to 7% increase).

What Is Proprioceptive Neuromuscular Facilitation (PNF), and How Is This Technique Used to Improve Flexibility?

PNF stretching increases ROM by inducing muscle relaxation through spinal reflex mechanisms. Using the *contract-relax technique*, your client first performs an isometric contraction of the muscle group being stretched, and then proceeds with the slow, static stretching (relaxation phase) of the muscle group. This technique is based on the concept of reciprocal inhibition. Theoretically, the isometric

contraction of the antagonists (muscle group being stretched) induces a reflex facilitation and contraction of the agonist, which suppresses the contractile activity in the antagonist during the slow, static stretching phase. The isometric contraction of the antagonists also stimulates the Golgi tendon organs, resulting in a reflex relaxation of the same muscle group. However, the isometric contraction may promote a lingering discharge in the same muscle which contributes to increased contractile activity in the muscle group during the relaxation (static stretching) phase of the contract-relax procedure (Moore and Hutton 1980).

Another type of PNF stretching is the *contract-relax with agonist contraction (CRAC) technique.* This method is identical to the contract-relax technique except that the stretching is assisted by a submaximal contraction of the opposing (agonist) muscle group. Theoretically, the voluntary contraction of the agonists induces additional inhibitory input to the antagonists (muscles being stretched) through reciprocal inhibition (Moore and Hutton 1980). The neuromuscular mechanisms underlying muscle stretch are extremely complicated and not fully understood. Simple explanations concerning the role of reciprocal inhibition during muscle stretch are inadequate. For example, recurrent collateral pathways from motoneurons of agonists have been shown to inhibit interneurons which normally reduce the excitation of alpha motoneurons of the antagonists during reciprocal inhibition. This results in an inhibition of inhibitory input to the antagonistic muscle groups (Hultborn, Illert, and Santini 1974).

How Are PNF Stretches Performed?

The following steps are recommended when using PNF stretching techniques to increase static flexibility:

Table 10.5 Comparison of Stretching Techniques			
Factor	Ballistic	Slow static	PNF[a]
Risk of injury	High	Low	Medium
Degree of pain	Medium	Low	High
Resistance to stretch	High	Low	Medium
Practicality (time and assistance needed)	Good	Excellent	Poor
Efficiency (energy consumption)	Poor	Excellent	Poor
Effective for increasing ROM[b]	Good	Good	Good

[a]Proprioceptive neuromuscular facilitation
[b]Range of motion

- Stretch the target muscle group by moving the joint to the end of its ROM.

- Isometrically contract the prestretched muscle group against an immovable resistance (such as a partner or wall) for 5 to 6 seconds.

- Relax the contracted muscle group as you or your partner statically stretch the muscle to a new point of limitation. With the contract-relax agonist contract technique, the opposing muscle group (agonist) contracts submaximally for 5 to 6 seconds to facilitate relaxation and further stretching of the target muscle group.

For example, to stretch the pectoral muscles, the individual assumes a sitting position on the floor with the arms horizontally extended. The pectoral muscles are isometrically contracted as the partner offers resistance to horizontal flexion. Following the isometric contraction, the partner applies a slow, static stretch as the horizontal extensors in the upper back are contracted submaximally.

Why Is Slow, Static Stretching Safer Than Ballistic Stretching?

Many exercise specialists recommend using slow, static stretching rather than ballistic stretching because there is less chance of injury and muscle soreness resulting from jerky, rapid movements. The ballistic technique uses a relatively fast, bouncing motion to produce stretch. The momentum of the moving body segment, rather than external force, pushes the joint beyond its present ROM. This technique appears to be counterproductive for increasing muscle stretch. Muscle spindles signal both changes in muscle length and speed of contraction. The spindle responds more to the speed of movement than to the muscle's length or position. In fact, muscle spindle activity is directly proportional to the speed of movement. Thus, ballistic or dynamic stretching evokes the stretch reflex, producing more contraction and resistance to stretch in the muscle group being stretched. This places strain on the muscle-tendon unit and may cause microscopic tearing of muscle fibers and connective tissue.

In slow, static stretching, your client stretches the muscle with the joint positioned at the end of its ROM. While maintaining this position, the client slowly applies torque to the muscle to stretch it further. Because the dynamic portion of the muscle spindle rapidly adapts to the lengthened position, the spindle discharge is decreased. This lessens reflex contraction of the muscle and allows the muscle to relax (viscoelastic stress relaxation) and to be stretched even further.

Is PNF Stretching Better Than Slow, Static Stretching?

Moore and Hutton (1980) compared the relative level of muscle relaxation achieved during static stretching and PNF stretching procedures. They noted that the CRAC method produced larger gains in hip flexion than either the contract-relax or static stretching methods. However, this technique produced greater electromyographic (EMG) activity in the hamstring muscle group and was ranked as the most uncomfortable in terms of perceived pain ratings. It also has been reported that the CRAC technique is more effective for improving ROM than the contract-relax technique (Alter 1996)).

A major disadvantage of the PNF technique is that the exercises, in some cases, cannot be performed alone. A partner is needed to resist movement during the isometric contraction phase and to apply external force to the muscle during the stretching phase. Thus, the amount of time required for both individuals to complete the flexibility exercises is increased.

The Exercise Prescription for Flexibility

When designing flexibility programs for your clients, follow the guidelines on the opposite page and be sure to address the following questions regarding various aspects of their exercise prescriptions.

How Many Exercises Should Be Included in a Flexibility Program?

A well-rounded program includes at least one exercise for each of the major muscle groups of the body. It is important to select exercises for problem areas such as the lower back, hips, and posterior thighs and legs. Use the results of the flexibility tests to identify specific muscle groups with relatively poor flexibility, and include more than one exercise for these muscle groups. The workout should take 15 to 30 minutes depending on the number of exercises to be performed. Appendix F.1 illustrates flexibility exercises for various regions of the body. For additional flexibility exercises see Anderson (1980) and Alter (1996).

Are Some Stretching Exercises Safer Than Others?

Some stretching exercises are not recommended for flexibility programs because they create excessive stress, thereby increasing your client's chance of musculoskeletal injuries—especially to the knee joints and low back regions. Appendix F.2 illustrates exercises that are contraindicated for flexibility programs and suggests alternative exercises you can prescribe to increase the flexibility of specific muscle groups.

What Is a Safe Intensity for Stretching Exercises?

The intensity of slow, static stretching and PNF stretching exercises should always be below the pain threshold of the individual. Some mild discomfort will occur, especially during the PNF exercises when the target muscle is contracted isometrically. However, the joint should not be stretched beyond its pain-free range of motion (ACSM 1995).

How Long Does Each Stretch Need to Be Held?

To date there is a limited amount of research concerning the optimal time that a static stretch should be sustained to improve ROM. In the past, some experts have suggested varying lengths of static stretch, ranging from 10 to 60 seconds (Beaulieu 1980). The ACSM (1995) recommends holding the stretched position only as long as it feels comfortable (usually 10 to 30 seconds).

Borms et al. (1987) compared the effects of 10, 20, and 30 seconds of static stretching on hip flexibility of women engaging in a 10-week (two sessions a week) static flexibility training program. They reported similar improvements in hip flexibility for all three groups, suggesting that a duration of 10 seconds of static stretching was sufficient for improving hip flexibility.

Another study compared the effect of three static stretching durations (15, 30, and 60 seconds) on the hip flexibility of men and women with "tight" hamstring muscles (Bandy and Irion 1994). The subjects participated in a 6-week static flexibility training program, stretching 5 times a week. The authors noted that 30 and 60 seconds of static stretching were more effective than stretching 15 seconds for increasing hip flexibility. They observed no significant difference between stretching for 30 seconds and for 60 seconds.

In light of these findings, it is recommended that the stretch be sustained at least 10 seconds during the initial stages of the static stretching program. As flexibility improves, the muscle group may be progressively overloaded by increasing the time that the stretched position is held, up to a maximum of 30 seconds for each repetition.

How Many Repetitions of Each Exercise Should Be Performed?

Beginners should start with 3 repetitions of each exercise. As flexibility improves, they may gradually increase the number of repetitions of each exercise to 5 in order to progressively overload the muscle group.

How Often Should Flexibility Exercises Be Performed?

Flexibility exercises should be performed at least 3 days a week but preferably daily (ACSM 1995). Flexibility exercises are an integral part of the warm-up and cool-down segments of aerobic exercise and resistance training workouts.

GUIDELINES FOR DESIGNING FLEXIBILITY PROGRAMS

Mode: Static or PNF stretching

Number of exercises: 10 to 12

Frequency: At least 3 days a week, preferably daily

Intensity: No stretching of a joint beyond its pain-free ROM

Time of stretch: 10 to 30 seconds

Repetitions: 3 to 5

Duration: 15 to 30 minutes per session

Instruct your clients engaging in stretching programs to adhere to the following guidelines (Kravitz and Heyward 1995):

CLIENT GUIDELINES FOR STRETCHING PROGRAMS

- Warm up before stretching to increase body temperature and ROM.

- Stretch all major muscle groups, as well as opposing muscle groups.

- Focus on the target muscles involved in the stretch, relax the target muscle, and minimize the movement of other body parts.

- Hold the stretch for 10 to 30 seconds.

- Stretch to the limit (endpoint) of the movement, not to the point of pain.

- Keep breathing slowly and rhythmically while holding the stretch.

- Stretch the target muscle groups in different planes to improve overall ROM at the joint.

DESIGNING LOW BACK CARE EXERCISE PROGRAMS

Low back pain frequently causes activity restrictions for middle-aged and older adults, disabling 3 to 4 million people each year. Improper alignment of the spinal column causes approximately 80% of all low back problems. A combination of stretching and strengthening exercises is often prescribed to correct this problem. Many people can achieve proper support and alignment of the pelvis and spinal column by using ROM exercises to prevent overtightness of the hip flexors, hamstrings, and low back extensors, and by doing strengthening exercises for the abdominal and low back muscles.

The following exercises are recommended for low back care. These exercises are described and illustrated in appendix F.1 and F.3.

- Pelvic tilt (supine-lying position) to stretch the abdominal muscles

- Knee-to-chest (supine-lying position) to stretch the hamstrings, buttock and low back muscles

- Trunk flex (on hands and knees) to stretch the back, abdominal, and hamstring muscles

- Curl-ups to strengthen the abdominal muscles

- Single leg extension (prone-lying position) to strengthen the hamstring and buttock muscles and to stretch the hip flexor muscles

- Controlled trunk extensions to strengthen the back extensors (do not hyperextend; instead, limit extension to the client's normal standing lumbar curvature)

HEALTHY BACK PRACTICES

Show your clients how they can prevent low back problems by using the following practices around the home and workplace (Sharkey 1990):

- Use the buttocks and leg muscles, instead of the low back muscles, when lifting heavy objects.

- Sleep on your side with the knees flexed and avoid sleeping on your back or stomach.

- Sit with your legs crossed or use a foot rest to keep one or both knees above your hips.

- While driving, keep the knees flexed and support the middle of the lower back.

- Stand with one foot on a stool when working at a counter for long periods of time.

- Avoid all activities that require hyperextension of the lower back.

Key Points

- Static flexibility is a measure of the total ROM at the joint.

- Dynamic flexibility is a measure of the torque or resistance to movement.

- Flexibility is highly joint-specific, and the ROM depends, in part, on the structure of the joint.

- Lack of physical activity is a major cause of inflexibility.

- A universal goniometer, flexometer, or inclinometer can be used to obtain direct measures of ROM.

- A yardstick and anthropometric tape measure can be used to obtain indirect measures of ROM.

- The principles of specificity and progressive overload must be applied to the design of flexibility exercise programs.

- Static, ballistic, and PNF stretching techniques are equally effective in increasing ROM. Ballistic stretching, however, increases the risk of injury and muscle soreness.

- A well-rounded flexibility program includes at least one exercise for each major muscle group of the body.

- The muscle group can be overloaded by progressively increasing the length of time that the stretched position is held (10 to 30 seconds) and the number of repetitions (3 to 5 repetitions) performed.

- Flexibility exercises should be performed at least 3 days a week, but preferably daily.

- Lack of flexibility is a major cause of low back problems.

- A combination of stretching and strengthening exercises for the abdominal and low back muscles is effective for preventing low back problems.

SOURCES FOR EQUIPMENT

Product	Manufacturer's Address
Flexometer	Country Technology Inc.
Inclinometer	P.O. Box 87
Sit-and-reach box	Gays Mills, WI 54631
Universal goniometer	Phone: (608) 735-4718

REFERENCES

Ahlback, S.O., and Lindahl, O. 1964. Sagittal mobility of the hip-joint. *Acta Orthopaedica Scandinavica* 34: 310-313.

Alter, M. J. 1996. *Science of flexibility and stretching.* Champaign, IL: Human Kinetics.

American College of Sports Medicine. 1995. *ACSM's guidelines for exercise testing and prescription.* Baltimore: Williams & Wilkins.

American Medical Association. 1988. *Guides to the evaluation of permanent impairment*, 3rd ed. Chicago, IL: Author.

Anderson, R. 1980. *Stretching.* Fullerton, CA: Shelter.

Bandy, W.D., and Irion, J.M. 1994. The effect of time on static stretch on the flexibility of the hamstring muscles. *Physical Therapy* 74: 845-851.

Beaulieu, J.E. 1980. *Stretching for all sports.* Pasadena, CA: Athletic Press.

Borms, J., Van Roy, P., Santens, J.P., and Haentjens, A. 1987. Optimal duration of static stretching exercises for improvement of coxo-femoral flexibility. *Journal of Sports Science* 5: 39-47.

Chapman, E.A., deVries, H.A., and Swezey, R. 1972. Joint stiffness: Effects of exercise on young and old men. *Journal of Gerontology* 27: 218-221.

Cotten, D.J. 1972. A comparison of selected trunk flexibility tests. *American Corrective Therapy Journal* 26: 24.

deVries, H.A. 1962. Evaluation of static stretching procedures for improvement of flexibility. *Research Quarterly* 33: 222-229.

Dickinson, R.V. 1968. The specificity of flexibility. *Research Quarterly* 39: 792-793.

Enwemeka, C.S. 1986. Radiographic verification of knee goniometry. *Scandinavian Journal of Rehabilitation Medicine* 18: 47-49.

Girouard, C.K., and Hurley, B.F. 1995. Does strength training inhibit gains in range of motion from flexibility training in older adults? *Medicine and Science in Sports and Exercise* 27: 1444-1449.

Greene, W.B., and Heckman, J.D. 1994. *The clinical measurement of joint motion.* Rosemont, IL: American Academy of Orthopaedic Surgeons.

Harris, M.L. 1969. A factor analytic study of flexibility. *Research Quarterly* 40: 62-70.

Hartley-O'Brien, S.J. 1980. Six mobilization exercises for active range of hip flexion. *Research Quarterly for Exercise and Sport* 51: 625-635.

Hoeger, W.W.K. 1989. *Lifetime physical fitness and wellness.* Englewood Cliffs, NJ: Morton.

Hoeger, W.W.K., and Hopkins, D.R. 1992. A comparison of the sit and reach and the modified sit and reach in the measurement of flexibility in women. *Research Quarterly for Exercise and Sport* 63: 191-195.

Hoeger, W.W.K., Hopkins, D.R., Button, S., and Palmer, T.A. 1990. Comparing the sit and reach with the modified sit and reach in measuring flexibility in adolescents. *Pediatric Exercise Science* 2: 156-162.

Holt, L.E., Travis, T.M., and Okita, T. 1970. Comparative study of three stretching techniques. *Perceptual and Motor Skills* 31: 611-616.

Hubley-Kozey, C.L. 1991. Testing flexibility. In J.D. MacDougall, H.A. Wenger, and H.J. Green, eds., *Physiological testing of the high-performance athlete*, 309-359. Champaign, IL: Human Kinetics.

Hultborn, H., Illert, M., and Santini, M. 1974. Disynaptic inhibition of the interneurons mediating the reciprocal Ia inhibition of motor neurones. *Acta Physiologica Scandinavica* 91: 14A-16A.

Jackson, A.W. and Baker, A.A. 1986. The relationship of the sit and reach test to criterion measures of hamstring and back flexibility in young females. *Research Quarterly for Exercise and Sport* 57: 183-186.

Jackson, A.W., and Lanford, N.J. 1989. The criterion-related validity of the sit-and-reach test: Replication and extension of previous findings. *Research Quarterly for Exercise and Sport* 60: 384-387.

Johns, R.J., and Wright, V. 1962. Relative importance of various tissues in joint stiffness. *Journal of Applied Physiology* 17: 824-828.

Kirby, R.L., Simms, F.C., Symington, V.J., and Garner, J.B. 1981. Flexibility and musculoskeletal symptomatology in female gymnasts and age-matched controls. *American Journal of Sports Medicine* 9: 160-164.

Kravitz, L., and Heyward, V.H. 1995. Flexibility training. *Fitness Management* 11(2): 32-38.

Leighton, J.R. 1955. An instrument and technique for measurement of range of joint motion. *Archives of Physical Medicine and Rehabilitation* 36: 571-578.

Mayer, T.G., Tencer, A.F., and Kristoferson, S. 1984. Use of noninvasive technique for quantification of spinal range-of-motion in normal subjects and chronic low back dysfunction patients. *Spine* 9: 588-595.

McCue, B.F. 1953. Flexibility of college women. *Research Quarterly* 24: 316-324.

McHugh, M.P., Magnusson, S.P., Gleim, G.W., and Nicholas, J.A. 1992. Viscoelastic stress relaxation in human skeletal muscle. *Medicine and Science in Sports and Exercise* 24: 1375-1382.

Mcrae, I.F., and Wright, V. 1969. Measurement of back movement. *Annals of Rheumatic Diseases* 28: 584-589.

Minkler, S., and Patterson, P. 1994. The validity of the modified sit-and-reach test in college-age students. *Research Quarterly for Exercise and Sport* 65: 189-192.

Moore, M.A., and Hutton, R.S. 1980. Electromyographic investigation of muscle stretching techniques. *Medicine and Science in Sports and Exercise* 12: 322-329.

Munroe, R.A., and Romance, T.J. 1975. Use of the Leighton flexometer in the development of a short flexibility test battery. *American Corrective Therapy Journal* 29: 22.

Norkin, C.C., and White, D.J. 1995. *Measurement of joint motion: A guide to goniometry.* Philadelphia: F.A. Davis.

Sell, K.E., Verity, T.M., Worrell, T.W., Pease, B.J., and Wigglesworth, J. 1994. Two measurement techniques for assessing subtalar joint position: A reliability study. *Journal of Orthopaedic and Sports Physical Therapy* 19: 162-167.

Sharkey, B.J. 1990. *Physiology of fitness,* 3rd ed. Champaign, IL: Human Kinetics.

Van Adrichem, J.A.M., and van der Krost, J.K. 1973. Assessment of flexibility of the lumbar spine: A pilot study in children and adolescents. *Scandinavian Journal of Rheumatology* 2: 87-91.

Wallin, D., Ekblom, B., Grahn, R., and Nordenborg, T. 1985. Improvement of muscle flexibility. A comparison between two techniques. *American Journal of Sports Medicine* 13: 263-268.

Wear, C.L. 1963. The relationship of flexibility measurements to length of body segments. *Research Quarterly* 34: 234-238.

Williams, R., Binkley, J., Bloch, R., Goldsmith, C.H., and Minuk, T. 1993. Reliability of the modified-modified Schober and double inclinometer methods for measuring lumbar flexion and extension. *Physical Therapy* 73: 26-37.

Worrell, T.W., Smith, T.L., and Winegardner, J. 1994. Effect of hamstring stretching on hamstring muscle performance. *Journal of Orthopaedic and Sports Physical Therapy* 20: 154-159.

Wright, V., and Johns, R.J. 1960. Physical factors concerned with the stiffness of normal and diseased joints. *Bulletin of Johns Hopkins Hospital* 106: 215-231.

CHAPTER 11

Assessing and Managing Stress

Key Questions

- What causes stress?
- How does the body respond and adapt to acute and chronic stress?
- What are the signs and symptoms of excessive stress?
- How is stress measured?
- What techniques may be used to effectively manage stress?
- What is the role of exercise in stress management?

Stress evokes a generalized physiological response of the body to physical, psychological, or environmental demands. Throughout life everyone encounters both good and bad changes which produce stress. For example, the death of a family member, the loss of a job, the birth of a child, and changes in one's eating or exercise habits are all potentially stressful events. People differ, however, in what they perceive as stressful and how they cope with stress-producing situations. It is important for each person to find ways to manage stress effectively, because constant stress or overstress may lead to disease or illness (Selye 1956).

This chapter discusses the body's response to stress and the role of exercise in alleviating stress. It also discusses techniques for assessing stress and neuromuscular tension, and methods of relaxation for relieving tension.

PHYSIOLOGICAL RESPONSE TO STRESS

Stressors may be physiological or psychological. Activities such as weightlifting, jogging, and swimming, as well as changes in temperature or altitude, are examples of physiological stressors. Psychological stressors include such life-event changes as a new job, family illness, or final examinations.

The body does not differentiate between physiological and psychological stressors. Instead, the immediate response of the body to stress is generalized, preparing the body to fight or flee from potentially threatening situations. The fight-or-flight response is characterized by increases in heart rate, breathing rate, body temperature, blood flow to muscles, sweating, oxygen utilization, and muscle tension.

These changes are mediated through the activation of the sympathetic nervous system and the adrenal glands. The glucocorticoids from the adrenal cortex promote fat utilization, protein catabolism, and carbohydrate conservation. The elevated blood glucose level supplies energy to the brain and nervous tissue and may increase the body's ability to resist stress (Lamb 1978). In addition, the glucocorticoids enhance the effect of the adrenal medulla hormones—norepinephrine and epinephrine (Sharkey 1990). These catecholamines produce physiological changes similar to those associated with neurotransmitters of the sympathetic nervous system.

Selye (1956) hypothesized three stages that describe the body's reaction to stress. In the first stage, known as the *alarm reaction*, the body perceives the stress and the fight-or-flight response is activated. In the second stage, *resistance and adaptation*, the body continues to resist and adapt to the stressor. If the stress is too intense or prolonged, the body may lose its ability to resist the stressor and enter the third, or *exhaustive*, stage, which is characterized by illness or even death in some cases.

STRESS AND DISEASE

Excessive stress from any source may lead to sickness or disease. Insomnia, diarrhea, loss of appetite, muscular tension, and headaches are physical symptoms of stress. Colitis, ulcers, hypertension, stroke, and coronary artery disease are also associated with excessive stress. Some of the psychological effects of excessive stress are anxiety, depression, decreased concentration, irritability, poor memory, and anger. In the workplace, signs of excessive stress are increased absenteeism, tardiness, accidents, and turnover, as well as poor communication among employees and decreased productivity.

Researchers are investigating the links among psychological stress, behavior profiles, and disease risk. Friedman and Rosenman (1974) identified behavior profiles that represent two extremes on a continuum. *Type A behavior* is characterized by an extreme need to achieve, competitiveness, impatience, overcommitment to work, explosive speech patterns, and aggressiveness. At the other extreme, the *Type B behavior* profile is characterized by a relaxed and easy-going nature. The Type A behavior pattern is positively associated with stress in black and white women (Adams-Campbell, Washburn, and Haile 1990) and with increased risk of coronary heart disease (CHD) in middle-class, white, American men. Researchers are investigating whether changing behavior patterns can reduce stress, the risk of CHD, and the recurrence of myocardial infarctions.

ASSESSMENT OF STRESS AND NEUROMUSCULAR TENSION

You can use data from questionnaires to assess the stress level and behavior characteristics of your clients. Computer software is available that generates a stress profile to help identify sources of stress for each individual. You also can use electromyography or manual tension tests to evaluate neuromuscular tension due to stress.

Stress

Questionnaires have been developed for self-assessment of stress (Orioli, Jaffe, and Scott 1987) and identification of overt characteristics associated with Type A behavior patterns (Jenkins, Rosenman, and Zyzanski 1974). The *StressMap Questionnaire* (Orioli et al. 1987) uses 21 scales divided into four parts to assess the following:

- environmental pressures,
- coping responses,
- inner thoughts and feelings, and
- signals of distress.

This comprehensive questionnaire provides a valid and reliable (r's ranging from 0.72 to 0.93) assessment of stress.

The *Jenkins Activity Survey* (JAS) (Jenkins et al. 1974) consists of 52 multiple choice questions and provides a Type A behavior standard score as well as three factor scores:

- speed and impatience,
- job involvement, and
- hard-driving behavior and competitiveness.

Various forms of the JAS have been validated for different groups, including employed men and women, housewives, college students, and retired persons. There are also many computerized health risk appraisals (HRA) you can use to evaluate the stress profiles of your clients.

Appendix G.1 includes an inventory to assess your client's sources of stress and coping strategies. Tests

1 through 3 measure vulnerability to stress due to frustration or inhibition, overload, and overly aggressive behavioral traits. Test 4 identifies the strategies used to cope with common sources of stress.

Neuromuscular Tension

Neuromuscular tension is associated with acute and chronic stress. The degree of tension in skeletal muscles increases as part of the fight-or-flight response to stress. Chronic or prolonged stress also may increase neuromuscular tension levels.

Electromyography (EMG) is the most valid method for measuring muscle activity at rest. There is a direct relationship between the frequency and amplitude of EMG signals and the degree of tension in the resting muscle. EMG equipment is relatively expensive, and the technique is time-consuming. Thus, for large groups, you should use alternative field techniques to evaluate muscular tension.

One such technique is the *Rathbone Manual Tension test* (Rathbone and Hunt 1965). This test assesses the muscular tension during passive movement of the wrist, elbow, shoulder, neck, hip, and knee joints (see appendix G.2). The validity of this test was established using EMG as the criterion for 11 muscle groups (r = 0.97). The test evaluates four manifestations of muscular tension:

1. Assistance—Client aids the tester in moving the body segment.

2. Resistance—Client resists the movement of the body segment.

3. Posturing—Client maintains the new position after the limb is released by the tester.

4. Perseveration—Client continues to move or repeats the movement of the body segment after it is released by the tester.

For each movement, you assign a numerical value which corresponds to the degree of tension observed in the limb:

0 = none

1 = slight

2 = moderate

3 = marked tension

In addition to manual symptoms, you can use visual signs to detect the presence of neuromuscular tension. Visual symptoms include frowning, twitching, fluttering eyelids, rapid breathing, tightness of the mouth, and repeated swallowing.

EXERCISE AND STRESS

Exercise is a physiological stressor which evokes an acute stress response, such as increased heart rate, blood pressure, breathing rate, blood flow to muscles, oxygen consumption, and metabolic rate. Intense and prolonged exercise (usually >30 minutes) increases the plasma levels of cortisol (Hartley et al. 1972; Shephard and Sidney 1975; Tharp 1975), epinephrine, and norepinephrine (Hartley et al. 1972; VonEuler 1974). It appears that a minimum exercise intensity of 60% $\dot{V}O_2$max is needed to produce these hormonal responses (Davies and Few 1973; Hartley 1975; VonEuler 1974).

The response patterns of corticosteroids and norepinephrine to exercise are partly dependent on the fitness status of the individual and may be modified by physical conditioning (Hartley et al. 1972; Hartley 1975; White, Ismail, and Bottoms 1976). The lower plasma corticosteroid and norepinephrine levels at a given submaximal work load in endurance-trained individuals suggest that they are better able to tolerate the physiological stress of exercise than are sedentary individuals.

Exercise also plays an important role in the management of psychological stress. Mental and emotional stress may lead to states of anxiety and depression. Vigorous exercise reduces state anxiety in both highly anxious and normally anxious men and women (Morgan 1973). Similarly, regular aerobic exercise appears to reduce symptoms of moderate depression (Falls, Baylor, and Dishman 1980) and to enhance psychological fitness. Highly trained, world-class athletes tend to be less anxious, depressed, and confused than the average person (Morgan 1979). Participation in exercise programs may improve mood states by reducing state anxiety and enhancing one's sense of vigor (Jin 1992). Many people who participate in a regular program of exercise report that they feel better after exercising (Falls et al. 1980). Thus, exercise appears to be an effective technique for reducing stress, coping with stress, and regulating mood behaviors (Anthony 1991; Severtsen and Bruya 1986; Thayer, Newman, and McClain 1994).

The underlying psychophysiological mechanisms, however, are not fully understood. Some factors that may explain, in part, the effectiveness of exercise for reducing psychological stress are the following:

• Exercise is a diversion which enables the person to relax due to a change in environment or routine.

- Exercise serves as an outlet to dissipate emotions such as anger, fear, and frustration.
- Exercise enhances one's self-concept and increases confidence in one's ability to deal with stress-producing situations.
- Exercise produces biochemical changes which alter psychological states. For example, a low level of norepinephrine is associated with depression. During exercise, plasma levels of norepinephrine increase, which may help to alleviate symptoms of depression (Falls et al. 1980). Exercise also may increase the levels of endorphins in the brain. These morphine-like substances have a narcotic effect which induce feelings of pleasure and wellness, such as the "runner's high" (Sharkey 1990).

RELAXATION TECHNIQUES

A number of relaxation techniques can relieve muscular tension and stress. The goal of these techniques is to elicit a relaxation response characterized by decreases in EMG activity, heart rate, blood pressure, breathing rate, and oxygen consumption. You can use physical, mental, or a combination of approaches to achieve the relaxation response.

Physical Approach

Aerobic exercise and the progressive relaxation technique (Jacobson 1978) are two methods that produce relaxation through the physical mode. Regular, aerobic exercise is effective for reducing psychological stress and increasing the body's resistance to many types of stressors. For tense individuals, low-intensity (30 to 60% maximum heart rate) rhythmic exercise, such as jogging, cycling, and walking, performed 5 to 30 minutes per day, lowers muscular tension levels at rest (deVries 1975). Participation in an aerobic exercise program enables one to reduce stress and tension while enjoying the cardiorespiratory, body composition, and weight control benefits of the exercise. Because of these multiple benefits, aerobic exercise is a highly recommended relaxation technique.

In the *progressive relaxation technique,* the client learns to identify muscular tension in the major muscle groups and to relax these muscles consciously. According to Jacobson (1978), progressive relaxation refers to the individual's ability to

- relax major muscle groups one after the other,
- relax each muscle group further and further, and
- progress toward a habit of effortless relaxation.

The relaxation response is developed by deliberately contracting and then relaxing ("letting it go") each muscle group, starting with the muscles of the feet and ending with the facial muscles. Daily practice of this technique is recommended to achieve effortless relaxation. For detailed information about the progressive relaxation technique, see Jacobson (1978).

Mental Approach

Meditation, imagery, biofeedback, and autogenic relaxation training use a mind-over-matter approach to relaxation (Curtis et al. 1985). Meditation produces a hypometabolic state in which oxygen consumption is reduced by 10 to 20% and heart rate is decreased 3 beats per minute on the average (Benson 1975). There is also an increase in alpha brain wave activity, which is indicative of a relaxed state. With this technique, relaxation is achieved through the continued repetition of a word or phrase known as a mantra.

The *Benson technique* (Benson 1975) also uses meditation to promote relaxation. Bahrke and Morgan (1978) noted that the Benson relaxation technique and aerobic exercise were equally effective in reducing state anxiety. The basic elements of this technique are

- quiet environment,
- comfortable position,
- repetition of a word or phrase, and
- passive, let-it-happen attitude.

Imagery is a form of autosuggestion or self-hypnosis that uses visual images to produce a relaxed state. Floating or sinking images are visualized and allow the individual temporary relief from tension, worry, and anxiety. A number of excellent sources deal with visualization to induce relaxation (Bry 1979; Curtis et al. 1985).

In *biofeedback,* the individual uses visual and auditory signals to control unconscious bodily functions such as blood pressure, body temperature, heart rate, and muscular tension. This technique can effectively reduce neuromuscular tension and promote relaxation. Detailed descriptions explaining how to use various methods of biofeedback training for relaxation are provided elsewhere (Basmajian 1983; Brown 1981; Curtis et al. 1985; Danskin and Crow 1981).

Autogenic relaxation training consists of a series of six mental exercises that are practiced several times daily to elicit the relaxation response (Benson 1975). Lying in a quiet room with the eyes closed, the client focuses on the following:

- sensation of heaviness in the limbs,
- sensation of warmth in the limbs,
- breathing,
- regulation of heart rate,
- feelings of coolness in the forehead, and
- passive, let-it-happen attitude.

Combination Approach

Some experts recommend a combination of aerobic exercise and meditation to reduce stress. Jin (1992) reported that the stress-reduction effect of Tai Chi was similar to that produced by moderate, brisk walking. Severtsen and Bruya (1986) noted that the combination of daily meditation and aerobic exercise increased ability to cope with stress. Likewise, Thayer, Newman, and McClain (1994) recommended a combination of relaxation, stress management, cognitive, and exercise techniques to self-regulate bad moods, to increase energy levels and vigor, and to reduce tension.

Hatha Yoga is a combination of physical and mental exercise that is sometimes used to achieve a state of total relaxation. Stretching exercises, poses, and breathing exercises are performed to relieve muscular tension. Mental relaxation is produced through concentration and autosuggestion techniques (Barney and Frauenglass 1980).

Key Points

- Stress is a state that evokes a generalized physiological response of the body to physical, psychological, or environmental demands.
- The immediate, generalized response of the body to physiological and psychological stressors is known as the fight-or-flight response.
- The physiological changes associated with the fight-or-flight response are mediated through the sympathetic nervous system and adrenal glands.
- The three stages of stress are alarm reaction, resistance, and exhaustion.
- Excessive stress may lead to illness, disease, or death.
- Type A behavior is associated with high levels of stress and an increased risk of coronary heart disease.
- The Jenkins Activity Survey may be used to assess Type A behavior patterns.
- Neuromuscular tension is associated with acute and chronic stress.
- Electromyography is a valid method of assessing tension levels in skeletal muscles.
- The Rathbone Manual Tension Test evaluates muscular tension during passive movements of body segments.
- Exercise is a physiological stressor that evokes an acute stress response.
- The hormonal response to exercise stress depends on the fitness status of the individual and may be modified by physical training.
- Exercise produces biochemical changes that may alter psychological states of anxiety and depression.
- Relaxation may be induced through physical and mental exercise.
- Aerobic exercise, progressive relaxation, meditation, imagery, biofeedback, autogenic relaxation training, Tai Chi, and yoga are effective relaxation techniques.

REFERENCES

Adams-Campbell, L.L., Washburn, R.A., and Haile, G.T. 1990. Physical activity, stress, and type A behavior in blacks. *Journal of the National Medical Association* 82: 701-705.

Anthony, J. 1991. Psychologic aspects of exercise. *Clinics in Sports Medicine* 10: 171-180.

Bahrke, M.S., and Morgan, W.P. 1978. Influence of acute physical activity and non-cultic meditation on state anxiety. *Cognitive Therapy and Research* 2: 323.

Barney, K., and Frauenglass, D. 1980. Introductory yoga. In W.L. DeGroot, ed., *Fitness and movement*, 137-167. Winston-Salem, NC: Hunter Publishing.

Basmajian, J. (Ed.) 1983. *Biofeedback: Principles and practice for clinicians*. Baltimore: Williams & Wilkins.

Benson, H. 1975. *The relaxation response*. New York: Morrow.

Brown, B. 1981. *Stress and the art of biofeedback*. New York: Bantam Books.

Bry, A. 1979. *Visualization—Directing the movies of your mind*. New York: Harper & Row.

Curtis, J.D., Detert, R.A., Schindler, J., and Zirkel, K. 1985. *Teaching stress management and relaxation skills: An instructor's guide*. La Crosse, WI: Coulee Press.

Danskin, D., and Crow, M. 1981. *Biofeedback: An introduction and guide*. Palo Alto, CA: Mayfield.

Davies, C.T.M., and Few, J.D. 1973. Effects of exercise on adrenocortical function. *Journal of Applied Physiology* 35: 887-891.

deVries, H.A. 1975. Physical education, adult fitness programs: Does physical activity promote relaxation? *Journal of Physical Education and Recreation* 46: 53-54.

Falls, H.B., Baylor, A.M., and Dishman, R.K. 1980. *Essentials of fitness*. Philadelphia: Saunders.

Friedman, M., and Rosenman, R.H. 1974. *Type A behavior and your heart*. New York: Knopf.

Hartley, L.H. 1975. Growth hormone and catecholamine response to exercise in relation to physical training. *Medicine and Science in Sports* 7: 34-36.

Hartley, L.H., Mason, J.W., Mougey, E.H., Wherry, F.E., Pennington, L.L., and Ricketts, P.T. 1972. Multiple hormonal responses to prolonged exercise in relation to physical training. *Journal of Applied Physiology* 33: 607-610.

Jacobson, E. 1978. *You must relax*. New York: McGraw-Hill.

Jenkins, C.D., Rosenman, R.H., and Zyzanski, S.J. 1974. Prediction of clinical coronary heart disease by a test for the coronary-prone behavior pattern. *New England Journal of Medicine* 290: 1271-1275.

Jin, P. 1992. Efficacy of Tai Chi, brisk walking, meditation, and reading in reducing mental and emotional stress. *Journal of Psychosomatic Research* 36: 361-370.

Lamb, D.R. 1978. *Physiology of exercise*. New York: Macmillan.

Morgan, W.P. 1973. Influence of acute physical activity on state anxiety. *NCPEAM Proceedings* 76: 113.

Morgan, W.P. 1979. Prediction of performance in athletics. In P. Klavora and J.V. Daniel, eds., *Coach, athlete, and the sports psychologist*, 173-186. Champaign, IL: Human Kinetics.

Orioli, E.M., Jaffe, D.T., and Scott, C.D. 1987. *StressMap*. New York: Newmarket.

Rathbone, J., and Hunt, V. 1965. *Corrective physical education*. Philadelphia: Saunders.

Selye, H. 1956. *The stress of life*. New York: McGraw-Hill.

Severtsen, B., and Bruya, M.A. 1986. Effects of meditation and aerobic exercise on EEG patterns. *Journal of Neuroscience Nursing* 18: 206-210.

Sharkey, B.J. 1990. *Physiology of fitness*. Champaign IL: Human Kinetics.

Shephard, R.J., and Sidney, K.H. 1975. Effects of physical exercise on plasma growth hormone and cortisol levels in human subjects. *Exercise and Sport Sciences Reviews* 3: 1-30.

Tharp, G.D. 1975. The role of glucocorticoids in exercise. *Medicine and Science in Sports* 7: 6-11.

Thayer, R.E., Newman, J.R., and McClain, T.M. 1994. Self-regulation of mood: Strategies for changing a bad mood, raising energy, and reducing tension. *Journal of Personality and Social Psychology* 67: 910-925.

VonEuler, U.S. 1974. Sympatho-adrenal activity in physical exercise. *Medicine and Science in Sports* 6: 165-173.

White, J.A., Ismail, A.H., and Bottoms, G.D. 1976. Effect of physical fitness on the adrenocortical response to exercise stress. *Medicine and Science in Sports* 8: 113-118.

List of Abbreviations

Terms

% BF	Relative body fat
AAHPERD	American Alliance for Health, Physical Education, Recreation and Dance
ACSM	American College of Sports Medicine
AHA	American Heart Association
ATP	Adenosine triphosphate
AV	Atrioventricular
BIA	Bioelectrical impedance analysis
BMI	Body mass index
BMR	Basal metabolic rate
BP	Blood pressure
BSA	Body surface area
BV	Body volume
BW	Body weight
C	Circumference
CDC	Centers for Disease Control
CHD	Coronary heart disease
CP	Creatine phosphate
CRAC	Contract–relax with agonist contraction
CSA	Cross-sectional area
CV	Cardiovascular
CVD	Cardiovascular disease
D	Distance
Db	Body density
DOMS	Delayed-onset muscle soreness
DXA	Dual-energy x-ray absorptiometry
E	Rate of energy expenditure
ECG	Electrocardiogram
EMG	Electromyography

Terms

F	Force
FFB	Fat-free body
FFM	Fat-free mass
FM	Fat mass
FRC	Functional residual lung capacity
GH	Growth hormone
GV	Volume of air in the gastro-intestinal tract
GXT	Graded exercise test
H	Horizontal component of metabolic work
HDL-C	High-density lipoprotein cholesterol
HR	Heart rate
HR max	Maximal heart rate
HR rest	Resting heart rate
HRA	Health risk appraisal
HRR	Heart rate range
HT	Standing height
HT^2/R	Resistance index
HW	Hydrostatic weighing
LDL-C	Low-density lipoprotein cholesterol
LPL	Lipoprotein lipase
MET	Metabolic equivalent
MRI	Magnetic resonance imaging
MVC	Maximal voluntary contraction
N	Sample size
NCEP	National cholesterol education program
NIDDM	noninsulin-dependent diabetes mellitis
NIH	National Institutes of Health
NIR	Near-infrared interactance

Terms

OD	Optical density
P	Power output
p	Specific resistivity
PAR-Q	Physical activity readiness questionnaire
PEI	Physical efficiency index
Q	Cardiac output
R	Resistance for bioimpedance analysis
R	Resting component of metabolic work
r	Pearson product-moment correlation
RDA	Recommended dietary allowance
rep	Repetition
RER	Respiratory exchange ratio
RM	Repetition maximum
R_{mc}	Multiple correlation coefficient
RMR	Resting metabolic rate
ROM	Range of motion
RPE	Rating of perceived exertion
RV	Residual lung volume
SEE	Standard error of estimate
SKF	Skinfold
SV	Stroke volume
TBW	Total body water
TC	Total cholesterol
TC/HDL-C	Ratio of total cholesterol to HDL-cholesterol
TLC	Total lung capacity
TLCNS	Total lung capacity, head not submerged
UWW	Underwater weighing
V	Vertical component of metabolic work
VC	Vital capacity
$\dot{V}O_2max$	Maximal oxygen uptake
$\dot{V}O_2$	Volume of oxygen consumed per minute
WHR	Waist-to-hip ratio
Xc	Reactance
YMCA	Young Men's Christian Association
Z	Impedance
ΣSKF	Sum of skinfolds

Units of Measure

bpm	beats per minute
C	Celsius
cc	cubic centimeter
cm	centimeter
dl	deciliter
F	Fahrenheit
ft-lb	foot-pound
g	gram
hr	hour
in	inch
kcal	kilocalorie
kg	kilogram
kgm	kilogram-meter
km	kilometer
L	liter
lb	pound
m	meter
meq	milli-equivalent
mg	milligram
min	minute
ml	milliliter
mmHg	millimeters of mercury
mm	millimeter
mph	miles per hour
Nm	newton-meter
rpm	revolutions per minute
sec	second
μg	microgram
μg RE	retinol equivalent
W	watt
yr	year
Ω	ohm

APPENDIX A

Health and Fitness Appraisal

APPENDIX A.1 GLOSSARY OF MEDICAL TERMINOLOGY

Medical Term	Common Term or Definition
Acquired immune deficiency syndrome (AIDS)	Disease characterized by a deficiency in the body's immune system, caused by human immunodeficiency virus (HIV)
Aneurysm	Dilation of a blood vessel wall causing a weakness in the vessel's wall; usually caused by atherosclerosis and hypertension
Angina pectoris	Chest pain
Aortic stenosis	Narrowing of the aortic valve that obstructs blood flow from the left ventricle into the aorta
Arrhythmia	Abnormal heart rhythm
Arteriosclerosis	Hardening of the arteries or thickening and loss of elasticity in the artery walls that obstructs blood flow; caused by deposits of fat, cholesterol, and other substances
Asthma	Respiratory disorder characterized by difficulty in breathing and wheezing due to constricted bronchi
Ataxia	Impaired ability to coordinate movement characterized by staggering gait or postural imbalance
Atherosclerosis	Buildup and deposition of fat and fibrous plaque in the inner walls of the coronary arteries
Atrial fibrillation	Cardiac dysrhythmia in which the atria quiver instead of pumping in an organized fashion
Atrial flutter	Type of atrial tachycardia in which the atria contract at rates of 230 to 380 beats per minute
Atrophy	A wasting or decrease in size of a body part
Bradycardia	Resting heart rate <60 beats per minute
Bronchitis	Acute or chronic inflammation of the bronchi of lungs
Cardiac arrest	Sudden loss of heart function usually caused by ventricular fibrillation
Cardiomyopathy	Any disease that affects the structure and function of the heart
Cirrhosis	Chronic, degenerative disease of the liver in which the lobes are covered with fibrous tissue; associated with chronic alcohol abuse
Claudication	Cramplike pain in the calves due to poor circulation to leg muscles
Congestive heart failure	Impaired cardiac pumping caused by myocardial infarction, ischemic heart disease, or cardiomyopathy
Cynanosis	Bluish discoloration of skin caused by lack of oxygenated hemoglobin in the blood
Diabetes	Complex disorder of carbohydrate, fat, and protein metabolism resulting from a lack of insulin secretion or defective insulin receptors
Dyspnea	Shortness of breath or difficulty breathing caused by certain heart conditions, anxiety, or strenuous exercise

Medical Term	Common Term or Definition
Edema	Accumulation of interstitial fluid in tissues such as pericardial sac and joint capsules
Embolism	Piece of tissue or thrombus that circulates in the blood until it lodges in a vessel
Emphysema	Pulmonary disease causing damage in alveoli and loss of lung elasticity
Glucose intolerance	Inability of body to metabolize glucose
Graves' disease	Disease associated with an overactive thyroid gland that secretes greater than normal amounts of thyroid hormones; also known as hyperthyroidism or thyrotoxicosis
Heart block	Interference in the normal conduction of electrical impulses that control normal contraction of the heart muscle; may occur at sino-atrial node, atrioventricular node, bundle of HIS, or at combination of these sites
Hepatitis	Inflammation of the liver characterized by jaundice and gastro-intestinal discomfort
Hypercholesterolemia	Excess of cholesterol in blood
Hyperlipidemia	Exess lipids in blood
Hypertension	High blood pressure
Hyperthyroidism	Overactive thyroid gland that secretes greater than normal amounts of thyroid hormones; also known as thyrotoxicosis or Graves' disease
Hypoglycemia	Low blood glucose level
Hypokalemia	Inadequate amount of potassium in the blood characterized by an abnormal ECG, weakness, and flaccid paralysis
Hypomagnesemia	Inadequate amount of magnesium in the blood resulting in nausea, vomiting, muscle weakness, and tremors
Hypothyroidism	Underactive thyroid gland that secretes lower than normal amounts of thyroid hormones; also known as myxedema
Hypoxia	Inadequate oxygen at the cellular level
Ischemia	Decreased supply of oxygenated blood to body part or organ
Ischemic heart disease	Pathologic condition of the myocardium caused by lack of oxygen to the heart muscle
McArdle's syndrome	Inherited metabolic disease characterized by inability to metabolize muscle glycogen, resulting in excessive amounts of glycogen stored in skeletal muscles
Murmur	Low-pitched fluttering or humming sound
Myocardial infarction	Heart attack
Myocarditis	Inflammation of the heart muscle caused by viral, bacterial, or fungal infection
Myxedema	Disease associated with an underactive thyroid gland that secretes lower than normal amounts of thyroid hormones; also known as hypothyroidism
Occlusion	Blockage of blood flow to body part or organ
Osteoarthritis	Degenerative disease of the joints characterized by excessive amounts of bone and cartilage in the joint
Osteoporosis	Disorder characterized by low bone mineral and bone density; occuring most frequently in postmenopausal women and sedentary individuals
Pallor	Unnatural paleness or absence of skin color
Palpitations	Racing or pounding of the heart
Pericarditis	Inflammation of the pericardium caused by trauma, infection, uremia, or heart attack
Prosthesis	An artificial replacement of a missing body part, such as artificial limbs and joints
Rheumatic heart disease	Condition in which the heart valves are damaged by rheumatic fever, contracted from a streptococcal infection (strep throat)
Rheumatoid arthritis	Chronic, destructive disease of the joints characterized by inflammation and thickening of the synovial membranes and swelling of the joints
Stroke	Rupture or blockage of blood flow to the brain caused by a blood clot or some other particle

Medical Term	Common Term or Definition
Syncope	Brief lapse in consciousness caused by lack of oxygen to the brain
Tachycardia	Resting heart rate >100 beats per minute
Thrombophlebitis	Inflammation of a vein often accompanied by formation of a blood clot
Thrombus	Lump of cellular elements of the blood attached to inner walls of an artery or vein, sometimes blocking blood flow through the vessel
Thyrotoxicosis	Overactive thyroid gland that secretes greater than normal amounts of thyroid hormones; also known as Graves' disease or hyperthyroidism
Uremia	Exessive amounts of urea and other nitrogen waste products in the blood associated with kidney failure
Valvular heart disease	Congenital disorder of a heart valve characterized by obstructed blood flow, valvular degeneration, and regurgitation of blood
Ventricular ectopy	Premature (out of sequence) contraction of the ventricles
Ventricular fibrillation	Cardiac dysrhythmia marked by rapid, uncoordinated, and unsynchronized contractions of the ventricles, so that no blood is pumped by the heart
Vertigo	Dizziness or inability to maintain normal balance in a standing or seated position

Physical Activity Readiness
Questionnaire - PAR-Q
(revised 1994)

APPENDIX A.2

PAR - Q & YOU

(A Questionnaire for People Aged 15 to 69)

Regular physical activity is fun and healthy, and increasingly more people are starting to become more active every day. Being more active is very safe for most people. However, some people should check with their doctor before they start becoming much more physically active.

If you are planning to become much more physically active than you are now, start by answering the seven questions in the box below. If you are between the ages of 15 or 69, the PAR-Q will tell you if you should check with your doctor before you start. If you are over 69 years of age, and you are not used to being very active, check with your doctor.

Common sense is your best guide when you answer these questions. Please read the questions carefully and answer each one honestly: check YES or NO.

YES	NO	
☐	☐	1. Has your doctor ever said that you have a heart condition <u>and</u> that you should only do physical activity recommended by a doctor?
☐	☐	2. Do you feel pain in your chest when you do physical activity?
☐	☐	3. In the past month, have you had chest pain when you were not doing physical activity?
☐	☐	4. Do you lose your balance because of dizziness or do you ever lose consciousness?
☐	☐	5. Do you have a bone or joint problem that could be made worse by a change in your physical activity?
☐	☐	6. Is your doctor currently prescribing drugs (for example, water pills) for your blood pressure or heart condition?
☐	☐	7. Do you know of <u>any other reason</u> why you should not do physical activity?

If you answered

YES to one or more questions

Talk with your doctor by phone or in person BEFORE you start becoming much more physically active or BEFORE you have a fitness appraisal. Tell your doctor about the PAR-Q and which questions you answered YES.

- You may be able to do any activity you want—as long as you start slowly and build up gradually. Or, you may need to restrict your activities to those which are safe for you. Talk with your doctor about the kinds of activities you wish to participate in and follow his/her advice.
- Find out which community programs are safe and helpful for you.

NO to all questions

If you answered NO honestly to <u>all</u> PAR-Q questions, you can be reasonably sure that you can:

- start becoming much more physically active—begin slowly and build up gradually. This is the safest and easiest way to go.
- take part in a fitness appraisal—this is an excellent way to determine your basic fitness so that you can plan the best way for you to live actively.

DELAY BECOMING MUCH MORE ACTIVE:

- if you are not feeling well because of a temporary illness such as a cold or a fever—wait until you feel better; or
- if you are or may be pregnant—talk to your doctor before you start becoming more active

Please note: If your health changes so that you then answer YES to any of the above questions, tell your fitness or health professional. Ask whether you should change your physical activity plan.

<u>Informed Use of the PAR-Q:</u> The Canadian Society for Exercise Physiology, Health Canada, and their agents assume no liability for persons who undertake physical activity, and if in doubt after completing this questionnaire, consult your doctor prior to physical activity.

You are encouraged to copy the PAR-Q but only if you use the entire form

Note: If the PAR-Q is being given to a person before he or she participates in a physical activity program or a fitness appraisal, this section may be used for legal or administrative purposes.

I have read, understood and completed this questionnaire. Any questions I had were answered to my full satisfaction.

NAME _____

SIGNATURE_____   DATE _____

SIGNATURE OF PARENT_____   WITNESS _____
or GUARDIAN (for participants under the age of majority)

APPENDIX A.3   RISKO: A HEART HEALTH APPRAISAL

	MEN		SCORE

1. Systolic blood pressure

If you *are not* taking anti-hypertensive medications and your blood pressure is . . .

124 or less	0 points
between 125 and 134	2 points
between 135 and 144	4 points
between 145 and 154	6 points
between 155 and 164	8 points
between 165 and 174	10 points
between 175 and 184	12 points
between 185 and 194	14 points
between 195 and 204	16 points
between 205 and 214	18 points
between 215 and 224	20 points

⇓

If you *are* taking anti-hypertensive medications and your blood pressure is . . .

120 or less	0 points
between 121 and 127	2 points
between 128 and 135	4 points
between 136 and 143	6 points
between 144 and 153	8 points
between 154 and 163	10 points
between 164 and 175	12 points
between 176 and 190	14 points
between 191 and 204	16 points
between 205 and 214	18 points
between 215 and 224	20 points

2. Blood Cholesterol

Locate the number of points for your total and HDL cholesterol in the table below.

SCORE

⇓

		HDL							
		25	30	35	40	50	60	70	80
	140	4	2	0	0	0	0	0	0
	160	5	3	2	0	0	0	0	0
	180	6	4	3	1	0	0	0	0
T	200	7	5	4	3	0	0	0	0
O	220	7	6	5	4	1	0	0	0
T	240	8	7	5	4	2	0	0	0
A	260	8	7	6	5	3	1	0	0
L	280	9	8	7	6	4	2	0	0
	300	9	8	7	6	4	3	1	0
	340	9	9	8	7	6	4	2	1
	400	10	9	9	8	7	5	4	3

3. Cigarette Smoking

SCORE

If you . . .

do not smoke	0 points
smoke less than a pack a day	2 points
smoke a pack a day	5 points
smoke two or more packs a day	9 points

4. Weight

Locate your weight category in the table below.

SCORE

		If you are in . . .		
		weight category A	0 points	
		weight category B	1 point	
		weight category C	2 points	

FT	IN	A	B	C
5	1	up to 162	163-250	251+
5	2	up to 167	168-257	258+
5	3	up to 172	173-264	265+
5	4	up to 176	177-272	273+
5	5	up to 181	182-279	280+
5	6	up to 185	186-286	287+
5	7	up to 190	191-293	294+
5	8	up to 195	196-300	301+
5	9	up to 199	200-307	308+
5	10	up to 204	205-315	316+
5	11	up to 209	210-322	323+
6	0	up to 213	214-329	330+
6	1	up to 218	219-336	337+
6	2	up to 223	224-343	344+
6	3	up to 227	228-350	351+
6	4	up to 232	233-358	359+
6	5	up to 238	239-365	366+
6	6	up to 241	242-372	373+

TOTAL SCORE

WOMEN

SCORE

1. Systolic blood pressure

If you *are not* taking anti-hypertensive medications and your blood pressure is . . .

124 or less	0 points
between 126 and 136	2 points
between 137 and 148	4 points
between 149 and 160	6 points
between 161 and 171	8 points
between 172 and 183	10 points
between 184 and 194	12 points
between 195 and 206	14 points
between 207 and 218	16 points

If you *are* taking anti-hypertensive medications and your blood pressure is . . .

117 or less	0 points
between 118 and 123	2 points
between 124 and 129	4 points
between 130 and 136	6 points
between 137 and 144	8 points
between 145 and 154	10 points
between 155 and 168	12 points
between 169 and 206	14 points
between 207 and 218	16 points

2. Blood Cholesterol

Locate the number of points for your total
and HDL cholesterol in the table below.

SCORE

⇓

		HDL							
		25	**30**	**35**	**40**	**50**	**60**	**70**	**80**
	140	2	1	0	0	0	0	0	0
	160	3	2	1	0	0	0	0	0
	180	4	3	2	1	0	0	0	0
T	**200**	4	3	2	2	0	0	0	0
O	**220**	5	4	3	2	1	0	0	0
T	**240**	5	4	3	3	1	0	0	0
A	**260**	5	4	4	3	2	1	0	0
L	**280**	5	5	4	4	2	1	0	0
	300	6	5	4	4	3	2	1	0
	340	6	5	5	4	3	2	1	0
	400	6	6	5	5	4	3	2	2

3. Cigarette Smoking

SCORE

⇓

If you . . .

do not smoke	0 points
smoke less than a pack a day	2 points
smoke a pack a day	5 points
smoke two or more packs a day	9 points

4. Weight

Locate your weight category in the table below.

SCORE

⇓

If you are in . . .

weight category A	0 points
weight category B	1 point
weight category C	2 points
weight category D	3 points

FT	IN	A	B	C	D
4	8	up to 139	140-161	162-184	185+
4	9	up to 140	141-162	163-185	186+
4	10	up to 141	142-163	164-187	188+
4	11	up to 143	144-166	167-190	191+
5	0	up to 145	146-168	169-193	194+
5	1	up to 147	148-171	172-196	197+
5	2	up to 149	150-173	174-198	199+
5	3	up to 152	153-176	177-201	202+
5	4	up to 154	155-178	179-204	205+
5	5	up to 157	158-182	183-209	210+
5	6	up to 160	161-186	187-213	214+
5	7	up to 165	166-191	192-219	220+
5	8	up to 169	170-196	197-225	226+
5	9	up to 173	174-201	202-231	232+
5	10	up to 178	179-206	207-238	239+
5	11	up to 182	183-212	213-242	243+
6	0	up to 187	188-217	218-248	249+
6	1	up to 191	192-222	223-254	255+

TOTAL SCORE

What Your Score Means

Note: If you're diabetic, you have a greater risk of heart disease. Add 7 points to your total score.

0 – 2   You have a low risk of heart disease for a person of your age and sex.

3 – 4   You have a low-to-moderate risk of heart disease for a person of your age and sex. That's good, but there's room for improvement.

5 – 7   You have a moderate-to-high risk of heart disease for a person of your age and sex. There's considerable room for improvement in some areas.

8 – 15   You have a high risk of developing heart disease for a person of your age and sex. There's lots of room for improvement in all areas.

16+   You have a very high risk of developing heart disease for a person of your age and sex. You should act now to reduce all your risk factors.

How to Reduce Your Risk

- Quit smoking for good.
- Have your blood pressure checked regularly
- Stay physically active
- Lose weight if necessary
- Reduce high blood cholesterol through your diet.

APPENDIX A.4   MEDICAL HISTORY QUESTIONNAIRE

Demographic Information

Last name	First name	Middle initial

Date of birth	Sex	Home phone

Address	City, state	Zip code

Work phone	Family physician

Section A

1. When was the last time you had a physical examination?

2. If you are allergic to any medications, foods, or other substances, please name them.

3. If you have been told that you have any chronic or serious illnesses, please list them.

4. Give the following information pertaining to to the last 3 times you have been hospitalized. *Note*: Women, do not list normal pregnancies.

	Hospitalization 1	Hospitalization 2	Hospitalization 3
Type of operation			
Month and year of hospitalization			
Hospital			
City and state			

Section B

During the past 12 months

1.	Has a physician prescribed any form of medication for you?	Yes	No
2.	Has your weight fluctuated more than a few pounds?	Yes	No
3.	Did you attempt to bring about this weight change through diet or exercise?	Yes	No
4.	Have you experienced any faintness, light-headedness, or blackouts?	Yes	No
5.	Have you occasionally had trouble sleeping?	Yes	No
6.	Have you experienced any blurred vision?	Yes	No
7.	Have you had any severe headaches?	Yes	No
8.	Have you experienced chronic morning cough?	Yes	No
9.	Have you experienced any temporary change in your speech pattern, such as slurring or loss of speech?	Yes	No
10.	Have you felt unusually nervous or anxious for no apparent reason?	Yes	No
11.	Have you experienced unusual heartbeats such as skipped beats or palpitations?	Yes	No
12.	Have you experienced periods in which your heart felt as though it were racing for no apparent reason?	Yes	No

At present

1. Do you experience shortness or loss of breath while walking with others your own age?   Yes   No

2. Do you experience sudden tingling, numbness, or loss of feeling in your arms, hands, legs, feet, or face?   Yes   No

3. Have you ever noticed that your hands or feet sometimes feel cooler than other parts of your body?   Yes   No

4. Do you experience swelling of your feet and ankles?   Yes   No

5. Do you get pains or cramps in your legs?   Yes   No

6. Do you experience any pain or discomfort in your chest?   Yes   No

7. Do you experience any pressure or heaviness in your chest?   Yes   No

8. Have you ever been told that your blood pressure was abnormal?   Yes   No

9. Have you ever been told that your serum cholesterol or triglyceride level was high?   Yes   No

10. Do you have diabetes?   Yes   No

    If yes, how is it controlled?

    ❐ Dietary means   ❐ Insulin injection   ❐ Oral medication   ❐ Uncontrolled

11. How often would you characterize your stress level as being high?

    ❐ Occasionally   ❐ Frequently   ❐ Constantly

12. Have you ever been told that you have any of the following illnesses?

    ❐ Myocardial infarction   ❐ Arteriosclerosis   ❐ Heart disease

    ❐ Coronary thrombosis   ❐ Rheumatic heart   ❐ Heart attack

    ❐ Coronary occlusion   ❐ Heart failure   ❐ Heart murmur

    ❐ Heart block   ❐ Aneurysm   ❐ Angina

Section C

Has any member of your immediate family been treated for or suspected to have had any of these conditions? Please identify their relationship to you (father, mother, sister, brother, etc.).

A. Diabetes

B. Heart disease

C. Stroke

D. High blood pressure

APPENDIX A.5   MEDICAL CLEARANCE

Patient's name _____   Date _____

Address _____   Age _____

_____

Phone _____

I consider the above individual to be:

_____ Normal   _____ Prone to coronary heart disease

_____ Cardiac patient _____ Other (explain)

Present physical

Etiologic diagnostic data
1. No heart disease
2. Rheumatic heart disease
3. Congenital heart disease
4. Hypertension
5. Ischemic heart disease
6. Other

Activity level
1. Very active
2. Normal
3. Limited
4. Very limited

ECG
1. Normal
2. Abnormal
3. Infarct

Rhythm
1. Sinus
2. Atrial fibrillation
3. Other

Specific cardiac diagnosis _____

Additional abnormalities you are aware of _____

Date of last complete physical examination _____

Present medication _____

Please fill in information if it is available:

1. Urine: sp gr _____ alb _____ glucose _____ micro_____
2. Complete blood count: Hbg _____ Hct _____ WBC _____ diff _____
3. ECG (12-lead) (enclose copy):
4. Blood pressure: systolic _____ mm Hg   Diastolic _____ mm Hg
5. Glucose _____ $mg \cdot dl^{-1}$
6. Cholesterol _____ $mg \cdot dl^{-1}$
7. Triglycerides _____ $mg \cdot dl^{-1}$

The above-named person is capable of participating in exercise laboratory evaluations under the guidance and supervision of an exercise leader.

Signed _____ MD

(Typed or print)

Name of physician _____

Address _____

Phone number _____

APPENDIX A.6   SAMPLE ECG TRACINGS

Directions: Use these ECG tracings to practice techniques described in chapter 2 for measuring heart rate from ECG recordings.

Date 1/27/1995   9:48A
Resting

3 Lead
ST Lead   V5   Level +0.7 Slope   +4 HR   65
Speed   MPH   Grade 0.0%
Filter on   Gain x1   25 mm/sec

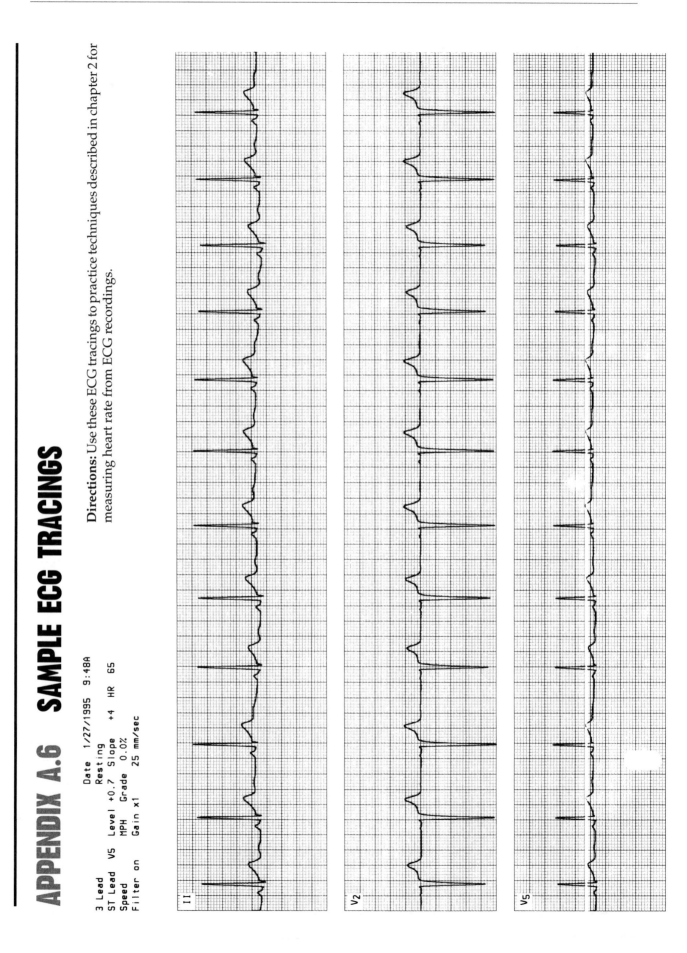

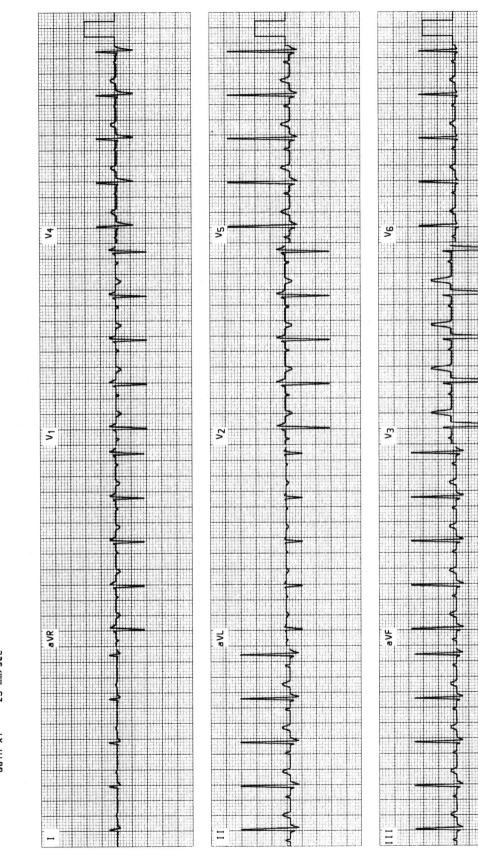

12 Lead Sml
ST Lead V5
Speed

Date 11/06/1996 11:44A
Resting
Level -0.1 Slope +4 HR 106
MPH Grade 0.0%
Gain x1   25 mm/sec

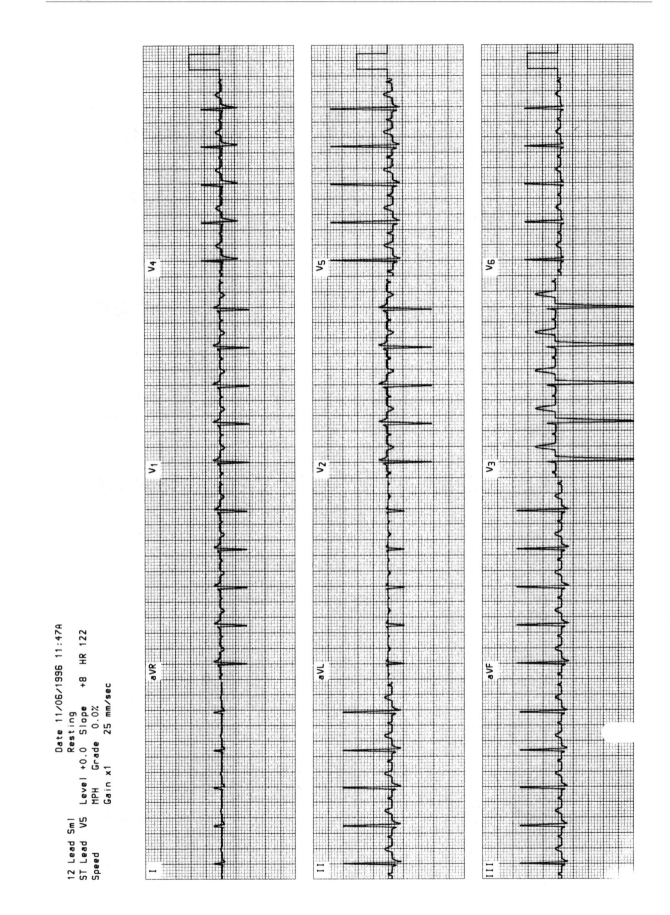

12 Lead Sml
ST Lead   V5
Speed

Date 11/06/1996 11:47A
        Resting
Level +0.0 Slope   +8 HR 122
MPH   Grade 0.0%
Gain x1   25 mm/sec

12 Lead Sml   Date 11/06/1996 11:48A
ST Lead V5   Resting
Speed   Level -0.1 Slope +2   HR 134
                       MPH Grade 0.0%
                       Gain x1   25 mm/sec

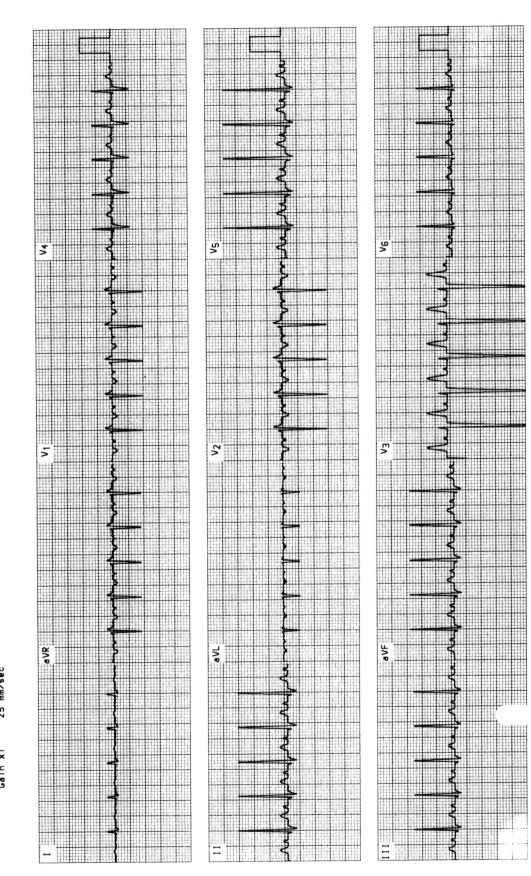

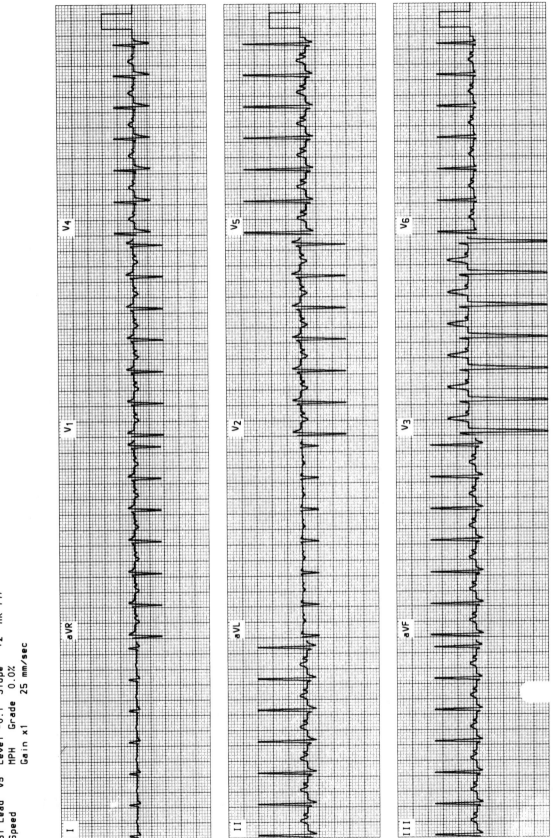

12 Lead Sml
ST Lead V5
Speed

Date 11/06/1996 11:49A
Resting
Level -0.1 Slope   +2 HR 147
MPH Grade 0.0%
Gain x1   25 mm/sec

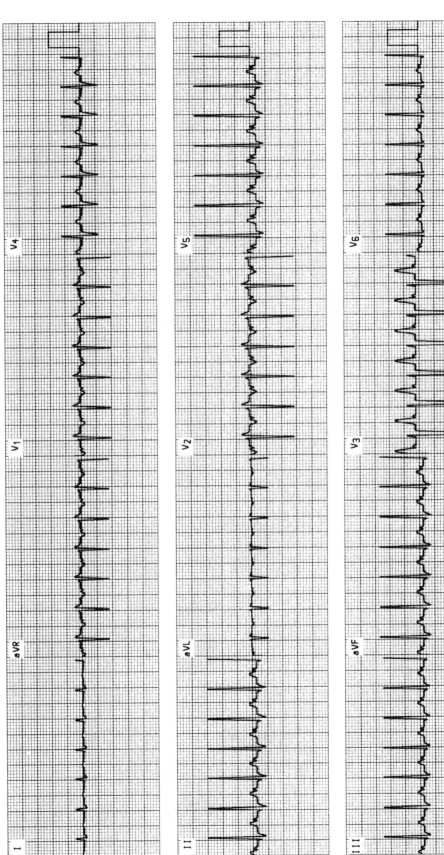

Date 11/06/1996 11:50A
Resting
12 Lead Sml
ST Lead V5   Level +0.1 Slope   +4 HR 155
Speed   MPH Grade 0.0%
              Gain x1   25 mm/sec

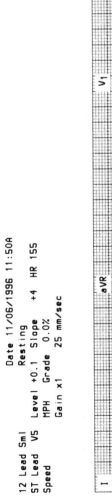

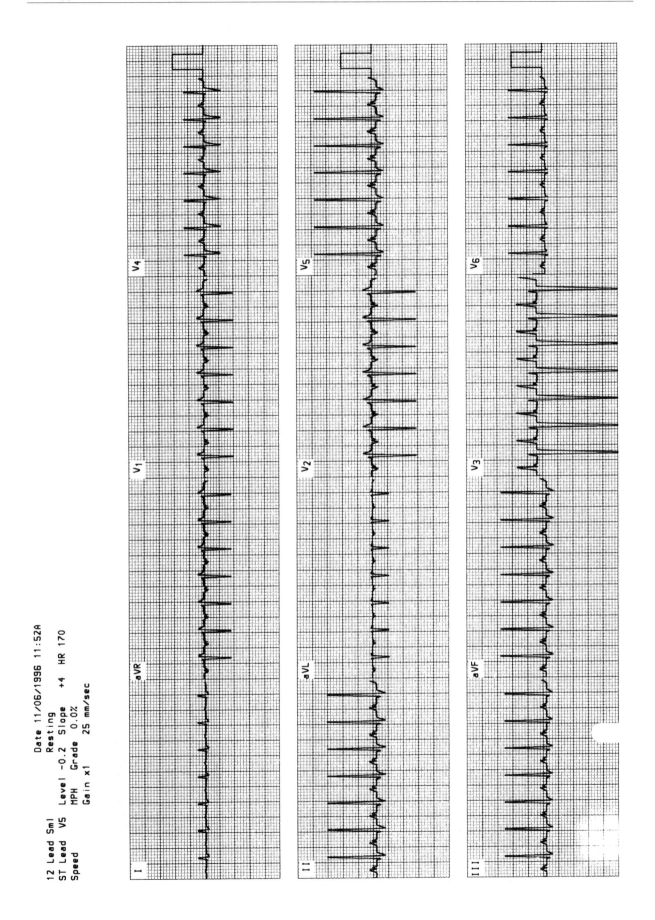

12 Lead Sml
ST Lead V5   Level -0.2 Slope +4 HR 170
Speed   MPH Grade 0.0%
Gain x1   25 mm/sec

Date 11/06/1996 11:52A
Resting

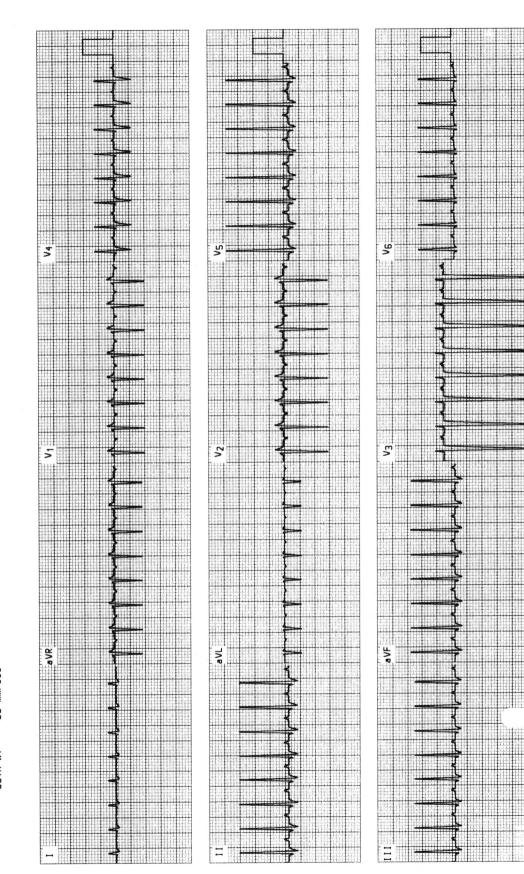

12 Lead Sml

ST Lead   V5

Speed

Date 11/06/1996 11:54A

Resting

Level -0.1 Slope   +4 HR 190

MPH   Grade 0.0%

Gain x1   25 mm/sec

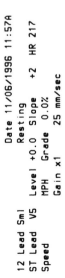

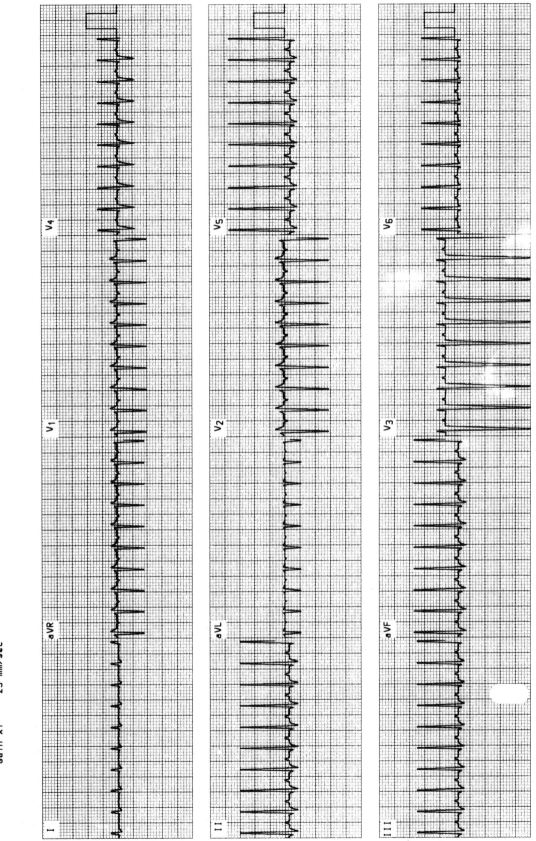

APPENDIX A.7   LIFESTYLE EVALUATION

Smoking habits

1. Have you ever smoked cigarettes, cigars, or a pipe?   Yes   No

2. Do you smoke presently?   Yes   No

     Cigarettes _____ a day

     Cigars _____ a day

     Pipefuls _____ a day

3. At what age did you start smoking? _____ years

4. If you have quit smoking, when did you quit? _____

Drinking habits

1. During the past month, on how many days did you drink alcoholic beverages?   _____

2. During the past month, how many times did you have 5 or more drinks per occasion?   _____

3. On the average, how many glasses of beer, wine, or cocktails do you consume a week?

     Beer _____ glasses or cans

     Wine _____ glasses

     Cocktails _____ glasses

     Other _____ glasses

Exercise habits

1. Do you exercise vigorously on a regular basis?   Yes   No

2. What activities do you engage in on a regular basis?

3. If you walk, run, or jog, what is the average number of miles you cover each workout? _____ miles

4. How many minutes on the average is each of your exercise workouts? _____ minutes

5. How many workouts a week do you participate in on the average? _____ workouts

6. Is your occupation

     _____ Inactive (e.g., desk job)

     _____ Light work (e.g., housework, light carpentry)

     _____ Heavy work (e.g., heavy carpentry, lifting)

7. Check those activities that you would prefer in a regular exercise program for yourself:

_____ Walking, running, or jogging	_____ Handball, racquetball, or squash
_____ Stationary running	_____ Basketball
_____ Jumping rope	_____ Swimming
_____ Bicycling	_____ Tennis
_____ Stationary cycling	_____ Aerobic dance
_____ Step aerobics	_____ Stairclimbing
_____ Other (specify)	

Dietary habits

1. What is your current weight? _____ lb _____ kg   height? _____ in.

2. What would you like to weigh? _____ lb _____ kg

3. What is the most you ever weighed as an adult? _____ lb _____ kg

4. What is the least you ever weighed as an adult? _____ lb _____ kg

5. What weight loss methods have you tried? _____

6. Which do you eat regularly?

    ❐ Breakfast   ❐ Midafternoon snack

    ❐ Midmorning snack   ❐ Dinner

    ❐ Lunch   ❐ After-dinner snack

7. How often do you eat out each week? _____ times

8. What size portions do you normally have?

    ❐ Small   ❐ Moderate   ❐ Large   ❐ Extra large   ❐ Uncertain

9. How often do you eat more than one serving?

    ❐ Always   ❐ Usually   ❐ Sometimes   ❐ Never

10. How long does it usually take you to eat a meal? _____ minutes

11. Do you eat while doing other activies (e.g., watching TV, reading, working)? _____

12. When you snack, how many times a week do you eat the following?

    Cookies, cake, pie _____   Candy _____   Diet soda _____

    Soft drinks _____   Doughnuts _____   Fruit _____

    Milk or milk beverage _____   Potato chips, pretzels, etc. _____

    Peanuts or other nuts _____   Ice cream _____

    Cheese and crackers _____   Other _____

13. How often do you eat dessert? _____ times a day _____ times a week

14. What dessert do you eat most often? _____

15. How often do you eat fried foods? _____ times a week

16. Do you salt your food at the table?   Yes   No

    ❐ Before tasting it   ❐ After tasting it

APPENDIX A.8   INFORMED CONSENT

In order to assess cardiovascular function, body composition, and other physical fitness components, the undersigned hereby voluntarily consents to engage in one or more of the following tests (check the appropriate boxes):

    ❐ Graded exercise stress test

    ❐ Body composition tests

    ❐ Muscle fitness tests

    ❐ Flexibility tests

Explanation of the Tests

The graded exercise test is performed on a bicycle ergometer or motor-driven treadmill. The work load is increased every few minutes until exhaustion or until other symptoms dictate that we terminate the test. You may stop the test at any time because of fatigue or discomfort.

The underwater weighing procedure involves being completely submerged in a tank or tub after fully exhaling the air from your lungs. You will be submerged for 3 to 5 seconds while we measure your underwater weight. This test provides an accurate assessment of your body composition.

For muscle fitness testing, you lift weights for a number of repetitions using barbells or exercise machines. These tests assess the strength and endurance of the major muscle groups in the body.

For evaluation of flexibility, you perform a number of movements so that we can measure the range of motion in your joints.

Risks and Discomforts

During the graded exercise test, certain changes may occur. These changes include abnormal blood pressure responses, fainting, irregularities in heartbeat, and heart attack. Every effort is made to minimize these occurrences. Emergency equipment and trained personnel are available to deal with these situations if they occur.

You may experience some discomfort during the underwater weighing, especially after you expire all the air from your lungs. However, this discomfort is momentary, lasting only 3 to 5 seconds. If this test causes you too much discomfort, an alternative procedure (e.g. skinfold, or bioelectrical impedance test) can be used to estimate your body composition.

There is a slight possibility of pulling a muscle or spraining a ligament during the muscle fitness and flexibility testing. In addition, you may experience muscle soreness 24 or 48 hours after testing. These risks can be minimized by performing warm-up exercises prior to taking the tests. If muscle soreness occurs, appropriate stretching exercises to relieve this soreness will be demonstrated.

Expected Benefits From Testing

These tests allow us to assess your physical working capacity and to appraise your physical fitness status. The results will be used to prescribe a safe, sound exercise program for you. Records are kept strictly confidential unless you consent to release this information.

Inquiries

Questions about the procedures used in the physical fitness tests are encouraged. If you have any questions or need additional information, please ask us to explain further.

Freedom of Consent

Your permission to perform these physical fitness tests is strictly voluntary. You are free to stop the tests at any point, if you so desire.

I have read this form carefully and I fully understand the test procedures that I will perform and the risks and discomforts. Knowing these risks and having had the opportunity to ask questions that have been answered to my satisfaction, I consent to participate in these tests.

| Date | Signature of client |

| Date | Signature of witness |

| Date | Signature of supervisor |

APPENDIX A.9   ANALYSIS OF SAMPLE CASE STUDY IN CHAPTER 5

1. <u>CHD risk profile</u>

This client has two major risk factors for CHD. Her total cholesterol (220 mg · dl^{-1}) is borderline high (200 to 230 mg · dl^{-1}) and her blood pressure (140/82 mmHg) is categorized as stage I, mild hypertension (140 to 159 mmHg). Also, her TC/HDL ratio (5.9) places her at higher risk (>5.0). She quit smoking cigarettes (1 pack a day) 3 years ago which is a step in the right direction. Following the NCEP's recommendation, (see figure 2.1 on page 19) you should encourage this client to have her LDL-C assessed to determine if she needs a cholesterol treatment program. Engaging in an aerobic exercise program should lower her systolic blood pressure. Her triglycerides and blood glucose levels are normal.

The client also has a number of secondary risk factors for developing CHD. She is not overweight, but her body fat is above average (28% BF). For optimal fitness the client should lose at least 3% BF. This could be accomplished by participating regularly in an aerobic exercise program and changing some of her eating behaviors. She should be encouraged to dine out less frequently and to eat three well-balanced meals a day. When dining out, she should select foods that are low in saturated fat, cholesterol, and sodium. This may help to lower her blood cholesterol and blood pressure.

The client is also at greater risk due to:

- the high stress associated with her job (police officer) and lifestyle (divorced parent raising two children),

- family history of cardiovascular disease, and

- physical inactivity (she does not exercise regularly outside of work-related physical activity).

2. Special considerations

The client has not exercised aerobically for the past six years, and she has gained 15 pounds during that time. It is likely that she will experience some discomfort when she starts her aerobic exercise program. Thus, it is important to initially prescribe low intensity exercise to minimize her physical discomfort.

You also need to consider her busy schedule to find a convenient time for her to exercise. She reports feeling dizzy after eating. This is most likely due to the fact that she is eating only one meal a day, and the insulin-surge after eating is lowering her blood glucose level. It is important to convince this client to start eating at least three meals a day to avoid this problem.

3. HR, BP, and RPE reponse to graded exercise test

The client's HR response to the graded exercise test was normal. The exercise HR increased during each stage of the exercise test. The maximal heart rate (190 bpm) was very close to her age-predicted maximal HR (220 − 28 = 192 bpm). The client's BP response to the graded exercise test was normal. The diastolic BP remained fairly constant (78 to 82 mmHg), and the systolic BP increased with each stage of the exercise test. The RPEs were normal. The ratings increased linearly with exercise intensity.

4. Functional aerobic capacity

The graded exercise test was voluntarily terminated by the client due to fatigue. This was most likely a maximal effort exercise test as indicated by the RPE (18) and the exercise heart rate (190 bpm) during the last stage of the graded exercise test. The treadmill speed and grade during the last stage of the protocol was 2.5 mph and 12%, respectively. This corresponds to a functional aerobic capacity of 7.0 METs or 24.5 ml · kg^{-1} · min^{-1}. According to the norms, this client's cardiorespiratory fitness level is poor for her age.

5. & 6. Training HRs

The graph of the client's HR and RPE responses to the graded exercise test is presented in Figure A.9.

Given the client's low cardiorespiratory fitness level and her lack of regular aerobic exercise, the initial minimal training intensity will be 50% $\dot{V}O_2$max (3.5 METs), gradually increasing to a maximum intensity of 75% $\dot{V}O_2$max (5.2 METS). The corresponding training HRs are 142 bpm (50% $\dot{V}O_2$max) and 170 bpm (75% $\dot{V}O_2$max). The HRs and RPEs corresponding to the relative exercise intensities are extrapolated from the graph.

%$\dot{V}O_2$max	METs	HR (bpm)	RPE
60%	4.2	155	12-13
70%	4.9	168	14
80%	5.6	175	15
85%	6.0	178	16

7. Speed calculations (ACSM formula for walking on level course)

To calculate walking speed corresponding to 60% of client's $\dot{V}O_2$max (.60 × 7 = 4.2 METs)

a. Convert METs into ml · kg^{-1} · min^{-1}.

$$4.2 \text{ METs} \times 3.5 \text{ ml} \cdot kg^{-1} \cdot min^{-1} = 14.7 \text{ ml} \cdot kg^{-1} \cdot min^{-1}$$

b. Substitute into ACSM walking equation and solve for speed (m · min⁻¹).

$$\dot{V}O_2max = \text{Horizontal Component} + \text{Resting Component}$$

$$14.7\ ml \cdot kg^{-1} \cdot min^{-1} = m \cdot min^{-1} \times 0.1 + 3.5\ ml \cdot kg^{-1} \cdot min^{-1}$$

$$11.2\ ml \cdot kg^{-1} \cdot min^{-1} = m \cdot min^{-1} \times 0.1$$

$$112\ m \cdot min^{-1} = speed$$

c. Convert speed (m · min⁻¹) into miles per hour.

$$(26.8\ m \cdot min^{-1} = 1\ mph)$$

$$112\ m \cdot min^{-1} / 26.8\ m/min^{-1} = 4.2\ mph$$

d. Convert miles per hour into minutes per mile walking pace.

$$60\ min \cdot hr^{-1} / 4.2\ mph = 14.28\ min \cdot mi^{-1}, \text{ or } 14{:}16\ (14\ min, 16\ sec\ per\ mile)$$

Follow these same steps to calculate walking speeds corresponding to 70% and 80% $\dot{V}O_2max$.

(**Answer:** 70% $\dot{V}O_2$ = 5.0 mph; 80% $\dot{V}O_2max$ = 6.0 mph)

8. Lifestyle modifications

- Eat three well-balanced meals a day.
- Avoid fried foods high in saturated fats, cholesterol, and sodium.
- Dine out less frequently and select restaurants offering healthy food choices (e.g., salad bar, grilled skinless chicken, or fish).
- Exercise aerobically at least 3 days a week.
- Try using relaxation techniques (e.g., stretching, progressive relaxation, mental imagery) to relax in the evening instead of drinking wine.

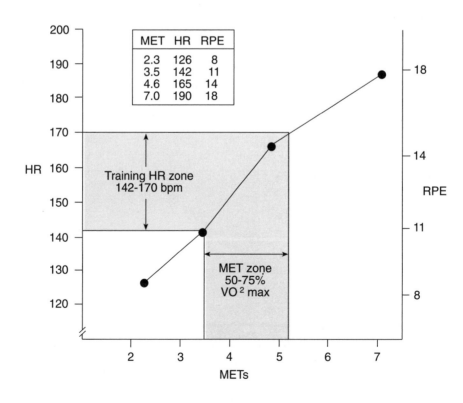

Figure A.9 Plotting heart rate vs METs for graded exercise test.

APPENDIX B

Cardiorespiratory Assessments

APPENDIX B.1 SUMMARY OF GXT AND CARDIO-RESPIRATORY FIELD TEST PROTOCOLS

Test Mode/Protocol	Population	Type	Method to estimate VO$_2$ max	Description (page)
Treadmill				
Balke	Active/sedentary men and women	Max or submax	Prediction equation Multistage equation/graphing	56
Modified Balke	Children	Max or submax	ACSM equations (walk/run) Multistage equations/graphing	77
	Elderly	Max or submax	Prediction equation Multistage equation/graphing	78
Bruce	Active/sedentary men and women	Max or submax	Prediction equation Multistage equation/graphing	56
	Cardiac patients	Max or submax	Prediction equation Multistage equation/graphing	56
Modified Bruce	High risk and elderly	Max or submax	ACSM walking equation Multistage equation/graphing	56
Ebbeling (single-stage walking)	Healthy adults (20-59 yr)	Submax	Prediction equation	66
George (single-stage jogging)	Healthy adults (18-28 yr)	Submax	Prediction equation	67
Latin & Elias (single-stage walking or jogging)	Healthy adults (19-40 yr)	Submax	Prediction equation	67
Naughton	Male cardiac patients	Max or submax	Prediction equation Multistage equation/graphing	57
Bicycle Ergometer				
Åstrand	Healthy adults	Max	ACSM leg ergometry equation	63
ACSM	Healthy adults	Submax	Multistage equation/graphing	68
Åstrand-Ryhming	Healthy adults	Submax	Nomogram	69

(continued)

APPENDIX B.1 *(CONTINUED)*

Fox	Healthy adults	Max or submax	ACSM leg ergometry equation Prediction equation	71
YMCA	Healthy adults	Submax	Multistage equation/graphing	67
McMaster	Children	Max or submax	ACSM leg ergometry equation Multistage equation/graphing	77

Test Mode/Protocol	Population	Type	Method to estimate VO$_2$ max	Description (page)
Bench Stepping				
Åstrand-Ryhming	Healthy adults	Submax	Nomogram	71
Nagle	Healthy adults	Max	ACSM stepping equation	65
Queen's college	Healthy adults (college age)	Submax	Prediction equation	71
Stairclimbing				
Howley	Healthy adults	Submax	Multistage equation/graphing	72
Rowing Ergometer				
Hagerman	Noncompetitive and unskilled rowers	Submax	Nomogram	72
Lakomy	Noncompetitive and skilled rowers	Submax	Nomogram	73
Distance run/walk				
1.0 mile run/walk	Children (8-17 yr)	Submax	Prediction equation	77
1.0 mile steady-state jog	Healthy adults (college age)	Submax	Prediction equation	75
1.5 mile run/walk	Healthy adults	Submax	Prediction equation	75
1.0 mile walk	Healthy adults	Submax	Prediction equation	75
12-minute run	Healthy adults	Submax	Prediction equation	75
15-minute run	Healthy adults	Submax	Prediction equation	72

APPENDIX B.2   ROCKPORT FITNESS CHARTS

Age-Gender Norms for the Rockport Walking Test

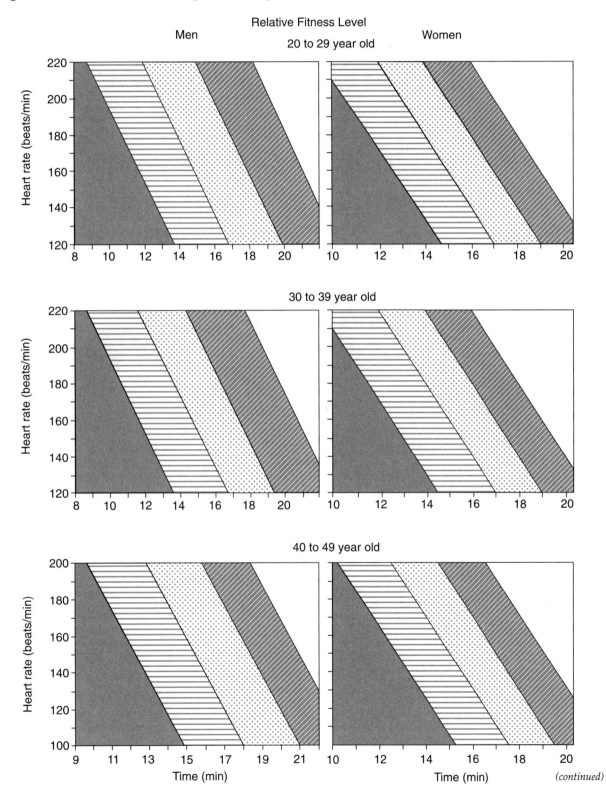

(continued)

APPENDIX B.2 *(CONTINUED)*

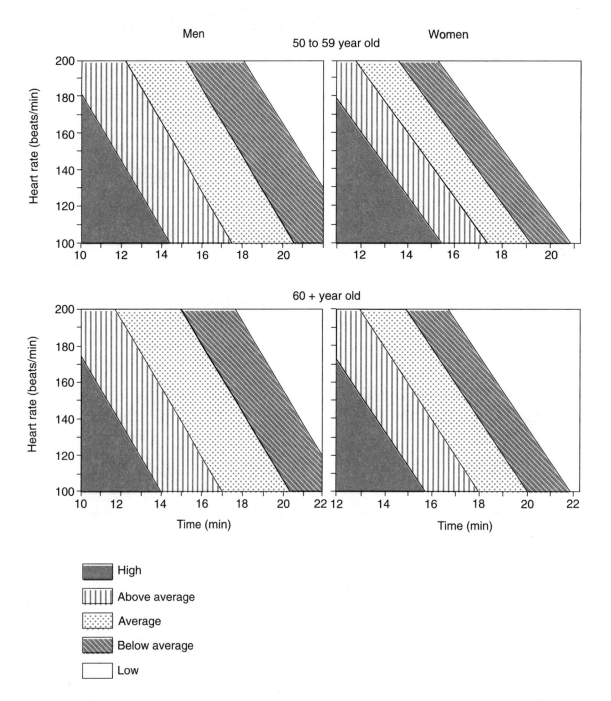

Reprinted with the permission of The Rockport Company, Inc.

APPENDIX B.3   STEP TEST PROTOCOLS

Harvard Step Test (Brouha 1943)

Age and sex: young men
Stepping rate: 30 steps · min⁻¹
Bench height: 20 in.
Duration of exercise: 5 minutes

Scoring procedures: Sit down immediately after exercise. The pulse rate is counted in 1/2-minute counts, from 1 to 1 1/2, 2 to 2 1/2, and 3 to 3 1/2 minutes after exercise. The three 1/2-minute pulse counts are summed and used in the following equation to determine physical efficiency index (PEI):

$$PEI = \frac{\textit{duration of exercise (sec)} \times \textbf{100}}{2 \times \text{sum of recovery HRs}}$$

You can evaluate the performance of college-age males using the following PEI classifications: <55 = poor, 55-64 = low average, 65-79 = average, 80-89 = good, and ≥90 = excellent.

Three-Minute Step Test (Hodgkins and Skubic 1963)

Age and sex: high school- and college-age women
Stepping rate: 24 steps · min⁻¹
Bench height: 18 in.
Duration of exercise: 3 minutes

Scoring procedures: Sit down immediately after exercise. The pulse rate is counted for 30 seconds after 1 minute of rest (1 to 1 1/2 minutes after exercise). Use the recovery pulse count in the following equation:

$$CV \text{ efficiency} = \frac{\textit{duration of exercise (sec)} \times \textbf{100}}{\text{recovery pulse} \times 5.6}$$

You can evaluate the performance of college-age women using the following classifications for CV efficiency: 0-27 = very poor, 28-38 = poor, 39-48 = fair, 49-59 = good, 60-70 = very good, and 71-100 = excellent.

OSU Step Test (Kurucz, Fox, & Mathews 1969)

Age and sex: men 19-56 yr
Stepping rate: 24 to 30 steps · min⁻¹
Bench height: split-level bench 15 and 20 in. high with an adjustable handbar
Duration of exercise: 18 innings, 50 seconds each

Phase I: 6 innings, 24 steps · min⁻¹, 15-in. bench

Phase II: 6 innings, 30 steps · min⁻¹, 15-in. bench

Phase III: 6 innings, 30 steps · min⁻¹, 20-in. bench

(Each inning consists of 30 seconds of stepping and 20 seconds of rest.)

Scoring procedures: Exactly five seconds into each rest period take a 10-second pulse count. Terminate the test when the heart rate reaches 150 bpm (25 counts × 6). The score is the inning during which the heart rate reaches 150 bpm.

Eastern Michigan University Step Test (Witten 1973)

Age and sex: college-age women
Stepping rate: 24 to 30 steps · min⁻¹
Bench height: tri-level bench 14 to 20 in.
Duration of exercise: 20 innings, 50 seconds each

Phase I: 5 innings, 24 steps · min⁻¹, 14-in. bench

Phase II: 5 innings, 30 steps · min⁻¹, 14 in. bench

Phase III: 5 innings, 30 steps · min^{-1}, 17-in. bench

Phase IV: 5 innings, 30 steps · min^{-1}, 20-in. bench

(Each inning consists of 30 seconds of stepping and 20 seconds of rest.)

Scoring procedures: Exactly five seconds into each rest period, take a 10-second pulse count. Terminate the test when the heart rate reaches 168 bpm (28 counts × 6). The score is the inning during which the heart rate reaches 168 bpm.

Cotten Revision of OSU Step Test (Cotten 1971)

Age and sex: high school- and college-age men
Stepping rate: 24 to 36 steps · min^{-1}
Bench height: 17 in.
Duration of exercise: 18 innings, 50 seconds each

Phase I: 6 innings, 24 steps · min^{-1}, 17-in. bench

Phase II: 6 innings, 30 steps · min^{-1}, 17-in. bench

Phase III: 6 innings, 36 steps · min^{-1}, 17-in. bench

(Each inning consists of 30 seconds of stepping and 20 seconds of rest.)

Scoring procedures: As for the OSU Step Test, the score is the inning during which to heart rate reaches 150 bpm (25 counts in 10 seconds). $\dot{V}O_2$max in ml · kg^{-1} · min^{-1} can be estimated using the following equation: $\dot{V}O_2$max = (1.69978 × step test score) – (0.06252 × BW in lb) + 47.12525.

Queens College Step Test (McArdle et al. 1972)

Age and sex: college-age women and men
Stepping rate: 22 steps · min^{-1} for women; 24 steps · min^{-1} for men
Bench height: 16 1/4 in.
Duration of exercise: 3 minutes

Scoring procedures: Remain standing after exercise. Beginning 5 seconds after the cessation of exercise, take a 15-second pulse count. Multiply the 15-second count by 4 to express the score in beats per minute (bpm). $\dot{V}O_2$max in ml · kg^{-1} · min^{-1} can be estimated using the following equations:

Women: $\dot{V}O_2$max = 65.81 – (0.1847 × HR)
Men: $\dot{V}O_2$max = 111.33 – (0.42 × HR)

REFERENCES

Brouha, L. 1943. The step test: A simple method of measuring physical fitness for muscular work in young men. *Research Quarterly* 14: 31-36.

Cotten, D.J. 1971. A modified step test for group cardiovascular testing. *Research Quarterly* 42: 91-95.

Hodgkins, J., and Skubic, V. 1963. Cardiovascular effiency test scores for college women in the United States. *Research Quarterly* 40: 454-461.

Kurucz, R., Fox, E.L., and Matthews, D.K. 1969. Construction of a submaximal cardiovascular step test. *Research Quarterly* 40: 115-122.

McArdle, W.D., Katch, F.I., Pechar, G.S., Jacobson, L., and Ruck, S. 1972. Reliability and interrelationships between maximal oxygen intake, physical working capacity and step-test scores in college women. *Medicine and Science in Sports* 4: 182-186.

Witten, C. 1973. Construction of a submaximal cardiovascular step test for college females. *Research Quarterly* 44: 46-50.

APPENDIX C

Muscular Fitness Exercises and Norms

APPENDIX C.1 AVERAGE STRENGTH, ENDURANCE, AND POWER VALUES FOR ISOKINETIC (OMNI-TRON) TESTS

Strength[a]	Young adult[b]	Older adult[c]	Weight trained[d]
Females			
Chest press	88.1	76.7	131.8
Lateral row	82.6	77.4	111.4
Shoulder press	32.9	30.4	60.1
Lateral pull-down	70.8	66.3	101.2
Knee extension	67.7	59.3	82.7
Knee flexion	51.5	43.3	64.3
Males			
Chest press	173.8	154.9	218.6
Lateral row	153.5	143.2	178.6
Shoulder press	69.2	62.4	102.6
Lateral pull-down	134.8	115.3	176.0
Knee extension	110.9	95.5	127.2
Knee flexion	75.9	67.3	89.9
			(continued)

Data courtesy of Hydra-Fitness, Belton, TX: 1988

[a]Values of strength measured in ft-lb at dial setting 10 on the Omni-tron

[b]Average age for females = 15.1 ± 2.6 years; for males = 15.8 ± 2.7 years.

[c]Average age for females = 38.2 ± 9.7 years; for males = 37.6 ± 9.6 years.

[d]Average age for females = 21.2 ± 2.0 years; for males = 20.6 ± 2.1 years.

APPENDIX C.1 (CONTINUED)   AVERAGE VALUES FOR OMNI-TRON

Endurance[a]	Young adult[b]	Older adult[c]	Weight trained[d]
Females			
Chest press	64.3	53.4	125.7
Lateral row	102.4	85.7	143.7
Shoulder press	28.1	25.1	56.3
Lateral pull-down	109.1	91.5	216.3
Knee extension	88.7	86.6	111.6
Knee flexion	114.3	89.2	148.2
Males			
Chest press	211.8	167.3	321.1
Lateral row	266.9	221.2	312.5
Shoulder press	112.4	94.2	170.9
Lateral pull-down	352.2	296.3	501.5
Knee extension	72.9	80.8	98.9
Knee flexion	83.5	84.2	130.9

Power[e]	Young adult[b]	Older adult[c]	Weight trained[d]
Females			
Chest press	86.3	73.7	163.0
Lateral row	121.3	113.6	156.3
Shoulder press	39.5	32.9	81.9
Lateral pull-down	165.4	128.4	254.1
Knee extension	101.9	73.4	122.5
Knee flexion	103.5	74.6	142.1
Males			
Chest press	264.9	228.4	392.3
Lateral row	302.4	268.4	345.0
Shoulder press	130.7	122.0	224.5
Lateral pull-down	430.9	354.7	550.9
Knee extension	198.4	159.4	233.5
Knee flexion	182.0	155.5	259.5

[a]Values of endurance measured in ft-lb at dial setting 3 on the Omni-tron [b]Average age for females = 15.1 ± 2.6 years; for males = 15.8 ± 2.7 years; [c]Average age for females = 38.2 ± 9.7 years; for males = 37.6 ± 9.6 years; [d]Average age for females = 21.2 ± 2.0 years; for males = 20.6 ± 2.1 years; [e]Values of power measured in ft-lb at dial setting 6 on the Omni-tron;

APPENDIX C.2   BASIC STATIC (ISOMETRIC) EXERCISES

Exercise 1:   Chest Push

Muscle groups: Shoulder and elbow flexors

Equipment: None

Description:

1. Lock hands together.
2. Keep forearms parallel to ground and hands close to chest.
3. Push hands together.

Exercise 2:   Shoulder Pull

Muscle groups: Shoulder and elbow flexors

Equipment: None

Description:

1. Using same position as in chest push, attempt to pull hands apart

Exercise 3:   Triceps Extension

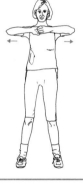

Muscle groups: Elbow extensors

Equipment: Towel or rope

Description:

1. Placing left hand over shoulder and right hand at small of back, grasp rope or towel behind back.
2. Attempt to pull towel upward with left hand.
3. Change position of hands.

Exercise 4:   Arm Curls

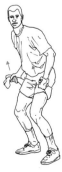

Muscle groups: Elbow flexors

Equipment: Towel or rope

Description:

1. Stand with knees flexed about 45°.
2. Place rope or towel behind thighs and grasp each end with hands shoulder-width apart.
3. Attempt to flex elbows.

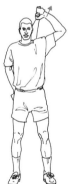

Exercise 5:   Ball Squeeze

Muscle groups: Wrist and finger flexors

Equipment: Tennis ball

Description:

1. Hold tennis ball firmly in hand and squeeze maximally.

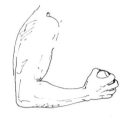

Exercise 6:   Leg and Thigh Extensions

Muscle groups: Hip and knee extensors

Equipment: Rope

Description:

1. Stand on rope with knees flexed.
2. Grasp rope firmly with hands at sides, elbows fully extended.
3. Keeping trunk erect, attempt to extend legs by lifting upward.

Exercise 7:   Leg Press

Muscle groups: Hip and knee extensors

Equipment: Doorway

Description:

1. Sit in doorway facing side of door frame.
2. Grasp door frame behind head.
3. Attempt to extend legs by pushing feet against door frame.

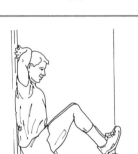

Exercise 8:   Leg Curl

Muscle groups: Knee flexors

Equipment: Dresser

Description:

1. Pull out lower dresser drawer slightly.
2. Lying prone, with knees flexed, hook heels under bottom of drawer.
3. Attempt to pull heels toward head.

Exercise 9:   Knee Squeeze or Pull

Muscle groups: Hip adductors or abductors

Equipment: Chair

Description:

1. Sitting on chair with forearms crossed and hands on inside of knees, attempt to squeeze knees together (adductors).
2. Same position but place hands on outside of knees; attempt to pull knees apart (abductors).

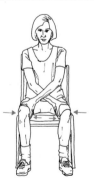

Exercise 10:   Pelvic Tilt

Muscle groups: Abdominals

Equipment: None

Description:

1. Supine with knees flexed and arms overhead.

2. Tighten abdominal muscles while pressing lower back into floor.

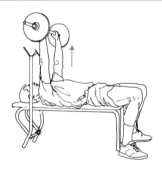

Exercise 11:   Gluteal Squeeze

Muscle groups: Hip extensors and abductors

Equipment: None

Description:

1. Lie prone with legs together and fully extended.

2. Tighten and squeeze the buttocks together.

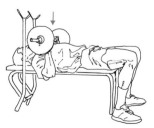

APPENDIX C.3   DYNAMIC RESISTANCE EXERCISES

Exercises in this section can be done with free weights or at an exercise station (for instance, on the Universal Gym). In many cases, the weights must be removed from a rack to begin a set and returned to the rack to end a set. An assistant ("spotter") should help with removal and return of the weights, if necessary.

CHEST AND SHOULDER REGIONS

Exercise 1: Bench Press

Muscle groups: Shoulder flexors and adductors; elbow extensors

Equipment: Barbell or bench press station

Starting position:

1. Pronated (overhand) grip—slightly wider than shoulder-width apart

2. Lying supine on bench, feet on floor astride bench

3. Hold bar at arm's length above chest.

Movement:

1. Lower the bar across chest.

2. Vigorously return to starting position.

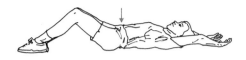

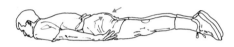

Exercise 2: Shoulder Shrugs

Muscle groups: Shoulder girdle elevators

Equipment: Barbell or bench press station

Starting position:

1. Pronated grip—slightly wider than shoulder-width apart, forearms extended, legs extended
2. Standing position, bar resting in front of thighs

Movement:

1. Lift and roll shoulders up and back.
2. Return to starting position.

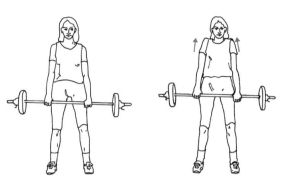

Exercise 3: Seated (Overhead) Press

Muscle groups: Shoulder flexors and abductors; elbow extensors

Equipment: Barbell or bench press station

Starting position:

1. Seated with feet on floor
2. Pronated grip—shoulder-width apart
3. Bar behind head

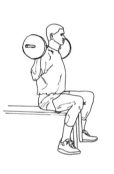
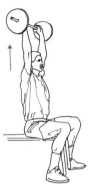

Movement:

1. Move the bar to overhead position until elbows are fully extended.
2. Return bar to base of neck.

Exercise 4: Upright Row

Muscle groups: Shoulder abductors and elbow flexors

Equipment: Barbell or curl station

Starting position:

1. Standing erect, feet apart
2. Overhand grip, hands close together near center of bar
3. Bar held at waist or hip level

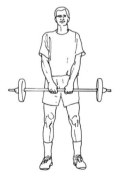
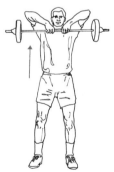

Movement:

1. Lift bar to chin level.
2. Keep elbows high and bar close to body.

UPPER AND LOWER BACK REGIONS

Exercise 1: Back Hypertension

Muscle groups: Trunk extensors

Equipment: Trunk lift station

Starting position:

1. Prone position with trunk unsupported over edge of support and flexed
2. Hands locked behind head

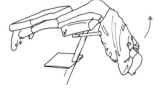
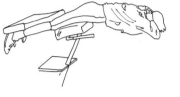

Movement:

1. Extended trunk so back is parallel to ground.
2. Return to starting position.

Exercise 2: Lat Pull-Down

Muscle groups: Shoulder extensors and adductors; elbow flexors

Equipment: Pull-down station

Starting position:

1. Sitting or kneeling on floor
2. Pronated grip—hands more than shoulder-width apart, elbows extended

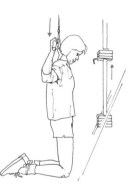

Movement:

1. Pull bar down to base of neck and shoulders.
2. Return to starting position.

Exercise 3: Bent-Over Row

Muscle groups: Shoulder extensors and elbow flexors

Equipment: Barbell or bench press station

Starting position:

1. Pronated grip wider than shoulder-width apart
2. Upper trunk parallel to floor
3. Feet spread shoulder-width apart

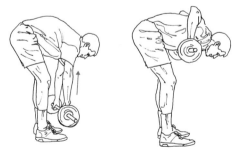

Movement:

1. Keeping trunk parallel to floor and knees extended, lift bar up to chest.
2. Return to starting position.

ABDOMINAL REGION

Exercise 1: Bent Knee Curl-Up

Muscle groups: Trunk flexors and hip flexors

Equipment: Sit-up station

Starting position:

1. Supine hook-lying position on incline board
2. Hands and additional weight plates folded across chest

Movement:

1. Keeping your middle and low back flat on the board, raise your head and shoulders off the board.
2. Return to starting position.

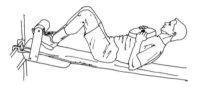

Exercise 2: Reverse Sit-Up

Muscle groups: Hip flexors and lower abdominals

Equipment: Sit-up station

Starting position:

1. Lying supine on incline board, knees extended
2. Grasp handle above foot rest.

Movement:

1. Flex hips, keeping legs straight, raise buttocks.
2. Return to starting position.

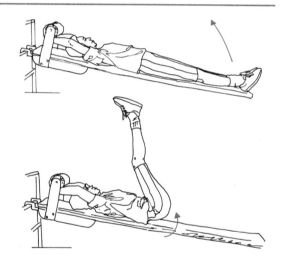

ARM REGION

Exercise 1: Arm Curl

Muscle groups: Elbow flexors

Equipment: Barbell or curl station

Starting position:

1. Standing with elbows extended fully and in front of thighs
2. Supinated grip—shoulder-width apart

Movement:

1. Flex the elbows, raising bar to chest; do not lean backward.
2. Return to starting position.

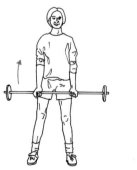
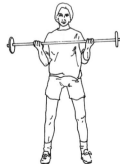

Exercise 2: Triceps Press-Down

Muscle groups: Elbow extensors

Equipment: Pull-down station

Starting position:

1. Standing with knees extended
2. Pronated grip, hands close together, elbows in close to body, bar about face level

Movement:

1. Fully extend elbows, pressing bar down.
2. Return to starting position.

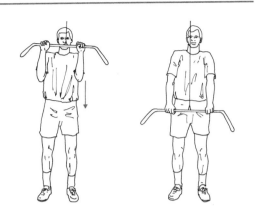

HIP AND THIGH REGIONS

Exercise 1: Leg Curl

Muscle groups: Knee flexors

Equipment: Leg machine

Starting position:

1. Prone on table, hook heels under support

Movement:

1. Flex knees keeping hips flat on table.
2. Return to starting position.

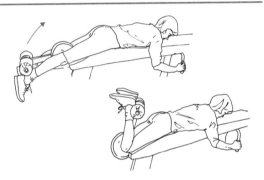

Exercise 2: Leg Extension

Muscle groups: Leg extensors

Equipment: Leg machine

Starting position:

1. Sitting on end of table with knees flexed at 90°, grasp sides of table.
2. Hook ankles under support.

Movement:

1. Fully extend knees, keeping trunk erect.
2. Return to starting position.

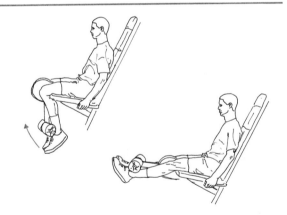

Exercise 3: Seated Leg Press

Muscle groups: Knee extensors and hip extensors

Equipment: Leg press station

Starting position:

1. Grasp handles on seat.
2. Place feet on foot rests.

Movement:

1. Fully extend legs and thighs.
2. Return to starting position.

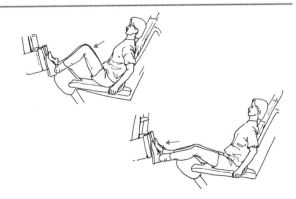

Exercise 4: Side Leg Raises

Muscle groups: Hip abductors or adductors

Equipment: Pulley station

Starting position:

1. Standing with side to pulley, hook ankle of either inside leg (for adductors) or outside leg (for abductors) to pulley.

Movement:

1. Fully adduct (abduct) the leg.
2. Return to starting position.

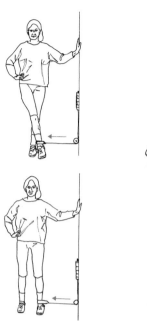

Exercise 5: Half Squat

Muscle groups: Hip, knee, and trunk extensors

Equipment: Barbell

Starting position:

1. Standing erect, feet shoulder-width apart, place bar on shoulders behind neck.
2. Use pronated grip and spread hands far apart on bar.

Movement:

1. Keeping back straight and head up, lower bar by flexing knees to 90°.
2. Return to starting position.

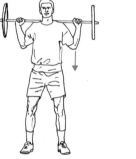
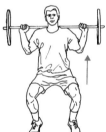

LEG REGION

Exercise 1: Toe (Heel) Raises

Muscle groups: Ankle plantar flexors

Equipment: Press station or barbell

Starting position:

1. Standing with balls of feet on board, feet apart, and knees extended
2. Grasp bar shoulder-width apart using pronated grip; rest bar on shoulders.

Movement:

1. Rise up on toes without moving shoulders.
2. Return, lowering heels to floor.

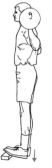
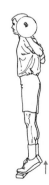

Body Composition Assessments

APPENDIX D.1   DENSITY OF WATER AT DIFFERENT TEMPERATURES

Temperature (°C)	Density (g · cc⁻¹)
21	0.9980
22	0.9978
23	0.9975
24	0.9973
25	0.9971
26	0.9968
27	0.9965
28	0.9963
29	0.9960
30	0.9957
31	0.9954
32	0.9951
33	0.9947
34	0.9944
35	0.9941
36	0.9937
37	0.9934
38	0.9930
39	0.9926
40	0.9922

Reprinted, with permission, from R.C. Weast (ed.), 1988-89, *CRC Handbook of Chemistry and Physics*, 69th ed. Copyright CRC Press, Boca Raton, Florida: © 1989, F-10.

APPENDIX D.2   PREDICTION EQUATIONS FOR RESIDUAL VOLUME (RV)

Population	Smoking history[a]	N	Equation[b]
Men			
Boren, Kory, and Syner (1966)	Mixed	422	$RV = 0.0115(Age) + 0.019(HT) - 2.24$ $R = .57$, $SEE = 0.53$ L
Women			
O'Brien & Drizd (1983)	Nonsmokers	926	$RV = 0.03(Age) + 0.0387(HT) - 0.73(BSA) - 4.78$ $R = .66$, $SEE = 0.49$ L
Black, Offord, and Hyatt (1974)	Mixed	110	$RV = 0.021(Age) + 0.023(HT) - 2.978$ $R = .70$, $SEE = 0.46$ L

[a]Mixed indicates that sample included both smokers and nonsmokers.

[b]For each equation, Age (in years); HT = height (in cm); BSA = body surface area (in m^2)

APPENDIX D.3 STANDARDIZED SITES FOR SKINFOLD MEASUREMENTS

Site	Direction of fold	Anatomical reference	Measurement
Chest	Diagonal	Axilla and nipple	Fold is taken between axilla and nipple as high as possible on anterior axillary fold with measurement taken 1 cm below fingers.
Subscapular	Diagonal	Inferior angle of scapula	Fold is along natural cleavage line of skin just inferior to inferior angle of scapula, with caliper applied 1 cm below fingers.
Midaxillary	Horizontal	Xiphisternal junction (point where costal cartilage of ribs 5-6 articulate with sternum, slightly above inferior tip of xiphoid process)	Fold is taken on midaxillary line at level of xiphisternal junction.
Suprailiac	Oblique	Iliac crest	Fold is grasped posteriorly to midaxillary line and superiorly to iliac crest along natural cleavage of skin with caliper applied 1 cm below fingers.
Abdominal	Horizontal	Umbilicus	Fold is taken 3 cm lateral and 1 cm inferior to center of the umbilicus.
Triceps	Vertical (midline)	Acromial process of scapula and olecranon process of ulna	Distance between lateral projection of acromial process and inferior margin of olecranon process is measured on lateral aspect of arm with elbow flexed 90° using a tape measure. Midpoint is marked on lateral side of arm. Fold is lifted 1 cm above marked line on posterior aspect of arm. Caliper is applied at marked level.
Biceps	Vertical (midline)	Biceps brachii	Fold is lifted over belly of the biceps brachii at the level marked for the triceps and on line with anterior border of the acromial process and the antecubital fossa. Caliper is applied 1 cm below fingers.
Thigh	Vertical (midline)	Inguinal crease and patella	Fold is lifted on anterior aspect of thigh midway between inguinal crease and proximal border of patella. Body weight is shifted to left foot and caliper is applied 1 cm below fingers.
Calf	Vertical (medial aspect)	Maximal calf circumference	Fold is lifted at level of maximal calf circumference on medial aspect of calf with knee and hip flexed to 90°.

Adapted from Harrison et al. (1988, pp. 55-70)

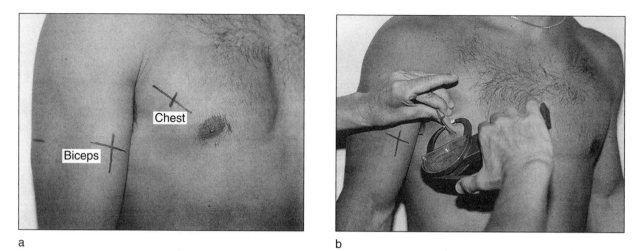

Figure D.3.1   (a) Site and (b) measurement of the chest skinfold. Photos courtesy of Linda K. Gilkey.

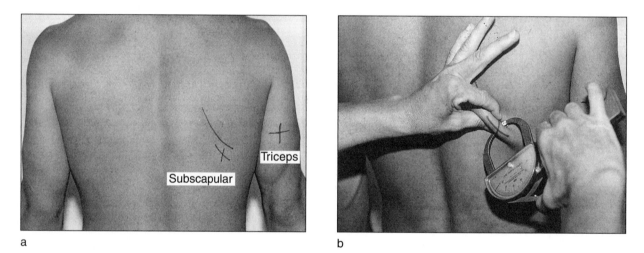

Figure D.3.2   (a) Site and (b) measurement of subscapular skinfold. Photos courtesy of Linda K. Gilkey.

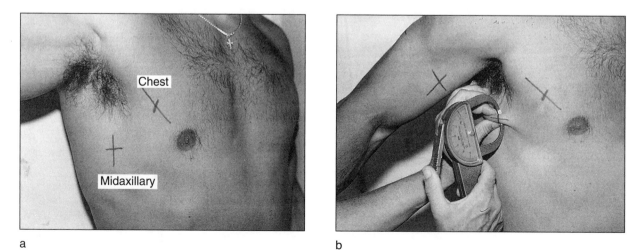

Figure D.3.3   (a) Site and (b) measurement of the midaxillary skinfold. Photos courtesy of Linda K. Gilkey.

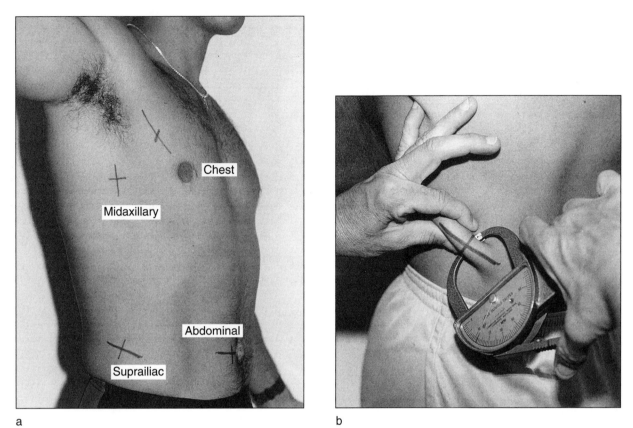

a   b

Figure D.3.4   (a) Site and (b) measurement of the suprailiac skinfold. Photos courtesy of Linda K. Gilkey.

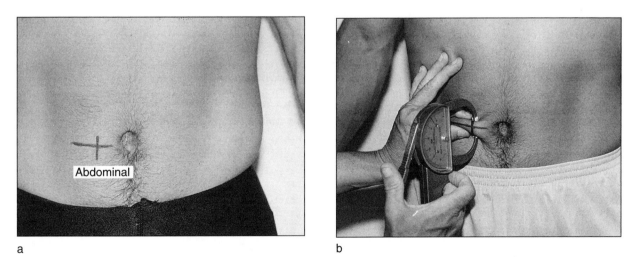

a   b

Figure D.3.5   (a) Site and (b) measurement of the abdominal skinfold. Photos courtesy of Linda K. Gilkey.

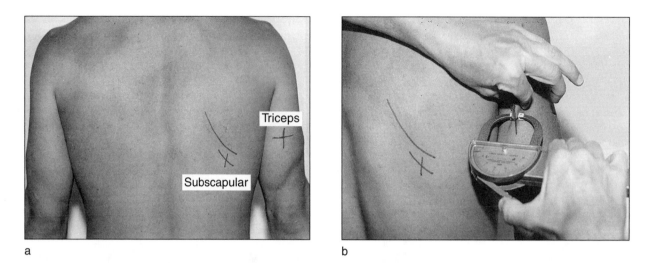

Figure D.3.6 (a) Site and (b) measurement of the triceps skinfold. Photos courtesy of Linda K. Gilkey.

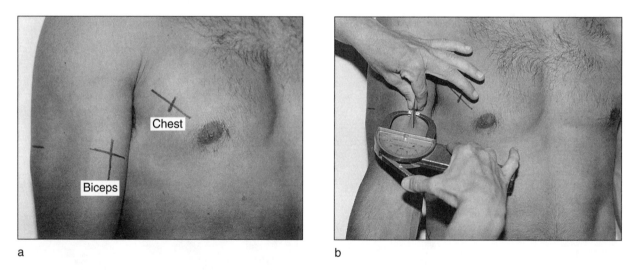

Figure D.3.7 (a) Site and (b) measurement of the biceps skinfold. Photos courtesy of Linda K. Gilkey.

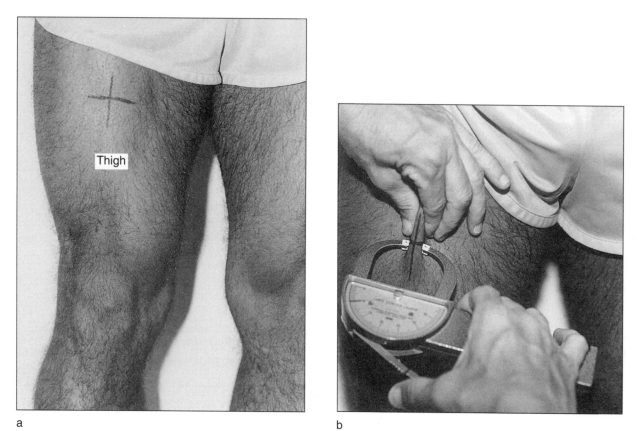

Figure D.3.8   (a) Site and (b) measurement of the thigh skinfold. Photos courtesy of Linda K. Gilkey.

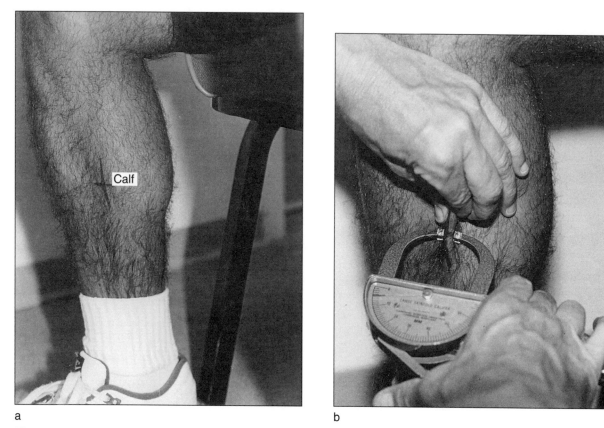

Figure D.3.9   (a) Site and (b) measurement of the calf skinfold. Photos courtesy of Linda K. Gilkey.

APPENDIX D.4   SKINFOLD SITES FOR JACKSON'S GENERALIZED SKINFOLD EQUATIONS

Site	Direction of fold	Anatomical reference	Measurement
Chest	Diagonal	Axilla and nipple	Fold is taken 1/2 the distance between the anterior axillary line and nipple for men and 1/3 of this distance for women.
Subscapular	Oblique	Vertebral border and inferior angle of scapula	Fold is taken on diagonal line coming from the vertebral border, 1-2 cm below the inferior angle.
Midaxillary	Vertical	Xiphoid process of sternum	Fold is taken at level of xiphoid process along the midaxillary line.
Suprailiac	Diagonal	Iliac crest	Fold is taken diagonally above the iliac crest along the anterior axillary line.
Abdominal	Vertical	Umbilicus	Fold is taken vertically 2 cm lateral to the umbilicus.

Adapted from Jackson and Pollock (1978) and Jackson, Pollock, and Ward (1980)

APPENDIX D.5   STANDARDIZED SITES FOR CIRCUMFERENCE MEASUREMENTS

Site	Anatomical reference	Position	Measurement
Neck	Laryngeal prominence "Adam's apple"	Perpendicular to long axis of neck	Apply tape with minimal pressure just inferior to the Adam's apple.
Shoulder	Deltoid muscles and acromion processes of scapula	Horizontal	Apply tape snugly over maximum bulges of the deltoid muscles, inferior to acromion processes. Record measurement at end of normal expiration.
Chest	Fourth costo-sternal joints	Horizontal	Apply tape snugly around the torso at level of fourth costo-sternal joints. Record at end of normal expiration.
Waist	Narrowest part of torso, level of the "natural" waist between ribs and iliac crest.	Horizontal	Apply tape snugly around the waist at level of narrowest part of torso. An assistant is needed to position tape behind the client. Take measurement at end of normal expiration.
Abdominal	Maximum anterior protuberance of abdomen, usually at umbilicus	Horizontal	Apply tape snugly around the abdomen at level of greatest anterior protuberance. An assistant is needed to position tape behind the client. Take measurement at the end of normal expiration.
Hip (*Buttocks*)	Maximum posterior extension of buttocks	Horizontal	Apply tape snugly around the buttocks. An assistant is needed to position tape on opposite side of body.
Thigh *proximal*	Gluteal fold	Horizontal	Apply tape snugly around thigh, just distal to the gluteal fold.
mid	Inguinal crease and proximal border of patella	Horizontal	With client's knee flexed 90° (right foot on bench), apply tape at level midway between inguinal crease and proximal border of patella.
distal	Femoral epicondyles	Horizontal	Apply tape just proximal to the femoral epicondyles.
Knee	Patella	Horizontal	Apply tape around the knee at mid-patellar level with knee relaxed in slight flexion.
Calf	Maximum girth of calf muscle	Perpendicular to long axis of leg	With client sitting on end of table, and legs hanging freely, apply tape horizontally around the maximum girth of calf.
Ankle	Malleoli of tibia and fibula	Perpendicular to long axis of leg	Apply tape snugly around minimum circumference of leg, just proximal to the malleoli.
Arm (*Biceps*)	Acromion process of scapula and olecranon process of ulna	Perpendicular to long axis of arm	With arms hanging freely at sides and palms facing thighs, apply tape snugly around the arm at level midway between the acromion process of scapula and olecranon process of ulna (as marked for triceps and biceps SKFs).
Forearm	Maximum girth of forearm	Perpendicular to long axis of forearm	With arms hanging down and away from trunk and forearm supinated, apply tape snugly around the maximum girth of the proximal part of the forearm.
Wrist	Styloid processes of radius and ulna	Perpendicular to long axis of forearm	With elbow flexed and forearm supinated, apply tape snugly around the wrist, just distal to the styloid processes of the radius and ulna.

Adapted from Callaway et al. (1988, pp. 41-53)

APPENDIX D.6   STANDARDIZED SITES FOR BONY BREADTH MEASUREMENTS

Site	Anatomical reference	Position	Measurement
Biacromial (*Shoulder*)	Lateral borders of acromion processes of scapula	Horizontal	With client standing, arms hanging vertically and shoulders relaxed downward and slightly forward, apply blades of anthropometer to lateral borders of acromion processes. Measurement is taken from the rear.
Chest	Sixth rib on midaxillary line or fourth costo-sternal joints anteriorly	Horizontal	With client standing, arms slightly abducted, apply the large spreading caliper tips lightly on the sixth ribs on the midaxillary line. Take measurement at end of normal expiration.
Bi-iliac (*Bicristal*)	Iliac crests	45° downward angle	With client standing, arms folded across the chest, apply anthropometer blades firmly at a 45° downward angle, at maximum breadth of iliac crest. Measurement is taken from rear.
Bitrochanteric	Greater trochanter of femur	Horizontal	With client standing, arms folded across the chest, apply anthropometer blade with considerable pressure to compress soft tissues. Measure maximum distance between the trochanters from the rear.
Knee	Femoral epicondyles	Diagonal or horizontal	With client sitting and knee flexed to 90°, apply caliper blades firmly on lateral and medial femoral epicondyles.
Ankle (*Bimalleolar*)	Malleoli of tibia and fibula	Oblique	With client standing and weight evenly distributed, place the caliper blades on the most lateral part of lateral malleolus and most medial part of medial malleolus. Measurement is taken on an oblique plane from the rear.
Elbow	Epicondyles of humerus	Oblique	With client's elbow flexed 90°, arm raised to the horizontal, and forearm supinated, apply the caliper blades firmly to the medial and lateral humeral epicondyles at an angle that bisects the right angle at the elbow.
Wrist	Styloid processes of radius and ulna, anatomical "snuff box"	Oblique	With client's elbow flexed 90°, upper arm vertical and close to torso, and forearm pronated, apply caliper tips firmly at an oblique angle to the styloid processes of the radius (at proximal part of anatomical snuff box) and ulna.

Adapted from Wilmore et al. (1988, pp. 28-38)

Energy Intake and Expenditure

Food code	Amount	Description

Number of servings _____

Food code: This is generally for our office use. For those with the food code list, however, use this space to more precisely describe your food item.

Amount: You can use common measures (cup, slice, etc.) or weight for your foods.

Food description: Be specific. For example, bread choices include soft and firm textures; vegetables may be raw, cooked fresh, frozen, or canned; meats should be lean only or lean with some fat; fruit juices are fresh, frozen, or canned; and cheese might be cream or skim, soft, hard, or cottage.

RDA Profile Information

Name: _____
      (please print)

Age: _____   Height: _____

Sex: Male _____   Weight: _____

       Female _____   Activity level: _____
                              (enter number from choices listed below)

       Pregnant _____

       Nursing _____

Most people engage in a variety of activities in a 24-hour period, and each activity can use a different amount of energy. Thus, any table of activity levels must depend on averages. Choose the level that represents your *normal daily average*.

1. Sedentary

   Inactive, sometimes under someone else's care. Energy level is for basal metabolism plus about 15% for minimal activities.

2. Lightly active

   Most professionals (lawyers, doctors, accountants, architects, etc.), office workers, shop workers, teachers, housewives with mechanical appliances, unemployed persons.

3. Moderately active

   Most persons in light industry, building workers (excluding heavy laborers), many farm workers, active students, department store workers, soldiers not in active service, commercial fishermen, housewives without mechanical household appliances.

4. Very active

   Full-time athletes, dancers, unskilled laborers, some agricultural workers (especially in peasant farming), forestry workers, army recruits, soldiers in active services, mine workers, steel workers.

5. Exceptionlly active

   Lumberjacks, blacksmiths, women construction workers, rickshaw pullers.

Courtesy of ESHA Research, 606 Juntura Way SE, Salem, OR 97302, phone: (503) 585-6242

APPENDIX E.2   SAMPLE COMPUTERIZED ANALYSIS OF FOOD INTAKE

Jane Doe   Personal Profile Report

Gender:	Female
Activity Level:	Lightly Active
Height:	5 ft 3 in
Weight:	132 lbs
Age:	25 yrs
BMI:	23.38

Recommended Daily Nutrients

Basic Components

Calories	2044		*
Protein	47.9	g	
Carbohydrates	296	g	**
Dietary Fiber	20	g	#
Fat - Total	68	g	**
Saturated Fat	20	g	**
Mono Fat	25	g	**
Poly Fat	23	g	**
Cholesterol	300	mg	

Vitamins

Vitamin A IU	4000	IU	
Vitamin A RE	800	RE	
Thiamin-B1	1.02	mg	
Riboflavin-B2	1.23	mg	
Niacin	13.49	NE	
Vitamin-B6	1.60	mg	
Vitamin-B12	2.00	mcg	
Biotin	65.00	mcg**	
Vitamin C	60.00	mg	

Vitamin D mcg	5.00	mcg	
Vit E-Alpha Equiv.	8.00	mg	
Folate	180.00	mcg	
Vitamin K	6.00	mcg	
Pantothenic	7.00	mg	**

Minerals

Calcium	800.00	mg	
Chromium	125.00	mcg**	
Copper	2.50	mg	**
Fluoride	2.75	mg	**
Iodine	150	mcg	
Iron	15	mg	
Magnesium	280	mg	
Manganese	3.50	mg	**
Molybdenum	163	mcg**	
Phosphorus	800	mg	
Potassium	3750	mg	
Selenium	55	mcg	
Sodium	2400	mg	
Zinc	12	mg	

*   Suggested Values within recommended ranges
**   Dietary Goals   # Fiber = 1 gram/100 kcal

The Food Processor® Nutrition Analysis program from ESHA Research, Salem, Oregon.

Daily Intake

June 23, 1997

Ratios and Percents

Source of Calories

	0	25	50	75	100

Nutrient	%	
Protein	19%	
Carbohydrates	58%	
Fat - Total	22%	
Alcohol	0%	

Source of Fat

	0	6	11	17	22

Nutrient	%	
Saturated (7 - 10%)	10%	
Mono Unsat (10 - 15%)	6%	
Poly Unsat (up to 10%)	4%	
Other/Missing	2%	

Exchanges

Bread / Starch:	8.0	Fruit:	4.6
Other Carbs / Sugar:	2.6	Vegetables:	3.8
Very Lean Meat / Protein:	4.5	Milk - Skim:	0.5
Lean Meat:	2.9	Fat:	5.4

Ratios

P : S (Poly / Saturated Fat)	0.39 : 1
Potassium : Sodium	1.61 : 1
Calcium : Phosphorus	0.53 : 1
CSI (Cholesterol / Saturated Fat Index)	28.21

Daily Intake

June 23, 1997

% comparison to: Jane Doe

Bar Graph

Nutrient	Value	Goal %	0	25	50	75	100
Basic Components							
Calories	1691.39	83%					
Protein	84.04 g	175%					
Carbohydrates	251.82 g	85%					
Dietary Fiber	20.71 g	101%					
Fat - Total	42.41 g	62%					
Saturated Fat	19.24 g	94%					
Mono Fat	11.86 g	47%					
Poly Fat	7.47 g	33%					
Cholesterol	175.49 mg	58%					
Vitamins							
Vitamin A RE	1326.90 RE	166%					
Thiamin-B1	1.79 mg	176%					
Riboflavin-B2	2.11 mg	171%					
Niacin-B3	37.54 mg	278%					
Vitamin-B6	3.37 mg	211%					
Vitamin-B12	2.55 mcg	127%					
Vitamin C	266.19 mg	444%					
Vitamin D mcg	7.07 mcg	141%					
Vit E-Alpha Equiv.	3.79 mg	47%					
Folate	440.36 mcg	245%					
Pantothenic Acid	4.87 mg	70%					
Minerals							
Calcium	665.59 mg	83%					
Copper	1.24 mg	49%					
Iron	12.83 mg	86%					
Magnesium	267.18 mg	95%					
Manganese	2.25 mg	64%					
Phosphorus	1254.53 mg	157%					
Potassium	3187.63 mg	85%					
Selenium	144.48 mcg	263%					
Sodium	1974.93 mg	82%					
Zinc	5.78 mg	48%					

Daily Intake

Spreadsheet

Amount	Food Item	Weight (g)	Cals	Prot (g)	Carb (g)	Fiber (g)	Fat-T (g)
1/2 cup	Orange Juice prepared from frozen	124.50	56.03	0.85	13.45	0.25	0.07
2 oz-wt	Kelloggs Corn Flakes Cereal	56.70	220.56	4.59	48.82	1.47	0.17
1 each	Banana--Medium size	118.00	108.56	1.22	27.61	2.83	0.57
1/2 cup	Skim Milk-Vitamin A Added	122.50	42.75	4.18	5.94	0	0.22
1 piece	Whole Wheat Bread-Toasted	25.00	69.25	2.73	12.93	1.85	1.20
2 tsp	Jelly	12.67	34.33	0.05	8.97	0.13	0.01
1 each	White Pita Pocket Bread 6 1/2"diameter	60.00	165.00	5.46	33.42	1.32	0.72
1/2 cup	Tuna Salad	102.50	191.67	16.40	9.65	0	9.49
1/4 cup	Alfalfa Sprouts-Raw	8.25	2.39	0.33	0.31	0.21	0.06
2 piece	Fresh Tomato Wedge(1/4 of Medium Tomato)	62.00	13.02	0.53	2.88	0.68	0.20
8 oz-wt	Diet soda pop - average assorted	226.80	0	0	0	0	0
1 each	Medium Apple w/Peel	138.00	81.42	0.26	21.11	3.73	0.50
4 oz-wt	Chicken light meat - roasted	113.40	173.50	30.73	0	0	4.62
1 each	Baked Potato w/skin - medium	122.00	132.98	2.82	30.74	2.93	0.12
1 oz-wt	Cheddar Cheese-Shredded	28.35	114.25	7.06	0.36	0	9.38
4 oz-wt	Broccoli Pieces-Steamed	113.40	31.75	3.39	5.95	3.40	0.40
1/2 cup	Rich Vanilla Ice Cream	74.00	178.34	2.59	16.58	0	11.99
1/2 cup	Fresh Strawberries-Slices-Cup	83.00	24.90	0.51	5.83	1.91	0.31
2 tbs	Frozen Dessert Topping-Semi Solid	9.38	29.81	0.12	2.17	0	2.37
1 cup	Brewed Coffee	237.00	4.74	0.24	0.95	0	0.01
1 tsp	White Granulated Sugar	4.17	16.13	0	4.16	0	0
	Totals	1841.61	1691.39	84.04	251.82	20.71	42.41

Amount	Food Item	Fat-S (g)	Fat-M (g)	Fat-P (g)	Chol (mg)	A-RE (RE)	B1 (mg)
1/2 cup	Orange Juice prepared from frozen	0.01	0.01	0.01	0	9.96	0.10
2 oz-wt	Kelloggs Corn Flakes Cereal	0.02	0.09	0.03	0	750.71	0.74
1 each	Banana--Medium size	0.22	0.05	0.11	0	9.44	0.05
1/2 cup	Skim Milk-Vitamin A Added	0.14	0.06	0.01	2.21	74.73	0.04
1 piece	Whole Wheat Bread-Toasted	0.26	0.47	0.28	0	0	0.08
2 tsp	Jelly	0.00	0.00	0.01	0	0.25	0.00
1 each	White Pita Pocket Bread 6 1/2"diameter	0.10	0.06	0.32	0	0	0.36
1/2 cup	Tuna Salad	1.58	2.96	4.22	13.32	27.67	0.03
1/4 cup	Alfalfa Sprouts-Raw	0.01	0.00	0.03	0	1.32	0.01
2 piece	Fresh Tomato Wedge(1/4 of Medium Tomato)	0.03	0.03	0.08	0	38.44	0.04
8 oz-wt	Diet soda pop - average assorted	0	0	0	0	0	0
1 each	Medium Apple w/Peel	0.08	0.02	0.14	0	6.90	0.02
4 oz-wt	Chicken light meat - roasted	1.24	1.75	1.05	85.05	9.07	0.07
1 each	Baked Potato w/skin - medium	0.03	0.00	0.05	0	0	0.13
1 oz-wt	Cheddar Cheese-Shredded	6.01	2.66	0.27	29.77	85.90	0.01
4 oz-wt	Broccoli Pieces-Steamed	0.06	0.03	0.19	0	165.79	0.07
1/2 cup	Rich Vanilla Ice Cream	7.39	3.45	0.45	45.14	136.16	0.03
1/2 cup	Fresh Strawberries-Slices-Cup	0.02	0.04	0.15	0	2.49	0.02
2 tbs	Frozen Dessert Topping-Semi Solid	2.05	0.15	0.05	0	8.06	0
1 cup	Brewed Coffee	0.00	0	0.00	0	0	0
1 tsp	White Granulated Sugar	0	0	0	0	0	0
	Totals	19.24	11.86	7.47	175.49	1326.90	1.79

The Food Processor® Nutrition Analysis program from ESHA Research, Salem, Oregon.

Daily Intake

June 23, 1997

Spreadsheet

Amount	Food Item	B2 (mg)	B3 (mg)	B6 (mg)	B12 (mcg)	Vit C (mg)	D-mcg (mcg)
1/2 cup	Orange Juice prepared from frozen	0.02	0.25	0.05	0	48.43	0
2 oz-wt	Kelloggs Corn Flakes Cereal	0.86	9.98	1.02	0	30.05	1.98
1 each	Banana--Medium size	0.12	0.64	0.68	0	10.74	0
1/2 cup	Skim Milk-Vitamin A Added	0.17	0.11	0.05	0.46	1.20	1.23
1 piece	Whole Wheat Bread-Toasted	0.05	0.97	0.05	0.00	0	0.05
2 tsp	Jelly	0.00	0.00	0.00	0	0.11	0
1 each	White Pita Pocket Bread 6 1/2"diameter	0.20	2.78	0.02	0	0	0
1/2 cup	Tuna Salad	0.07	6.87	0.08	1.23	2.25	3.31
1/4 cup	Alfalfa Sprouts-Raw	0.01	0.04	0.00	0	0.68	0
2 piece	Fresh Tomato Wedge(1/4 of Medium Tomato)	0.03	0.39	0.05	0	11.84	0
8 oz-wt	Diet soda pop - average assorted	0	0	0	0	0	0
1 each	Medium Apple w/Peel	0.02	0.11	0.07	0	7.87	0
4 oz-wt	Chicken light meat - roasted	0.11	11.91	0.61	0.35	0	0.34
1 each	Baked Potato w/skin - medium	0.04	2.01	0.42	0	15.74	0
1 oz-wt	Cheddar Cheese-Shredded	0.11	0.02	0.02	0.23	0	0.09
4 oz-wt	Broccoli Pieces-Steamed	0.13	0.69	0.16	0	89.70	0
1/2 cup	Rich Vanilla Ice Cream	0.12	0.06	0.03	0.27	0.52	0.07
1/2 cup	Fresh Strawberries-Slices-Cup	0.05	0.19	0.05	0	47.06	0
2 tbs	Frozen Dessert Topping-Semi Solid	0	0	0	0	0	0
1 cup	Brewed Coffee	0	0.53	0	0	0	0
1 tsp	White Granulated Sugar	0.00	0	0	0	0	0
	Totals	2.11	37.54	3.37	2.55	266.19	7.07

Amount	Food Item	E-aTE (mg)	Fola (mcg)	Panto (mg)	Calc (mg)	Copp (mg)	Iron (mg)
1/2 cup	Orange Juice prepared from frozen	0.24	54.53	0.20	11.21	0.05	0.12
2 oz-wt	Kelloggs Corn Flakes Cereal	0.14	200.15	0.10	1.70	0.04	3.58
1 each	Banana--Medium size	0.32	22.54	0.31	7.08	0.12	0.37
1/2 cup	Skim Milk-Vitamin A Added	0.05	6.37	0.40	150.68	0.01	0.05
1 piece	Whole Wheat Bread-Toasted	0.23	9.75	0.10	20.25	0.08	0.93
2 tsp	Jelly	0	0.13	0.02	1.01	0.00	0.03
1 each	White Pita Pocket Bread 6 1/2"diameter	0.02	14.40	0.24	51.60	0.10	1.57
1/2 cup	Tuna Salad	0.97	7.48	0.27	17.42	0.15	1.02
1/4 cup	Alfalfa Sprouts-Raw	0.00	2.97	0.05	2.64	0.01	0.08
2 piece	Fresh Tomato Wedge(1/4 of Medium Tomato)	0.24	9.30	0.15	3.10	0.05	0.28
8 oz-wt	Diet soda pop - average assorted	0	0	0	0	0	0
1 each	Medium Apple w/Peel	0.44	3.86	0.08	9.66	0.06	0.25
4 oz-wt	Chicken light meat - roasted	0.30	3.40	1.03	14.74	0.05	1.22
1 each	Baked Potato w/skin - medium	0.06	13.42	0.68	12.20	0.37	1.66
1 oz-wt	Cheddar Cheese-Shredded	0.10	5.16	0.12	204.40	0.01	0.19
4 oz-wt	Broccoli Pieces-Steamed	0.54	68.27	0.58	54.32	0.05	1.00
1/2 cup	Rich Vanilla Ice Cream	0	3.70	0.27	86.58	0.02	0.04
1/2 cup	Fresh Strawberries-Slices-Cup	0.12	14.69	0.28	11.62	0.04	0.32
2 tbs	Frozen Dessert Topping-Semi Solid	0.02	0	0	0.59	0.00	0.01
1 cup	Brewed Coffee	0	0.24	0.00	4.74	0.02	0.12
1 tsp	White Granulated Sugar	0	0	0	0.04	0.00	0.00
	Totals	3.79	440.36	4.87	665.59	1.24	12.83

Daily Intake

June 23, 1997

Spreadsheet

Amount	Food Item	Magn (mg)	Mang (mg)	Phos (mg)	Potas (mg)	Sel (mcg)	Sod (mg)
1/2 cup	Orange Juice prepared from frozen	12.45	0.02	19.92	236.55	0.25	1.25
2 oz-wt	Kelloggs Corn Flakes Cereal	6.80	0.05	35.72	52.16	2.89	580.04
1 each	Banana--Medium size	34.22	0.18	23.60	467.28	1.18	1.18
1/2 cup	Skim Milk-Vitamin A Added	13.97	0.00	123.73	203.35	1.23	63.09
1 piece	Whole Wheat Bread-Toasted	24.25	0.65	64.50	70.75	10.25	148.00
2 tsp	Jelly	0.76	0.02	0.63	8.11	0.25	4.56
1 each	White Pita Pocket Bread 6 1/2"diameter	15.60	0.29	58.20	72.00	18.00	321.60
1/2 cup	Tuna Salad	19.47	0.04	182.45	182.45	70.01	412.05
1/4 cup	Alfalfa Sprouts-Raw	2.23	0.02	5.78	6.52	--	0.50
2 piece	Fresh Tomato Wedge(1/4 of Medium Tomato)	6.82	0.07	14.88	137.64	0.25	5.58
8 oz-wt	Diet soda pop - average assorted	0	0	90.72	34.02	0	113.40
1 each	Medium Apple w/Peel	6.90	0.06	9.66	158.70	0.41	0
4 oz-wt	Chicken light meat - roasted	26.08	0.02	246.08	267.62	28.92	57.83
1 each	Baked Potato w/skin - medium	32.94	0.28	69.54	509.96	1.95	9.76
1 oz-wt	Cheddar Cheese-Shredded	7.88	0.00	145.15	27.90	4.03	176.05
4 oz-wt	Broccoli Pieces-Steamed	28.35	0.25	74.73	367.42	--	30.62
1/2 cup	Rich Vanilla Ice Cream	8.14	0.01	70.30	117.66	4.00	41.44
1/2 cup	Fresh Strawberries-Slices-Cup	8.30	0.24	15.77	137.78	0.75	0.83
2 tbs	Frozen Dessert Topping-Semi Solid	0.17	0.01	0.72	1.71	--	2.37
1 cup	Brewed Coffee	11.85	0.06	2.37	127.98	0.11	4.74
1 tsp	White Granulated Sugar	0	0.00	0.08	0.08	0.01	0.04
	Totals	267.18	2.25	1254.53	3187.63	144.48	1974.93

Amount	Food Item	Zinc (mg)
1/2 cup	Orange Juice prepared from frozen	0.06
2 oz-wt	Kelloggs Corn Flakes Cereal	0.16
1 each	Banana--Medium size	0.19
1/2 cup	Skim Milk-Vitamin A Added	0.49
1 piece	Whole Wheat Bread-Toasted	0.55
2 tsp	Jelly	0.01
1 each	White Pita Pocket Bread 6 1/2"diameter	0.50
1/2 cup	Tuna Salad	0.57
1/4 cup	Alfalfa Sprouts-Raw	0.08
2 piece	Fresh Tomato Wedge(1/4 of Medium Tomato)	0.06
8 oz-wt	Diet soda pop - average assorted	0
1 each	Medium Apple w/Peel	0.06
4 oz-wt	Chicken light meat - roasted	0.88
1 each	Baked Potato w/skin - medium	0.39
1 oz-wt	Cheddar Cheese-Shredded	0.88
4 oz-wt	Broccoli Pieces-Steamed	0.45
1/2 cup	Rich Vanilla Ice Cream	0.30
1/2 cup	Fresh Strawberries-Slices-Cup	0.11
2 tbs	Frozen Dessert Topping-Semi Solid	0.00
1 cup	Brewed Coffee	0.05
1 tsp	White Granulated Sugar	0.00
	Totals	5.78

The Food Processor® Nutrition Analysis program from ESHA Research, Salem, Oregon.

APPENDIX E.3   PHYSICAL ACTIVITY LOG

Name _____ Date _____

Day and date	Activity	Duration (min)	×	kcal/min	= Total (kcal)

APPENDIX E.4   COMPENDIUM OF PHYSICAL ACTIVITIES

Code	METs[a]	Activity	Description
01009	8.5	Bicycling	Bicycling, BMX or mountain
01010	4.0	Bicycling	Bicycling, general, <10 mph, leisure, to work or for pleasure (T 115)[b]
01020	6.0	Bicycling	Bicycling 10-11.9 mph, leisure, slow, light effort
01030	8.0	Bicycling	Bicycling 12-13.9 mph, leisure, moderate effort
01040	10.0	Bicycling	Bicycling 14-15.9 mph, racing or leisure, fast, vigorous effort
01050	12.0	Bicycling	Bicycling 16-19 mph, racing/not drafting or >19 mph drafting, very fast, racing general
01060	16.0	Bicycling	Bicycling >20 mph, racing, not drafting
01070	5.0	Bicycling	Unicycling
02010	5.0	Conditioning exercise	Bicycling, stationary, general
02011	3.0	Conditioning exercise	Bicycling, stationary, 50 watts, very light effort
02012	5.5	Conditioning exercise	Bicycling, stationary, 100 watts, light effort
02013	7.0	Conditioning exercise	Bicycling, stationary, 150 watts, moderate effort
02014	10.5	Conditioning exercise	Bicycling, stationary, 200 watts, vigorous effort
02015	12.5	Conditioning exercise	Bicycling, stationary, 250 watts, very vigorous effort
02020	8.0	Conditioning exercise	Calisthenics (e.g., pushups, pullups, situps), heavy, vigorous effort
02030	4.5	Conditioning exercise	Calisthenics, home exercise, light or moderate effort, general (T 150) (example: back exercises), going up and down from floor
02040	8.0	Conditioning exercise	Circuit training, general
02050	6.0	Conditioning exercise	Weight lifting (free weight, nautilus, or universal-type), power lifting or body building, vigorous effort (T 210)
02060	5.5	Conditioning exercise	Health club exercise, general (T 160)
02065	6.0	Conditioning exercise	Stair-treadmill ergometer, general
02070	9.5	Conditioning exercise	Rowing, stationary ergometer, general
02071	3.5	Conditioning exercise	Rowing, stationary, 50 watts, light effort
02072	7.0	Conditioning exercise	Rowing, stationary, 100 watts, moderate effort
02073	8.5	Conditioning exercise	Rowing, stationary, 150 watts, vigorous effort
02074	12.0	Conditioning exercise	Rowing, stationary, 200 watts, very vigorous effort
02080	9.5	Conditioning exercise	Ski machine, general
02090	6.0	Conditioning exercise	Slimnastics
02100	4.0	Conditioning exercise	Stretching, hatha yoga
02110	6.0	Conditioning exercise	Teaching aerobic exercise class
02120	4.5	Conditioning exercise	Water aerobics, water calisthenics
02130	3.0	Conditioning exercise	Weight lifting (free, nautilus, or universal-type), light or moderate effort, light workout, general
02135	1.0	Conditioning exercise	Whirlpool, sitting

(continued)

APPENDIX E.4 *(CONTINUED)*

Code	METs[a]	Activity	Description
03010	6.0	Dancing	Aerobic, ballet or modern, twist
03015	6.0	Dancing	Aerobic, general
03020	5.0	Dancing	Aerobic, low impact
03021	7.0	Dancing	Aerobic, high impact
03025	4.5	Dancing	General
03030	5.5	Dancing	Ballroom, fast (disco, folk, square) (T 125)
03040	3.0	Dancing	Ballroom, slow (e.g., waltz, foxtrot, slow dancing)
04001	4.0	Fishing and hunting	Fishing, general
04010	4.0	Fishing and hunting	Digging worms, with shovel
04020	5.0	Fishing and hunting	Fishing from river bank and walking
04030	2.5	Fishing and hunting	Fishing from boat, sitting
04040	3.5	Fishing and hunting	Fishing from river bank, standing (T 660)
04050	6.0	Fishing and hunting	Fishing in stream, in waders (T 670)
04060	2.0	Fishing and hunting	Fishing, ice, sitting
04070	2.5	Fishing and hunting	Hunting, bow and arrow or crossbow
04080	6.0	Fishing and hunting	Hunting, deer, elk, large game (T 710)
04090	2.5	Fishing and hunting	Hunting, duck, wading
04100	5.0	Fishing and hunting	Hunting, general
04110	6.0	Fishing and hunting	Hunting, pheasants or grouse (T 680)
04120	5.0	Fishing and hunting	Hunting, rabbit, squirrel, prairie chick, raccoon, small game (T 690)
04130	2.5	Fishing and hunting	Pistol shooting or trap shooting, standing
05010	2.5	Home activities	Carpet sweeping, sweeping floors
05020	4.5	Home activities	Cleaning, heavy or major (e.g., wash car, wash windows, mop, clean garage), vigorous effort
05030	3.5	Home activities	Cleaning, house or cabin, general
05040	2.5	Home activities	Cleaning, light (dusting, straightening up, vacuuming, changing linen, carrying out trash), moderate effort
05041	2.3	Home activities	Washing dishes—standing or in general (not broken into stand/walk components)
05042	2.3	Home activities	Washing dishes; clearing dishes from table—walking
05050	2.5	Home activities	Cooking or food preparation—standing or sitting or in general (not broken into stand/walk components)
05051	2.5	Home activities	Serving food, setting table—implied walking or standing
05052	2.5	Home activities	Cooking or food preparation—walking
05055	2.5	Home activities	Putting away groceries (e.g., carrying groceries, shopping without a grocery cart)
05056	8.0	Home activities	Carrying groceries upstairs
05060	3.5	Home activities	Food shopping with or without a grocery cart, walking
05065	2.0	Home activities	Non-food shopping, standing
05066	2.3	Home activities	Non-food shopping, walking
05070	2.3	Home activities	Ironing
05080	1.5	Home activities	Sitting—knitting, sewing, light wrapping (presents)
05090	2.0	Home activities	Implied standing—folding laundry, folding or hanging clothes, putting clothes in washer or dryer, packing suitcase
05095	2.3	Home activities	Implied walking—putting away clothes, gathering clothes to pack, putting away laundry

Code	Category	METs	Description
05100	Home activities	2.0	Making bed
05110	Home activities	5.0	Maple syruping/sugar bushing (including carrying buckets, carrying wood)
05120	Home activities	6.0	Moving furniture, household
05130	Home activities	5.5	Scrubbing floors, on hands and knees
05140	Home activities	4.0	Sweeping garage, sidewalk, or outside of house
05145	Home activities	7.0	Moving household items, carrying boxes
05146	Home activities	3.5	Standing—packing/unpacking boxes, occasional lifting of household items, light—moderate effort
05147	Home activities	3.0	Implied walking—putting away household items—moderate effort
05150	Home activities	9.0	Moving household items upstairs, carrying boxes or furniture
05160	Home activities	2.5	Standing—light (pump gas, change light bulb, etc.)
05165	Home activities	3.0	Walking—light, non-cleaning (readying to leave, shut/lock doors, close windows, etc.)
05170	Home activities	2.5	Sitting—playing with child(ren)—light
05171	Home activities	2.8	Standing—playing with child(ren)—light
05175	Home activities	4.0	Walk/run—playing with child(ren)—moderate
05180	Home activities	5.0	Walk/run—playing with child(ren)—vigorous
05185	Home activities	3.0	Child care: sitting/kneeling—dressing, bathing, grooming, feeding, occasional lifting of child—light effort
05186	Home activities	3.5	Child care: standing—dressing, bathing, grooming, feeding, occasional lifting of child—light effort
06010	Home repair	3.0	Airplane repair
06020	Home repair	4.5	Automobile body work
06030	Home repair	3.0	Automobile repair
06040	Home repair	3.0	Carpentry, general, workshop (T 620)
06050	Home repair	6.0	Carpentry, outside house (T 640), installing rain gutters, building fire outside
06060	Home repair	4.5	Carpentry, finishing or refinishing cabinets or furniture
06070	Home repair	7.5	Carpentry, sawing hardwood
06080	Home repair	5.0	Caulking, chinking log cabin
06090	Home repair	4.5	Caulking, except log cabin
06100	Home repair	5.0	Cleaning gutters
06110	Home repair	5.0	Excavating garage
06120	Home repair	5.0	Hanging storm windows
06130	Home repair	4.5	Laying or removing carpet
06140	Home repair	4.5	Laying tile or linoleum
06150	Home repair	5.0	Painting, outside home (T 650)
06160	Home repair	4.5	Painting, papering, plastering, scraping inside house, hanging sheet rock, remodeling (T 630)
06170	Home repair	3.0	Putting on and removing tarp—sailboat
06180	Home repair	6.0	Roofing
06190	Home repair	4.5	Sanding floors with a power sander
06200	Home repair	4.5	Scraping and painting sailboat or powerboat
06210	Home repair	5.0	Spreading dirt with a shovel
06220	Home repair	4.5	Washing and waxing hull of sailboat, car, powerboat, airplane
06230	Home repair	4.5	Washing fence
06240	Home repair	3.0	Wiring, plumbing
07010	Inactivity, quiet	0.9	Lying quietly, reclining (watching television), lying quietly in bed—awake
07020	Inactivity, quiet	1.0	Sitting quietly (riding in a car, listening to a lecture or music, watching television or a movie)
07030	Inactivity, quiet	0.9	Sleeping
07040	Inactivity, quiet	1.2	Standing quietly (standing in a line)
07050	Inactivity, light	1.0	Reclining—writing
07060	Inactivity, light	1.0	Reclining—talking or talking on phone
07070	Inactivity, light	1.0	Reclining—reading

(continued)

APPENDIX E.4 *(CONTINUED)*

Code	METs[a]	Activity	Description
08010	5.0	Lawn and garden	Carrying, loading, or stacking wood, loading/unloading or carrying lumber
08020	6.0	Lawn and garden	Chopping wood, splitting logs
08030	5.0	Lawn and garden	Clearing land, hauling branches
08040	5.0	Lawn and garden	Digging sandbox
08050	5.0	Lawn and garden	Digging, spading, filling garden (T 590)
08060	6.0	Lawn and garden	Gardening with heavy power tools, tilling a garden (see Occupation, Shoveling)
08080	5.0	Lawn and garden	Laying crushed rock
08090	5.0	Lawn and garden	Laying sod
08095	5.5	Lawn and garden	Mowing lawn, general
08100	2.5	Lawn and garden	Mowing lawn, riding mower (T 550)
08110	6.0	Lawn and garden	Mowing lawn, walk, hand mower (T 570)
08120	4.5	Lawn and garden	Mowing lawn, walk, power mower (T 590)
08130	4.5	Lawn and garden	Operating snow blower, walking
08140	4.0	Lawn and garden	Planting seedlings, shrubs
08150	4.5	Lawn and garden	Planting trees
08160	4.0	Lawn and garden	Raking lawn (T 600)
08170	4.0	Lawn and garden	Raking roof with snow rake
08180	3.0	Lawn and garden	Riding snow blower
08190	4.0	Lawn and garden	Sacking grass, leaves
08200	6.0	Lawn and garden	Shoveling snow, by hand (T 610)
08210	4.5	Lawn and garden	Trimming shrubs or trees, manual cutter
08215	3.5	Lawn and garden	Trimming shrubs or trees, power cutter
08220	2.5	Lawn and garden	Walking, applying fertilizer or seeding a lawn
08230	1.5	Lawn and garden	Watering lawn or garden, standing or walking
08240	4.5	Lawn and garden	Weeding, cultivating garden (T 580)
08245	5.0	Lawn and garden	Gardening, general
08250	3.0	Lawn and garden	Implied walking/standing—picking up yard, light
09010	1.5	Miscellaneous	Sitting—card playing, playing board games
09020	2.0	Miscellaneous	Standing—drawing (writing), casino gambling
09030	1.3	Miscellaneous	Sitting—reading, book, newspaper, etc.
09040	1.8	Miscellaneous	Sitting—writing, desk work
09050	1.8	Miscellaneous	Standing—talking or talking on the phone
09055	1.5	Miscellaneous	Sitting—talking or talking on the phone
09060	1.8	Miscellaneous	Sitting—studying, general, including reading and/or writing
09065	1.8	Miscellaneous	Sitting—in class, general, including note-taking or class discussion
09070	1.8	Miscellaneous	Standing—reading
10010	1.8	Music playing	Accordion
10020	2.0	Music playing	Cello
10030	2.5	Music playing	Conducting

Code	Category	METs	Activity
10040	Music playing	4.0	Drums
10050	Music playing	2.0	Flute (sitting)
10060	Music playing	2.0	Horn
10070	Music playing	2.5	Piano or organ
10080	Music playing	3.5	Trombone
10090	Music playing	2.5	Trumpet
10100	Music playing	2.0	Violin
10110	Music playing	2.0	Woodwind
10120	Music playing	2.0	Guitar, classical, folk (sitting)
10125	Music playing	3.0	Guitar, rock and roll band (standing)
10130	Music playing	4.0	Marching band, playing an instrument, baton twirling (walking)
10135	Music playing	3.5	Marching band, drum major (walking)
11010	Occupation	4.0	Bakery, general
11020	Occupation	2.3	Bookbinding
11030	Occupation	6.0	Building road (including hauling debris, driving heavy machinery)
11035	Occupation	2.0	Building road, directing traffic (standing)
11040	Occupation	3.5	Carpentry, general
11050	Occupation	8.0	Carrying heavy loads, such as bricks
11060	Occupation	8.0	Carrying moderate loads up stairs, moving boxes (16-40 pounds)
11070	Occupation	2.5	Chambermaid, making bed (nursing)
11080	Occupation	6.5	Coal mining, drilling coal, rock
11090	Occupation	6.5	Coal mining, erecting supports
11100	Occupation	6.0	Coal mining, general
11110	Occupation	7.0	Coal mining, shoveling coal
11120	Occupation	5.5	Construction, outside, remodeling
11130	Occupation	3.5	Electrical work, plumbing
11140	Occupation	8.0	Farming, baling hay, cleaning barn, poultry work
11150	Occupation	3.5	Farming, chasing cattle
11160	Occupation	2.5	Farming, driving harvester
11170	Occupation	2.5	Farming, driving tractor
11180	Occupation	4.0	Farming, feeding small animals
11190	Occupation	4.5	Farming, feeding cattle
11200	Occupation	8.0	Farming, forking straw bales, cleaning corral or barn
11210	Occupation	3.0	Farming, milking by hand
11220	Occupation	1.5	Farming, milking by machine
11230	Occupation	5.5	Farming shoveling grain
11240	Occupation	12.0	Fire fighter, general
11245	Occupation	11.0	Fire fighter, climbing ladder with full gear
11246	Occupation	8.0	Fire fighter, hauling hoses on ground
11250	Occupation	17.0	Forestry, ax chopping, fast
11260	Occupation	5.0	Forestry, ax chopping, slow
11270	Occupation	7.0	Forestry, barking trees
11280	Occupation	11.0	Forestry, carrying logs
11290	Occupation	8.0	Forestry, felling trees
11300	Occupation	8.0	Forestry, general
11310	Occupation	5.0	Forestry, hoeing
11320	Occupation	6.0	Forestry, planting by hand
11330	Occupation	7.0	Forestry, sawing by hand
11340	Occupation	4.5	Forestry, sawing, power

(continued)

APPENDIX E.4 *(CONTINUED)*

Code	METs[a]	Activity	Description
111350	9.0	Occupation	Forestry, trimming trees
11360	4.0	Occupation	Forestry, weeding
11370	4.5	Occupation	Furriery
11380	6.0	Occupation	Horse grooming
11390	8.0	Occupation	Horse racing, galloping
11400	6.5	Occupation	Horse racing, trotting
11410	2.6	Occupation	Horse racing, walking
11420	3.5	Occupation	Locksmith
11430	2.5	Occupation	Machine tooling, machining, working sheet metal
11440	3.0	Occupation	Machine tooling, operating lathe
11450	5.0	Occupation	Machine tooling, operating punch press
11460	4.0	Occupation	Machine tooling, tapping and drilling
11470	3.0	Occupation	Machine tooling, welding
11480	7.0	Occupation	Masonry, concrete
11485	4.0	Occupation	Masseur, masseuse (standing)
11490	7.0	Occupation	Moving, pushing heavy objects, 75 lbs or more (desks, moving van work)
11500	2.5	Occupation	Operating heavy duty equipment/automated, not driving
11510	4.5	Occupation	Orange grove work
11520	2.3	Occupation	Printing (standing)
11525	2.5	Occupation	Police, directing traffic (standing)
11526	2.0	Occupation	Police, driving a squad car (sitting)
11527	1.3	Occupation	Police, riding in a squad car (sitting)
11528	8.0	Occupation	Police, making an arrest (standing)
11530	2.5	Occupation	Shoe repair, general
11540	8.5	Occupation	Shoveling, digging ditches
11550	9.0	Occupation	Shoveling, heavy (more than 16 pounds/minute)
11560	6.0	Occupation	Shoveling, light (less than 10 pounds/minute)
11570	7.0	Occupation	Shoveling, moderate (10 to 15 pounds/minute)
11580	1.5	Occupation	Sitting—light office work, in general (chemistry lab work, light). Use hand tools, watch repair or micro-assembly, light assembly/repair.
11585	1.5	Occupation	Sitting—meetings, general, and/or with talking involved
11590	2.5	Occupation	Sitting—moderate (heavy levers, riding mower/forklift, crane operation)
11600	2.5	Occupation	Standing—light (bartending, store clerk, assembling, filing, photocopying, putting up Christmas tree)
11610	3.0	Occupation	Standing—light/moderate (assembling/repairing of heavy parts, welding, stocking, auto repair, packing boxes for moving, etc.), patient care (as in nursing)
11620	3.5	Occupation	Standing—moderate (assembling at fast rate, lifting 50 lbs, hitch/twisting ropes)
11630	4.0	Occupation	Standing—moderate/heavy (lifting more than 50 lbs, masonry, painting, paper hanging)
11640	5.0	Occupation	Steel mill, fettling

Code	Category	METs	Description
11650	Occupation	5.5	Steel mill, forging
11660	Occupation	8.0	Steel mill, hand rolling
11670	Occupation	8.0	Steel mill, merchant mill rolling
11680	Occupation	11.0	Steel mill, removing slag
11690	Occupation	7.5	Steel mill, tending furnace
11700	Occupation	5.5	Steel mill, tipping molds
11710	Occupation	8.0	Steel mill, working in general
11720	Occupation	2.5	Tailoring, cutting
11730	Occupation	2.5	Tailoring, general
11740	Occupation	2.0	Tailoring, hand sewing
11750	Occupation	2.5	Tailoring, machine sewing
11760	Occupation	4.0	Tailoring, pressing
11766	Occupation	6.5	Truck driving, loading and unloading truck (standing)
11770	Occupation	1.5	Typing, electric, manual, or computer
11780	Occupation	6.0	Using heavy power tools such as pneumatic tools (jackhammers, drills, etc.)
11790	Occupation	8.0	Using heavy tools (not power) such as shovel, pick, tunnel bar, spade
11791	Occupation	2.0	Walking on job, less than 2.0 mph (in office or lab area), very slow
11792	Occupation	3.5	Walking on job, 3.0 mph, in office, moderate speed, not carrying anything
11793	Occupation	4.0	Walking on job, 3.5 mph, in office, brisk speed, not carrying anything
11795	Occupation	3.0	Walking, 2.5 mph, slowly and carrying light objects less than 25 pounds
11800	Occupation	4.0	Walking, 3.0 mph, in office, moderate speed, carrying light objects less than 25 pounds
11810	Occupation	4.5	Walking, 3.5 mph, briskly and carrying objects less than 25 pounds
11820	Occupation	5.0	Walking or walking down stairs or standing, carrying objects about 25 to 49 pounds
11830	Occupation	6.5	Walking or walking down stairs or standing, carrying objects about 50 to 74 pounds
11840	Occupation	7.5	Walking or walking down stairs or standing, carrying objects about 75 to 99 pounds
11850	Occupation	8.5	Walking or walking down stairs or standing, carrying objects about 100 pounds or over
11870	Occupation	3.0	Working in scene shop, theater actor, backstage employee
12010	Running	6.0	Jog/walk combination (jogging component of less than 10 minutes) (T 180)
12020	Running	7.0	Jogging, general
12030	Running	8.0	Running, 5 mph (12 min/mile)
12040	Running	9.0	Running, 5.2 mph (11.5 min/mile)
12050	Running	10.0	Running, 6 mph (10 min/mile)
12060	Running	11.0	Running, 6.7 mph (9 min/mile)
12070	Running	11.5	Running, 7 mph (8.5 min/mile)
12080	Running	12.5	Running, 7.5 mph (8 min/mile)
12090	Running	13.5	Running, 8 mph (7.5 min/mile)
12100	Running	14.0	Running, 8.6 mph (7 min/mile)
12110	Running	15.0	Running, 9 mph (6.5 min/mile)
12120	Running	16.0	Running, 10 mph (6 min/mile)
12130	Running	18.0	Running, 10.9 mph (5.5 min/mile)
12140	Running	9.0	Running, cross country
12150	Running	8.0	Running, general (T 200)
12160	Running	8.0	Running, in place
12170	Running	15.0	Running, up stairs
12180	Running	10.0	Running, on a track, team practice
12190	Running	8.0	Running, training, pushing wheelchair, marathon wheeling
12195	Running	3.0	Running, wheeling, general

(continued)

APPENDIX E.4 (CONTINUED)

Code	METs[a]	Activity	Description
12130	18.0	Running	Running, 10.9 mph (5.5 min/mile)
12140	9.0	Running	Running, cross country
12150	8.0	Running	Running, general (T 200)
12160	8.0	Running	Running, in place
12170	15.0	Running	Running, up stairs
12180	10.0	Running	Running, on a track, team practice
12190	8.0	Running	Running, training, pushing wheelchair, marathon wheeling
12195	3.0	Running	Running, wheeling, general
13000	2.5	Self care	Standing—getting ready for bed, in general
13009	1.0	Self care	Sitting on toilet
13010	2.0	Self care	Bathing (sitting)
13020	2.5	Self care	Dressing, undressing (standing or sitting)
13030	1.5	Self care	Eating (sitting)
13035	2.0	Self care	Talking and eating or eating only (standing)
13040	2.5	Self care	Sitting or standing—grooming (washing, shaving, brushing teeth, urinating, washing hands, doing make-up)
13050	4.0	Self care	Showering, toweling off (standing)
14010	1.5	Sexual activity	Active, vigorous effort
14020	1.3	Sexual activity	General, moderate effort
14030	1.0	Sexual activity	Passive, light effort, kissing, hugging
15010	3.5	Sports	Archery (non-hunting)
15020	7.0	Sports	Badminton, competitive (T 450)
15030	4.5	Sports	Badminton, social singles and doubles, general
15040	8.0	Sports	Basketball, game (T 490)
15050	6.0	Sports	Basketball, non-game, general (T 480)
15060	7.0	Sports	Basketball, officiating (T 500)
15070	4.5	Sports	Basketball, shooting baskets
15075	6.5	Sports	Basketball, wheelchair
15080	2.5	Sports	Billiards
15090	3.0	Sports	Bowling (T 390)
15100	12.0	Sports	Boxing, in ring, general
15110	6.0	Sports	Boxing, punching bag
15120	9.0	Sports	Boxing, sparring
15130	7.0	Sports	Broomball
15135	5.0	Sports	Children's games (hopscotch, 4-square, dodge ball, playground apparatus, t-ball, tetherball, marbles, jacks, arcade games)
15140	4.0	Sports	Coaching: football, soccer, basketball, swimming, etc.
15150	5.0	Sports	Cricket (batting, bowling)
15160	2.5	Sports	Croquet
15170	4.0	Sports	Curling
15180	2.5	Sports	Darts, wall or lawn
15190	6.0	Sports	Drag racing, pushing or driving a car

15200	Sports	6.0	Fencing
15210	Sports	9.0	Football, competitive
15230	Sports	8.0	Football, touch, flag, general (T 510)
15235	Sports	2.5	Football or baseball, playing catch
15240	Sports	3.0	Frisbee playing, general
15250	Sports	3.5	Frisbee, ultimate
15255	Sports	4.5	Golf, general
15260	Sports	5.5	Golf, carrying clubs (T 090)
15270	Sports	3.0	Golf, miniature, driving range
15280	Sports	5.0	Golf, pulling clubs (T 080)
15290	Sports	3.5	Golf, using power cart (T 070)
15300	Sports	4.0	Gymnastics, general
15310	Sports	4.0	Hacky sack
15320	Sports	12.0	Handball, general (T 520)
15330	Sports	8.0	Handball, team
15340	Sports	3.5	Hand gliding
15350	Sports	8.0	Hockey, field
15360	Sports	8.0	Hockey, ice
15370	Sports	4.0	Horseback riding, general
15380	Sports	3.5	Horseback riding, saddling horse, grooming horse
15390	Sports	6.5	Horseback riding, trotting
15400	Sports	2.5	Horseback riding, walking
15410	Sports	3.0	Horseshoe pitching, quoits
15420	Sports	12.0	Jai alai
15430	Sports	10.0	Judo, jujitsu, karate, kick boxing, tae kwan do
15440	Sports	4.0	Juggling
15450	Sports	7.0	Kickball
15460	Sports	8.0	Lacrosse
15470	Sports	4.0	Moto-cross
15480	Sports	9.0	Orienteering
15490	Sports	10.0	Paddleball, competitive
15500	Sports	6.0	Paddleball, casual, general (T 460)
15510	Sports	8.0	Polo
15520	Sports	10.0	Racketball, competitive
15530	Sports	7.0	Racketball, casual, general (T 470)
15535	Sports	11.0	Rock climbing, ascending rock
15540	Sports	8.0	Rock climbing, rapelling
15550	Sports	12.0	Rope jumping, fast
15551	Sports	10.0	Rope jumping, moderate, general
15552	Sports	8.0	Rope jumping, slow
15560	Sports	10.0	Rugby
15570	Sports	3.0	Shuffleboard, lawn bowling
15580	Sports	5.0	Skateboarding
15590	Sports	7.0	Skating, roller (T 360)

(continued)

APPENDIX E.4 (CONTINUED)

Code	METs[a]	Activity	Description
15600	3.5	Sports	Sky diving
15605	10.0	Sports	Soccer, competitive
15610	7.0	Sports	Soccer, casual, general (T 540)
15620	5.0	Sports	Softball or baseball, fast or slow pitch, general (T 440)
15630	4.0	Sports	Softball, officiating
15640	6.0	Sports	Softball, pitching
15650	12.0	Sports	Squash (T 530)
15660	4.0	Sports	Table tennis, ping pong (T 410)
15670	4.0	Sports	Tai chi
15675	7.0	Sports	Tennis, general
15680	6.0	Sports	Tennis, doubles (T 430)
15690	8.0	Sports	Tennis, singles (T 420)
15700	4.0	Sports	Trampoline
15710	4.0	Sports	Volleyball, competitive, in gymnasium (T 400)
15720	3.0	Sports	Volleyball, non-competitive, 6-9 member team, general
15725	8.0	Sports	Volleyball, beach
15730	6.0	Sports	Wrestling (one match = 5 minutes)
15731	7.0	Sports	Wallyball, general
16010	2.0	Transportation	Automobile or light truck (not a semi) driving
16020	2.0	Transportation	Flying airplane
16030	2.5	Transportation	Motor scooter, motorcyle
16040	6.0	Transportation	Pushing plane in and out of hangar
16050	3.0	Transportation	Driving heavy truck, tractor, bus
17010	7.0	Walking	Backpacking, general (T 050)
17020	3.5	Walking	Carrying infant or 15-pound load (e.g., suitcase), level ground or down stairs
17025	9.0	Walking	Carrying load up stairs, general
17026	5.0	Walking	Carrying 1- to 15-lb load, up stairs
17027	6.0	Walking	Carrying 16- to 24-lb load, up stairs
17028	8.0	Walking	Carrying 25- to 49-lb load, up stairs
17029	10.0	Walking	Carrying 50- to 74-lb load, up stairs
17030	12.0	Walking	Carrying 74+ lb load, up stairs
17035	7.0	Walking	Climbing hills with 0 to 9-pound load
17040	7.5	Walking	Climbing hills with 10- to 20-pound load
17050	8.0	Walking	Climbing hills with 21- to 42-pound load
17060	9.0	Walking	Climbing hills with 42+ pound load
17070	3.0	Walking	Down stairs
17080	6.0	Walking	Hiking, cross country (T 040)
17090	6.5	Walking	Marching, rapidly, military
17100	2.5	Walking	Pushing or pulling stroller with child
17110	6.5	Walking	Race walking
17120	8.0	Walking	Rock or mountain climbing (T 060)

Code	Category	METs	Activity
17130	Walking	8.0	Up stairs, using or climbing up ladder (T 030)
17140	Walking	4.0	Using crutches
17150	Walking	2.0	Walking, less than 2.0 mph, level ground, strolling, household walking, very slow
17160	Walking	2.5	Walking, 2.0 mph, level, slow pace, firm surface (T 020)
17161	Walking	2.5	Walk from house to car or bus, from car or bus to go places, from car or bus to and from worksite, to neighbor's or family's house
17170	Walking	3.0	Walking, 2.5 mph, firm surface
17180	Walking	3.0	Walking, 2.5 mph, downhill
17190	Walking	3.5	Walking, 3.0 mph, level, moderate pace, firm surface, walking for social reasons or for pleasure, walking with children (pushing a stroller or general walking)
17200	Walking	4.0	Walking, 3.5 mph, level, brisk, firm surface, walking for exercise
17210	Walking	6.0	Walking, 3.5 mph, uphill
17220	Walking	4.0	Walking, 4.0 mph, level, firm surface, very brisk pace
17230	Walking	4.5	Walking, 4.5 mph, level, firm surface, very, very brisk
17250	Walking	3.5	Walking, for pleasure, work break
17260	Walking	5.0	Walking, grass track
17270	Walking	4.0	Walking, to work or class (T 015)
17280	Walking	2.5	Walking, to and from outhouse
18010	Water activities	2.5	Boating, power
18020	Water activities	4.0	Canoeing, on camping trip (T 270)
18030	Water activities	7.0	Canoeing, portaging
18040	Water activities	3.0	Canoeing, rowing, 2.0-3.9 mph, light effort
18050	Water activities	7.0	Canoeing, rowing, 4.0-5.9 mph, moderate effort
18060	Water activities	12.0	Canoeing, rowing, >6 mph, vigorous effort
18070	Water activities	3.5	Canoeing, rowing, for pleasure, general (T 250)
18080	Water activities	12.0	Canoeing, rowing, in competition, or crew or sculling (T 260)
18090	Water activities	3.0	Diving, springboard or platform
18100	Water activities	5.0	Kayaking
18110	Water activities	4.0	Paddle boating
18120	Water activities	3.0	Sailing, boat and board sailing, windsurfing, ice sailing, general (T 235)
18130	Water activities	5.0	Sailing, in competition
18140	Water activities	3.0	Sailing, sunfish/laser/hobby cat, keel boats, ocean sailing, yachting
18150	Water activities	6.0	Skiing, water (T 220)
18160	Water activities	7.0	Skimobiling
18170	Water activities	12.0	Skindiving or scuba diving as frogman
18180	Water activities	16.0	Skindiving, fast
18190	Water activities	12.5	Skindiving, moderate
18200	Water activities	7.0	Skindiving, scuba diving, general (T 310)
18210	Water activities	5.0	Snorkeling (T 320)
18220	Water activities	3.0	Surfing, body or board
18230	Water activities	10.0	Swimming laps, freestyle, fast, vigorous effort
18240	Water activities	8.0	Swimming laps, freestyle, slow, moderate, or light effort
18250	Water activities	8.0	Swimming, backstroke, general
18260	Water activities	10.0	Swimming, breaststroke, general

(continued)

APPENDIX E.4 (CONTINUED)

Code	METs[a]	Activity	Description
18270	11.0	Water activities	Swimming, butterfly, general
18280	11.0	Water activities	Swimming, crawl, fast (75 yards/minute), vigorous effort
18290	8.0	Water activities	Swimming, crawl, slow (50 yards/minute), moderate or light effort
18300	6.0	Water activities	Swimming, lake, ocean, river (T 280, T 295)
18310	6.0	Water activities	Swimming, leisurely, not lap swimming, general
18320	8.0	Water activities	Swimming, sidestroke, general
18330	8.0	Water activities	Swimming, synchronized
18340	10.0	Water activities	Swimming, treading water, fast vigorous effort
18350	4.0	Water activities	Swimming, treading water, moderate effort, general
18360	10.0	Water activities	Water polo
18365	3.0	Water activities	Water volleyball
18370	5.0	Water activities	Whitewater rafting, kayaking, or canoeing
19010	6.0	Winter activities	Moving ice house (setting up/drilling holes, etc.)
19020	5.5	Winter activities	Skating, ice, 9 mph or less
19030	7.0	Winter activities	Skating, ice, general (T 360)
19040	9.0	Winter activities	Skating, ice, rapidly, more than 9 mph
19050	15.0	Winter activities	Skating, speed, competitive
19060	7.0	Winter activities	Ski jumping (climbing up or carrying skis)
19075	7.0	Winter activities	Skiing, general
19080	7.0	Winter activities	Skiing, cross country, 2.5 mph, slow or light effort, ski walking
19090	8.0	Winter activities	Skiing, cross country, 4.0-4.9 mph, moderate speed and effort, general
19100	9.0	Winter activities	Skiing, cross country, 5.0-7.9 mph, brisk speed, vigorous effort
19110	14.0	Winter activities	Skiing, cross country, >8.0 mph, racing
19130	16.5	Winter activities	Skiing, cross country, hard snow, uphill, maximum
19150	5.0	Winter activities	Skiing, downhill, light effort
19160	6.0	Winter activities	Skiing, downhill, moderate effort, general
19170	8.0	Winter activities	Skiing, downhill, vigorous effort, racing
19180	7.0	Winter activities	Sledding, tobogganing, bobsledding, luge (T 370)
19190	8.0	Winter activities	Snow shoeing
19200	3.5	Winter activities	Snowmobiling

From Ainsworth, B. et al. 1993. "Compendium of physical activities: Classification of energy costs of human physical activities." *Medicine and Science in Sports and Exercise* 25: 71-80. Reprinted by permission.

[a]1 MET = 1 kcal · kg[-1] · hr[-1]. To calculate kcal · min[-1], multiply the client's body weight (in kg) by the MET value and divide this value by 60.

[b]The number in parentheses refers to the physical activity codes used in the Minnesota Leisure Time Physical Activity Questionnaire (LTPA).

APPENDIX F

Flexibility and Low Back Care Exercises

APPENDIX F.1 SELECTED FLEXIBILITY EXERCISES

ANTERIOR THIGH REGION

Muscle Groups: Quadriceps and Hip Flexors

Exercise 1

Description: From a standing position, raise one foot toward hips and grasp ankle. Pull leg upward toward buttocks.

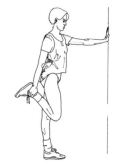

Exercise 2

Description: Lying on your side, flex the knee and grasp the ankle. Press the foot into the hand and squeeze the pelvis forward. Do not pull the foot.

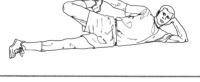

Exercise 3

Description: In a prone position, flex the knee and grasp ankle or foot with both hands. Do not pull on the foot. Keep knees on the floor and do not arch the back.

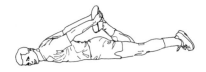

POSTERIOR THIGH REGION

Muscle Groups: **Hamstrings and Hip Extensors**

Exercise 1

Description: In a supine position, grasp knee and pull knee toward chest, then flex head to knee.

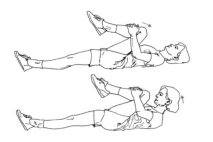

Exercise 2

Description: From a long-sitting position, grasp ankles and flex trunk to legs.

Exercise 3

Description: From a standing position, place your foot on a low step, keep the knee flexed slightly, and bend from the hips until you feel the stretch.

Exercise 4

Description: From a sitting position, with one knee flexed, flex the trunk keeping the spine extended until you feel tension.

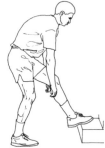
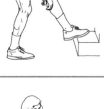

Exercise 5

Description: From a lying position, with one leg extended and the other leg flexed, grasp leg with both hands and flex thigh to trunk.

GROIN REGION (MEDIAL THIGH REGION)

Muscle Groups: Hip Adductors

Exercise 1

Description: From a tailor-sitting position, with soles of feet together, place hands on inside of knees and push downward slowly.

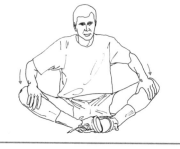

Exercise 2

Description: From a straddle-standing position, flex one knee and hip, lowering body closer to floor.

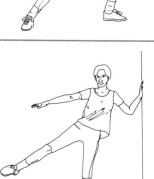

Exercise 3

Description: Standing on one leg while supporting yourself against wall or chair abduct hip, keeping leg straight. Have partner grasp ankle and passively stretch the muscle further.

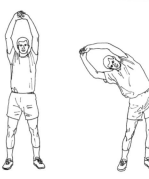

LATERAL THIGH-TRUNK REGION

Muscle Groups: Hip Abductors and Trunk Lateral Flexors

Exercise 1

Description: From standing position, with arms overhead, clasp hands together and laterally flex trunk to side no more than 20°.

Exercise 2

Description: From a crossed-leg sitting position, rotate trunk to the right. Place hands on right side of thigh and pull. Repeat to opposite side.

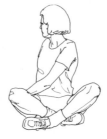

POSTERIOR LEG REGION

Muscle Group: Plantar Flexors

Exercise 1

Description: Assume front-leaning position against wall with one foot ahead of the other. Flex hip, knee, and ankle to lower body closer to ground, keeping feet flat on floor.

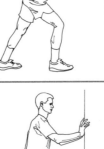

Exercise 2

Description: Standing with balls of feet on stairs, curb, or wood block, lower heels to floor.

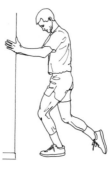

ANTERIOR LEG REGION

Muscle Group: Dorsiflexors

Exercise 1

Description: Standing with ankle of the non-supporting leg fully extended, stretch the dorsiflexors by slowly flexing the knee of the supporting leg.

UPPER AND LOWER BACK REGIONS

Muscle Group: Trunk Extensors

Exercise 1

Description: Sit with legs crossed and arms relaxed. Tuck chin and curl forward attempting to touch forehead to knees.

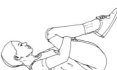

Exercise 2

Description: In a supine position, with knees flexed, grasp thighs below the knee caps and bring knees to chest. Flattten lower back to floor.

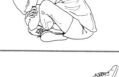

Exercise 3

Description: From a kneeling position, bring chin to chest. Contract abdomen and buttocks muscles while rounding lower back.

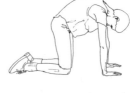

ANTERIOR CHEST, SHOULDER, AND ABDOMINAL REGIONS

Muscle Groups: Shoulder Flexors and Adductors, Trunk Flexors

Exercise 1

Description: In a prone position, push up until elbows are fully extended. Keep pelvis and hips on floor.

Exercise 2

Description: Grasp towel or rope with both hands. Rotate arms overhead behind trunk.

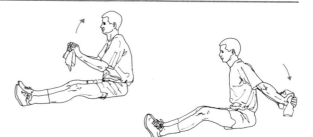

Exercise 3

Description: Clasp hands together behind trunk with elbows extended. Slowly raise arms upward.

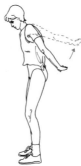

APPENDIX F.2   EXERCISE DO's AND DON'Ts

DON'T: Neck Hyperextension

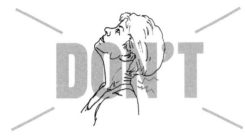

DON'T: Head Throws in a Crunch

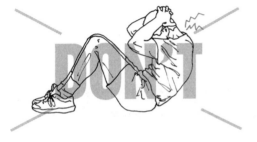

DON'T: Unsupported Hip/Trunk Flexion

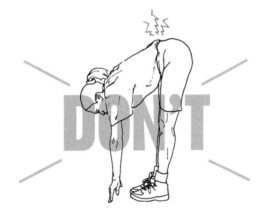

DON'T: The Plow

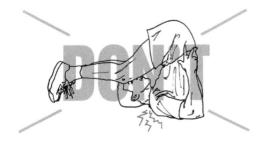

DO: Neck Lateral Flexion

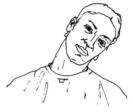

DO: Partial Sit-Up (see Appendix F.3, p. 311)

DO: Seated Hip/Trunk Flexion (see Appendix F.1, Exercise 4, p. 304)

DO: Camel (see Appendix F.3, p. 311)

DON'T: Swan Lifts

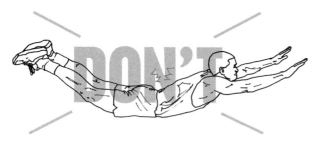

DO: Trunk Extensions

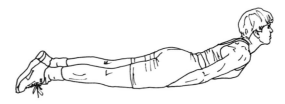

DON'T: V-Sits

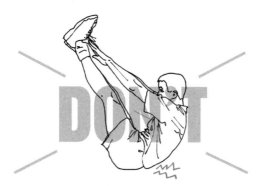

DO: Partial Sit-Up (see Appendix F.3, p. 311)

DON'T: Leg Lifts With Trunk Hyperextended

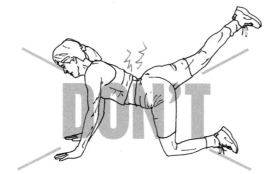

DO: Leg Lifts With Trunk and Leg in Straight Line

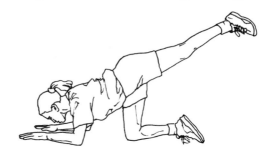

DON'T: Hamstring Stretch—Leg on Bar

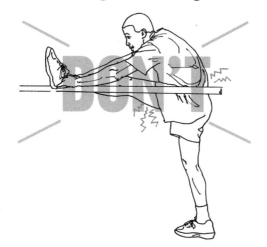

DO: Hamstring Stretch—Knee to Chest (see Appendix F.1, Exercise 5, p. 304)

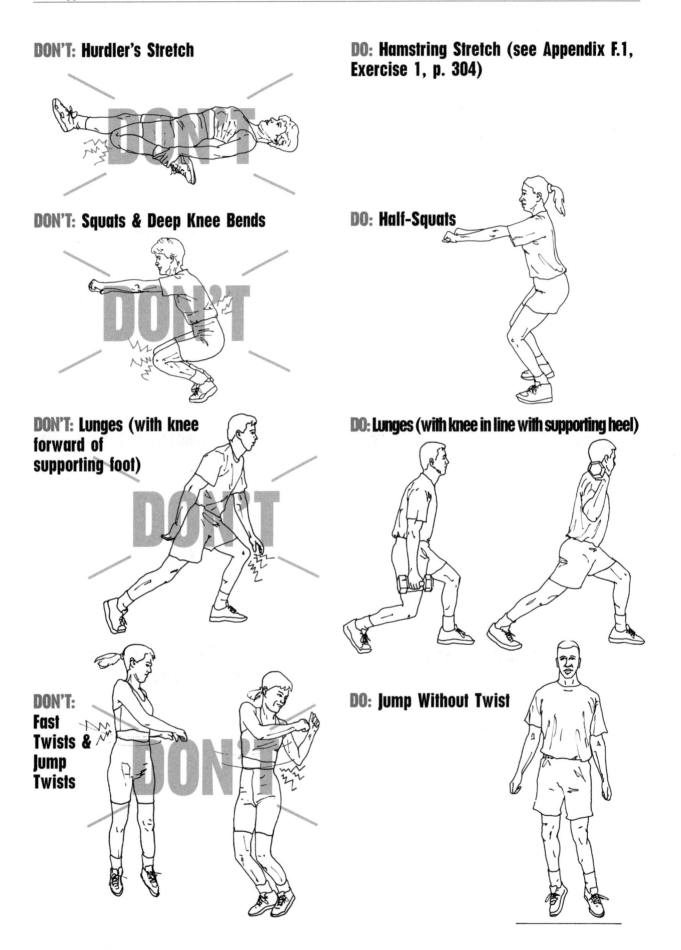

DON'T: Hurdler's Stretch

DO: Hamstring Stretch (see Appendix F.1, Exercise 1, p. 304)

DON'T: Squats & Deep Knee Bends

DO: Half-Squats

DON'T: Lunges (with knee forward of supporting foot)

DO: Lunges (with knee in line with supporting heel)

DON'T: Fast Twists & Jump Twists

DO: Jump Without Twist

APPENDIX F.3   EXERCISES FOR LOW BACK CARE

Pelvic Tilt (stretches abdominal muscles)

Lie on your back with knees bent, feet flat on the floor, and arms at your sides. Flatten the small of your back against the floor. (Your hips will tilt upward.) Hold.

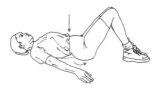

Double Knee to Chest (stretches hip, buttock, and lower back muscles)

Lie on your back with knees bent, feet flat on the floor, and arms at your sides. Raise both knees, one at a time, to your chest and hold with your hands. Lower your legs, one at a time, to the floor and rest briefly.

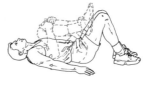

Trunk Flex (stretches back, abdominal, and leg muscles)

On your hands and knees, tuck in your chin and arch your back. Slowly sit back on your heels, letting your shoulders drop toward the floor. Hold.

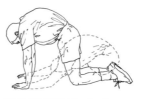

Cat and Camel (strengthens back and abdominal muscles)

On your hands and knees with your head parallel to the floor, arch your back and then let it slowly sag toward the floor. Try to keep your arms straight.

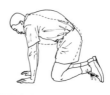

Partial Sit-Up (strengthens abdominal muscles)

Lie on your back with knees bent, feet flat on the floor, and arms crossed over your chest. Keeping your middle and lower back flat on the floor, raise your head and shoulders off the floor, and hold. Gradually increase your holding time.

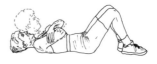

Single Leg Extension (strengthens hip and buttock muscles, and stretches abdominal and leg muscles)

Lie on your stomach with your arms folded under your chin. Slowly lift one leg—not too high—without bending it, while keeping your pelvis flat on the floor. Slowly lower your leg and repeat with the other leg.

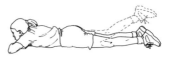

Notes

APPENDIX G

Stress Assessment

APPENDIX G.1 STRESS INVENTORY AND COPING STRATEGIES

Test 1

Purpose: To assess the degree of stress due to frustration and inhibition.

Directions: For each statement, circle the number corresponding to the degree it describes your behavior.

Scoring: Add each vertical column of numbers you have circled. Then add column totals horizontally to get your total score. A total score greater than 25 suggests vulnerability to this source of stress.

Statement	Almost always true	Usually true	Usually false	Almost always false
1. When I can't do something "my way," I simply adjust and do it the easiest way.	1	2	3	4
2. I get upset when someone in front of me drives slowly.	4	3	2	1
3. It bothers me when my plans are dependent upon others.	4	3	2	1
4. Whenever possible, I tend to avoid large crowds.	4	3	2	1
5. I am uncomfortable when I have to stand in long lines.	4	3	2	1
6. Arguments upset me.	4	3	2	1
7. When my plans don't flow smoothly, I become anxious.	4	3	2	1
8. I require a lot of space in which to live and work.	4	3	2	1
9. When I am busy at some task, I hate to be disturbed.	4	3	2	1
10. I believe that "all good things are worth waiting for."	1	2	3	4
Total =	____ +	____ +	____ +	____

From D.A. Girdano and G.S. Everly, *Controlling Stress and Tension: A Holistic Approach* © 1979 by Allyn and Bacon. Reprinted by permission.

Test 2

Purpose: To assess your vulnerability to overload.

Directions: For each statement, circle the number corresponding to how often you exhibit that behavior or feeling.

Scoring: Same as Test 1. A total score greater than 25 suggests vulnerability to this source of stress.

Question	Almost always	Very often	Seldom	Never
1. Find yourself with insufficient time to complete your work?	4	3	2	1
2. Find yourself becoming confused and unable to think clearly because too many things are happening at once?	4	3	2	1
3. Wish you had help to get everything done?	4	3	2	1
4. Feel your boss or professor expects too much from you?	4	3	2	1
5. Feel your family and friends expect too much from you?	4	3	2	1
6. Find your work infringing on your leisure hours?	4	3	2	1
7. Find yourself doing extra work to set an example for those around you?	4	3	2	1
8. Find yourself doing extra work to impress your superiors?	4	3	2	1
9. Have to skip a meal so that you can get work completed?	4	3	2	1
10. Feel that you have too much responsibility?	4	3	2	1
Total =	____ +	____ +	____ +	____

Test 3

Purpose: To measure compulsive, time-urgent, and aggressive behavioral traits.

Directions: For each statement, circle the number corresponding to how often you exhibit that behavior.

Scoring: Same as Test 1. A total score greater than 25 suggests the presence of one or more of these behavioral traits.

Statement	Almost always true	Usually true	Usually False	Almost always false
1. I hate to wait in lines.	4	3	2	1
2. I often find myself racing against the clock to save time.	4	3	2	1
3. I become upset if I think something is taking too long.	4	3	2	1
4. When under pressure, I tend to lose my temper.	4	3	2	1
5. My friends tell me that I tend to lose my temper.	4	3	2	1
6. I seldom like to do anything unless I can make it competitive.	4	3	2	1
7. When something must be done, I'm the first to begin even though the details may still need to be worked out.	4	3	2	1
8. When I make a mistake, it is usually because I've rushed into something without giving it enough thought and planning.	4	3	2	1
9. Whenever possible, I try to do two things at once, such as eating while working or planning while driving or bathing.	4	3	2	1
10. When I go on a vacation, I usually take along some work to do just in case I get a chance.	4	3	2	1
Total =	____ +	____ +	____ +	____

Test 4

Purpose: To indicate strategies you use to cope with common sources of stress.

Directions: Follow the instructions given for each item.

Scoring: >115 pts = excellent
     61-114 pts = good
     50-60 pts = adequate
     <50 pts = inadequate

1. Give yourself 10 points if you feel that you have a supportive family.

2. Give yourself 10 points if you actively pursue a hobby.

3. Give yourself 10 points if you belong to some social or activity group that meets at least once a month (other than with your family).

4. Give yourself 15 points if you are within 5 pounds of your ideal body weight, considering your height and bone structure.

5. Give yourself 15 points if you practice some form of deep relaxation at least three times a week. Deep relaxation exercises include meditation, imagery, yoga, and so on.

6. Give yourself 5 points for each time you exercise 30 minutes or longer during an average week.

7. Give yourself 5 points for each nutritionally balanced and wholesome meal you consume during an average day.

8. Give yourself 5 points if you do something that you really enjoy just for yourself during an average week.

9. Give yourself 10 points if you have some place in your home that you can go in order to relax or be alone.

10. Give yourself 10 points if you practice time management techniques in your daily life.

11. Subtract 10 points for each pack of cigarettes you smoke during one average day.

12. Subtract 5 points for each evening during an average week that you take any form of medication or chemical (including alcohol) to help you sleep.

13. Subtract 10 points for each day during an average week that you consume any form of medication or chemical substance (including alcohol) to reduce your anxiety or just calm you down.

14. Subtract 5 points for each evening during an average week that you bring work home—work that was meant to be done at your place of employment.

APPENDIX G.2 RATHBONE MANUAL TENSION TEST

Purpose: This test was developed to assess neuromuscular tension in the wrist, elbow, shoulder, knee, hip, and neck joints at rest. Neuromuscular tension is measured during passive movement of the joints throughout the range of motion using a 4-point scale. 0 = no tension, 1 = slight tension, 2 = moderate tension, 3 = marked tension detected.

Tension Factors: Four tension factors are evaluated and scored:

1. Assistance—the client anticipated the movement and aids the testor in moving the body segment.
2. Resistance—the client resists the passive movement of the joint, limiting the range of motion or making the limb seem heavier than usual.
3. Posturing—the client maintains a static position against the pull of gravity when support of the limb by the tester is removed.
4. Perseveration—the client repeats the movement of the body segment after it is released by the tester.

Procedure:

1. The client assumes a relaxed, back-lying position on a padded table or mat.
2. To test each joint, support the client's body segment and passively rotate the body segment through the range of motion (e.g., flexion, extension, abduction, adduction, and circumduction of the shoulder joint) in a flowing, rhythmical manner.
3. Move the wrist, elbow, and shoulder joints while supporting the client's forearm and hand.
4. Move knee and hip joints while supporting the client's thigh and lower leg.
5. Move the neck by holding the client's head posterolaterally with both hands.
6. Use the 4-point scale to evaluate each tension factor for both right and left body segments. Record scores on the data sheet.

Data Sheet

Joint	Assistance R/L	Resistance R/L	Posturing R/L	Perseveration R/L
Wrist	_____	_____	_____	_____
Elbow	_____	_____	_____	_____
Shoulder	_____	_____	_____	_____
Knee	_____	_____	_____	_____
Hip	_____	_____	_____	_____
Neck	_____	_____	_____	_____
Total	_____	_____	_____	_____

Scoring: Score each joint movement for assistance, resistance, posturing, and perseveration on a 0 to 3 scale. Use the following hints for scoring: *assistance*—the client aids in lifting the limb; *resistance*—the client does not "let go," but offers opposition; *posturing*—when the limb is lifted and then released, it does not fall, but floats down or stays in the new position; *perseveration*—the client independently continues a motion.

Adapted from Rathbone and Hunt (1965).

Index

Page numbers in italics are figures and tables.

A

abbreviations, 229-230
abdominal region exercises, 270, 307
accommodating resistance, 114
activities, compendium of, 291-302
acute inflammation theory, 138-139
aerobic capacity, 136-137. *See also* $\dot{V}O_2$max
aerobic exercise
    and body fat, 197
    classification of modalities, 85
    dance, 93
    intensity of, 198
    riding, 94
    and steady-state HR response, *86*
    vs. resistance training, 194
aerobic training
    continuous mode of, 93-94
    discontinuous mode of, 94-95
    methods and modes, 92-93
age
 and body fat, 178
    and cardiorespiratory fitness, 76-78
    and flexibility, 204-205
    and 1-RM testing, 117-118
    push-up test norms for, *116*
    and resistance training, 130, 134
    and skeletal muscle, 136
American College of Sports Medicine (ACSM)
    bicycle ergometer submaximal test, 68-69, *70*
    exercise prescription guidelines of, 84
    exercise testing guidelines of, *27*
    physical activity statement by, 2
    resistance training guidelines of, *124*
anaeroid manometers, 21
android obesity, 178
anorexia nervosa, 178
anterior chest region exercises, 307
anterior leg region exercises, 306
anterior thigh region exercises, 303
anthropometric body composition measurement, 164-165
    measurement error in, 169-170
    standardized procedures for, 165-169
    techniques, 165

arm curl exercise, 265, 270
arm exercises, 270-271
Åstrand bicycle ergometer maximal test, 63
Åstrand-Rhyming bicycle ergometer submaximal test, 68-69
Åstrand-Rhyming step test protocol, 71
atherosclerosis, 5
autogenic relaxation training, 227

B

back
    exercises for, 269, 307
    healthy practices for, 220
    strength testing for, 108-109
back hypertension exercise, 269
Balke treadmill protocol, 56
ball squeeze exercise, 266
basal metabolic rate (BMR), 179
bench press exercise, 267
bench stepping
    with aerobics, 93
    maximal exercise tests for, 64-65
    submaximal exercise tests with, 71
Benson relaxation technique, 227
bent knee curl-up exercise, 270
bent-over row exercise, 269
biaxial joints, 204
bicycle ergometers
    maximal exercise tests with, 58-64
    submaximal exercise tests with, 67-71
    test guidelines for, 61-63
    test protocols for, *62*
binge/purge syndrome, 178
bioelectrical impedance method (BIA), 159-160
    measurement errors in, 162-164
    prediction equations for, *161*
    standardized testing procedures for, 162
    technique for, 160
biofeedback, 226-227
blood, variable normal values, *20*
blood pressure. *See also* hypertension
    assessment of, 20-22
    classification of, *17*
    error in measurement, 22
blood profile, 20
BMI (body mass index), 164, *167*

BMR (basal metabolic rate), 179
body composition
   classification of measures, 145-146
   exercise prescription for, 198-199
   field methods for assessment, 152-159
   improvement of, 197-199
   laboratory assessment of, 148-151
   models of, 146-148
body density (Db)
   conversion to body-fat percentage, *147*
   skinfold relationship to, *153*
body fat
   and aerobic exercise, 197
   conversion from Db (body density), *147*
   standards for men and women, *146*
body mass index (BMI), 164, *167*
body weight
   and cardiorespiratory fitness, 193-194
   sample calculation of healthy, *187*
bone fractures, 8, 178
bone health, 137
bony breadth measurements, 169-170, 281
Bruce treadmill protocol, 56
bulimia, 178

C
caloric expenditure, 187-189
caloric intake, 186-187
carbohydrates, 182
   common sources of, *192*
   dietary necessity of, 195
cardiac arrhythmia, 178
cardiorespiratory exercise
   physiological changes from, 91
   workout essentials of, 92
cardiorespiratory fitness
   and body weight, 193-194
   classification of, 48
   exercise evaluation, 48-49
   field test prediction equations for, *72*
   field tests for, 73-76, 257-258
   for older adults and children, 76-78
   testing procedures for, 49-51
cardiovascular disease (CVD), 4-5
certification, 42-44
CHD (coronary heart disease), 5
chest and shoulder exercises, 267-268
chest push exercise, 265
cholesterol
   classification of, *17*
   evaluation guidelines for, *19*
   profile of, 18-20
cigarette smoking, 7-8
circuit resistance training, 94-95, 126-127
circumference measurements, 281
clinical exercise testing procedures, 51-52
comprehensive health evaluation, 15
concentric contractions, 105-106
connective tissue damage, 8, 138
coronary heart disease (CHD), 5, *6, 16*

CVD (cardiovascular disease), 4-5
cycling, 93, 97, 98
D
Db (body density)
   conversion to body-fat percentage, *147*
   skinfold relationship to, *153*
delayed-onset muscle soreness (DOMS), 137-139
diabetes, *6, 8*
diet
   and cholesterol levels, 20
   comparison to dietary goals, *183*
   weight gain analysis and planning, 197
   weight loss analysis and planning, 190-192
   well-balanced, 182-186
dietary fat, 183, *192*
Dietary Guidelines for Americans (U.S. Department of
   Health and Human Services 1995), 180
diminishing returns, principle of, 39, 122
disease
   risk classification of, 16-17
   signs and symptoms of, 15-16
   and stress, 224
distance run tests, for cardiorespiratory fitness, 75
DOMS (delayed-onset muscle soreness), 137-139
dual-energy x-ray absorptiometry, 151
dynamic contractions, 105
dynamic endurance tests, 115-116
dynamic flexibility, 203
dynamic muscle testing
   with constant- and variable-resistance, 110-112
   for endurance, 111-112
   endurance battery for, *113*
   with isokinetic and omnikinetic exercise, 112-115
dynamic resistance training, 123-127
   exercises for, 267-272
   guidelines for, *124*
   vs. isokinetic training, 129
   vs. static resistance training, 128-129
dynamic strength tests, 110-111, 115
dynamometers, *108, 114*
E
eccentric contractions, 106
edema, 178
elbow breadth norms, *169*
electrocardiogram (ECG)
   electrode placement for, *26, 27*
   monitoring guidelines for, 23-26
   sample tracings, 242-250
electromyography (EMG), 225
energy balance, 179
energy expenditure, 187-189
   for selected activities, *190*
energy intake, 186-187
equipment sources
   for body composition assessment, 171-172
   for cardiorespiratory fitness testing, 78
   for flexibility testing, 221
   for health evaluation, 29
for muscular fitness testing, 119-120

exercise. *See also* personalized exercise programs
  adherence to programs, 41-42, *43*
  benefits of, 193-194
  design of programs, 38-39
  do's and dont's of, 308-310
  frequency for body-fat loss, 197-198
  instruction for dynamic resistance, 267-272
  instruction for flexibility, 303-307
  instruction for isometric, 265-267
  order of, 125-126
  progression of, 41
  and resting metabolic rate (RMR), 193-194
  role in disease prevention, *2*
  and stress, 225-226
  types of, 194-195
exercise and physical activity pyramid, *4*
exercise-induced muscle hypertrophy, 135-136
exercise intensity
  for aerobics, 198
  comparison of methods for prescribing, *90*
  definition of, 123
  guidelines for, 124-125
  heart rate (HR) method, 88-90
  high *vs.* low, 194
  MET method, 87-88
  rating of perceived exertion (RPE) method, 90
  for stretching, 219
  variations for, 126
exercise prescription
  for body composition, 198-199
  duration of exercise, 90-91
  for flexibility, 218-219
  frequency of exercise, 91
  guidelines for, 83-84, *84*
  intensity of exercise, 87-90
  modes of exercise, 84-87
  rate of progression, 91
  science of, 39-41
  stages of progression, 92
  for weight gain, 197
  for weight loss, 193
exercise specialists, 31-32
  certification and licensure of, 42-44
exercise testing, 26-27
  contraindications to, 28
  principles of, 52

F
fad diets, 195-196
fat. *See* body fat; dietary fat
flexibility
  definition and nature of, 203-204
  exercise prescription for, 218-219
  exercises for, 303-307
  factors affecting, 204-205
  guidelines for program design, 219
  program design for, 215-219
flexibility testing, 205-215
flexometer testing, 207, *212*
fluid-electrolyte imbalances, 178

food guide pyramid, *192*
food intake, sample computerized analysis, 285-289
food record form, 283
Fox bicycle ergometer maximal test protocol, 63-64
Fox single-stage bicycle ergometer test, 71
frequency, of exercise
  for body-fat loss, 197-198
  guidelines for, 91, 125, 126
functional aerobic capacity. *See* $\dot{V}O_2$max

G
gender
  and flexibility, 205
  push-up test norms for, *116*
  and skeletal muscle, 135-136
genetics, and obesity, 180
gluteal squeeze exercise, 266
goniometer
  measurement procedures with, *208-211*
  test procedures for, 206-207
Graded Exercise Test (GXT), 26-28
  administration procedures for, 49-50
  for children, *77*
  summary of protocols, 257-258
grip testing, 107
groin region exercises, 305
gynoid obesity, 178

H
half squat exercise, 272
Hatha Yoga, 227
health evaluation, 14-28
heart health appraisal (RISKO), 235-238
heart rate
  assessment of, 22-23
  auscultation assessment of, 23
  and Graded Exercise Test (GXT), 26-28
  methods, of exercise intensity assessment, 88-90
  monitors and ECG recordings, 23-26
  palpation assessment of, 23
  pulse rate measurement, 74
  target heart rate zone, plotting, *88*
high-fat diets, 196
high-protein diets, 196
hip and thigh exercises, 271-272
hydrostatic weighing, 148-151
hypercholesterolemia, 7
hyperlipidemia, *6*, 7
hypertension, 5-7. *See also* blood pressure
  risk factors for, *6*
  treatments for, 20
hypokinetic diseases, 2

I
imagery, 226
inclinometer testing, 207, *213*
individual variability, principle of, 38-39, 122
informed consent, 28-29, 253-254
initial values, principle of, 38, 122
intensity. *See* exercise intensity
interval training, 94

isokinetic contractions, definition of, 107
isokinetic tests, *115,* 263-264
isokinetic training, 127
    guidelines for, *128*
    vs. dynamic resistance training, 129
isometric contractions, definition of, 105
isometric muscle testing
    with cable tensiometers, 109
    with dynamometers, 107-109
isometric training, 123, 265-267
isotonic contractions, definition of, 106

J
Jenkins Activity Survey (Jenkins, Rosenman, and
    Zyzanski), 224
jogging, 93, 97-99
jogging test, 75
joints
    classification by structure and function, *204*
    integrity of, 137

K
Karvonen method, of exercise intensity assessment,
    88-90
knee squeeze exercise, 266

L
laboratory tests
    for body composition, 148-151
    for health evaluation, 18
lateral-thigh trunk region exercises, 305-306
lat pull-down exercise, 269
lean body mass, 193, 198
leg and thigh extension exercise, 266
leg curl exercise, 266, 271
leg ergometry equation, ACSM, 62-63
leg exercises, 272
leg extension exercise, 271
leg press exercise, 266
leg strength testing, 108
licensure, 42-44
lifestyle
    changes to, 180-181
    evaluation of, 28, 251-253
lipoprotein profile, 18-20
low back
    exercise programs for, 220
    exercises for, 303-307, 311
low back pain, *6,* 9
low-carbohydrate diets, 195
lower-body obesity, 178
lumbosacral flexion, measurement of, *213*

M
macronutrients
    common sources of, *192*
    energy yields of, *179*
maximal exercise tests
    with bench stepping, 64-65
    with bicycle ergometers, 58-64
    with treadmills, 53-58
measurements, standardized sites for, 275-281

medial thigh region exercises, 305
medical clearance, 18, 241
medical history questionnaire, 18, 238-240
medical terminology, 231-233
metabolic calculations, *54,* 55
metabolic equivalents (METs)
    and exercise intensity assessment, 87-88
    of physical activities, 291-302
    treadmill estimates for common protocols, *59*
minerals, *184,* 185
modified Bruce treadmill protocol, 56
multicomponent body composition model, 147
multimodal exercise, 99-102
muscle. *See also* skeletal muscle
    balance, assessment of, 118
    contractions, types of, *106*
    fibers and resistance training, 135
muscle hypertrophy, 135, 136
muscular endurance, definition of, 105
muscular fitness testing, 107-115
    additional considerations for, 117-119
    with calisthenics, 115-116
    measurement error in, 116-117
muscular soreness, 137-139
musculoskeletal disorders, 8-9

N
Nagle, Balke, and Naughton Maximal Step Test
    Protocol, 65
National Cholesterol Education Program (NCEP),
    18-20
near-infrared interactance method (NIR), 170-171
negative energy balance, 179
neuromuscular tension, 225
nomograms
    for Åstrand-Rhyming test, *70*
    for Balke GXT, *60*
    for body-fat percentage, *156*
    for body mass index (BMI), *167*
    for Bruce GXT, *60*
    to predict body surface area (BSA), *188*
    for $\dot{V}O_2$max in skilled rowers, *74*
    for $\dot{V}O_2$max in unskilled rowers, *73*
    for waist-to-hip circumference ratio (WHR), *168*
    noninsulin-dependent diabetes mellitus
    (NIDDM), 8

O
obesity, 8, 177
    based on body mass index (BMI), *167*
    causes of, 178-181
    definition of, 178
    risk factors for, *6*
    types of, 178
omnikinetic test protocols, *115*
Omni-tron tests, 263-264
1-RM testing, 110
    bench press, *111*
    of children and older adults, 117-118
    leg press, *111*
    strength-to-body weight ratios for, *112*

order of exercise, 125-126
osteoarthritis, 8
osteopenia, 178
osteoporosis, *6, 8,* 178
overload principle, 38, 122
overweight, 8
    causes of, 178-181
    definition of, 178

P

PAR-Q (Physical Activity Readiness Questionnaire), 14, 234
pelvic tilt exercise, 266
periodization
    definition of, 126
    guidelines for, *127*
personalized exercise programs
    case study of, 95-97, 254-256
    samples of, 97-102
physical activity
    and cholesterol levels, 20
    compendium of, 291-302
    and coronary heart disease (CHD), 5
    example of moderate amounts, 3
    and flexibility, 205
    health and disease overview, 1-4
    health benefits of, 3
    and hypertension, 5-7
    and lipid profiles, 7
    log form for, 290
    role in disease prevention, *4*
Physical Activity Readiness Questionnaire (PAR-Q), 14, 234
physical examination, and medical clearance, 18
physical fitness components, 32
    measures of, *35*
    types of training for, *40*
physical fitness testing, 33-34
    administration and interpretation of, 37-38
    evaluating prediction equations, 34-37
PNF (proprioceptive neuromuscular facilitation), 217-218
positive energy balance, 179
posterior leg region exercises, 306
posterior thigh region exercises, 304
prediction equations
    for bioelectrical impedance method (BIA), *161*
    for cardiorespiratory fitness, *72*
    for circumference and skeletal diameter, *166*
    evaluation of, 34-37
    for residual volume (RV), 274
    for skinfold measurement, *155*
progression, principle of, 38, 122
progressive relaxation technique, 227
proprioceptive neuromuscular facilitation (PNF), 217-218
protein, 182-183
    common sources of, *192*

psychological factors, of obesity, 180
pulse rate measurement, 74
push-up test, age-gender norms for, *116*

Q

Queen's College step test protocol, 71
quick weight-loss diets, 195-196

R

range of motion (ROM)
    average values for, *211*
    measurement with flexometer, *212*
    measurement with universal goniometer, *206*
Rathbone manual tension test, 225, 316
rating of perceived exertion (RPE)
    exercise intensity assessment by, 90
    scales of, 50
recommended daily allowance (RDA), *184,* 284
relaxation techniques, 226-227
renal disorders, 178
repetitions, definition of, 123
reproductive disorders, 178
resistance training
    biochemical effects of, 136
    and body fat, 198
    for children, 133-134
    comparison of methods, 127-129
    exercise order samples for, *126*
    morphological effects of, 134-136
    neurological effects of, 137
    for older adults, 134
    principles of, 122
    program development for, 129-133
    questions about, 139-140
    sample program for bodybuilder, 132-133
    sample program for novice, 131
    sample program for older adult, 130
    types of, 122-127
    vs. aerobic exercise, 194
resting blood pressure, measurement of, 21-22
resting metabolic rate (RMR), 179
    estimation of, 187-189
    and exercise, 193-194
reverse sit-up exercise, 270
reversibility, principle of, 39, 122
risk factors
    for coronary heart disease (CHD), 5, *16*
    for various diseases, *6*
RISKO: heart health appraisal, 235-238
Rockport fitness charts, 259-260
ROM (range of motion). *See* range of motion (ROM)
rowing ergometer submaximal test protocol, 72-73
running tests, 75

S

seated leg press exercise, 271
seated (overhead) press exercise, 268
sets
    definition of, 123
    guidelines for, 125

shoulder pull exercise, 265
shoulder region exercises, 307
shoulder shrug exercise, 268
side leg raise exercise, 272
sit-and-reach (modified) test, 211-215, *214, 215*
sit-and-reach (standard) test, 207-211
skeletal muscle
    damage to, 138
    effects of resistance training, 135-136
    and gender, 135-136
    metabolic profile of, 136
    in older adults, 136
skin distraction test, 215, *216*
skinfold measurement, 152-154
    measurement errors in, 157-159
    prediction equations for, *155*
    sites for Jackson's generalized equations, 280
    standardized testing procedures for, 154
    standard sites for, 275-279
    technique for, 154-157
smoking, 7-8
specificity principle, 38, 122
sphygmomanometers, 21-22
spot-reduction exercises, 194-195
stairclimbing submaximal test protocol, 72
standardized sites, for measurements, 275-281
static contractions, definition of, 105
static flexibility, 203
    direct measurement of, 206-207
    indirect measurement of, 207-215
static (isometric) training, 123, 265-267
static resistance training, 128-129
static strength norms, *109*
step ergometry, 93-94
stepping equation, ACSM, 64
step tests
    for cardiorespiratory fitness, 76
    protocols for, 261-262
strength
    definition of, 105
    in relation to knee joint angle, *106*
    testing modes of, *107*
stress
    assessment of, 224-225
    and disease, 224
    and exercise, 225-226
    inventory and coping strategies, 312-315
    physiological response to, 223-224
Stress Map Questionnaire (Orioli, Jaffe, and Scott),
    224
stress relaxation, 204
stretching
    comparison of techniques, *217*, 218
    intensity of exercises, 219
    modes of, 217-218
submaximal exercise tests
    addition modes of, 71-73
    with bench stepping, 71
    with bicycle ergometers, 67-71
    with treadmills, 65-67

T
Tai Chi, 227
target heart rate zone, plotting, *88*
terminology, 105-107, 231-233
testing, for physical fitness, 33-34, 37-38
toe (heel) raise exercise, 272
training volume
    definition of, 123
    variations for, 126
treadmills
    exercise test protocols, *57*
    maximal exercise tests with, 53-58
    MET estimates for common protocols, *59*
    population-specific equations for protocols, *59*
    submaximal exercise tests with, 65-67
triaxial joints, 204
triceps extension exercise, 265
triceps press-down exercise, 271
triglycerides, classification of, *17*
twelve-lead electrocardiogram (ECG), 24-26
two-component body composition model, 146-147

U
uniaxial joints, 204
universal goniometer
measurement procedures with, *208-211*
test procedures for, 206-207
upper-body obesity, 178
upright row exercise, 268

V
vitamins, 183-185
$\dot{V}O_2$max, 47-48, *69*
equations for, *54*, 55

W
waist-to-hip circumference ratio (WHR), 164, *168*
walking, 93
walking tests, 75-76
warm up, and flexibility, 205
water
    density at different temperatures, 273
    in diet, 185-186
weight management
principles and practices, 181-182
program design for, 186-189
and resistance training, 137
weight gain overview, 179-180
weight-gain programs for, 196-197
weight-loss programs, *191*
weight-loss programs for, 189-195
weight resistance exercise, 122

Y
YMCA bench press, test norms, *113*
YMCA bicycle ergometer submaximal test, 67-68

About the Author

An internationally recognized expert in exercise science, Dr. Vivian Heyward has conducted extensive research on physical fitness and body composition assessment. In addition to three previous texts, she's published more than four dozen articles on the subject. Dr. Heyward has given presentations for professional organizations and institutions at the regional, national, and international levels; she has also conducted workshops for nutritionists, health promotion and fitness professionals, physical therapists, nurses, and other allied health professionals.

Since receiving her PhD from the University of Illinois in 1974, Dr. Heyward has been a professor of exercise science at the University of New Mexico, where she has addressed the gap between research and practice in the field. Her career has been characterized by awards and distinctions, including multiple teaching awards and visiting scholar lectureships. Most recently, Dr. Heyward received the University of Illinois' Distinguished Alumni Award. She has also received recent research grants from NIH and OMRON Healthcare Corp.

A resident of Albuquerque, New Mexico, Dr. Heyward enjoys weightlifting, mountain biking, hiking, and wood carving. She is a Fellow of the American College of Sports Medicine and the American Society of Clinical Nutrition.

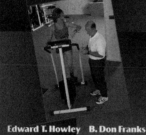
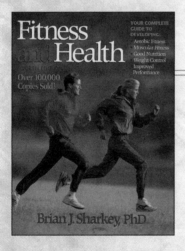